THE GOLD'S GYM®

ENCYCLOPEDIA OF BODYBUILDING

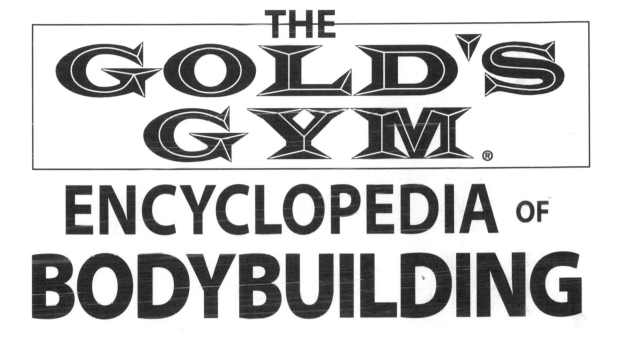

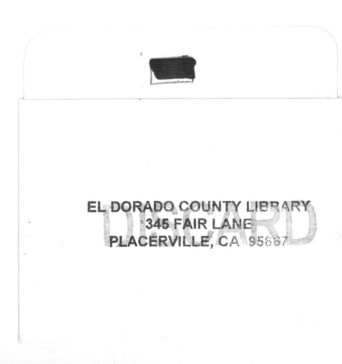

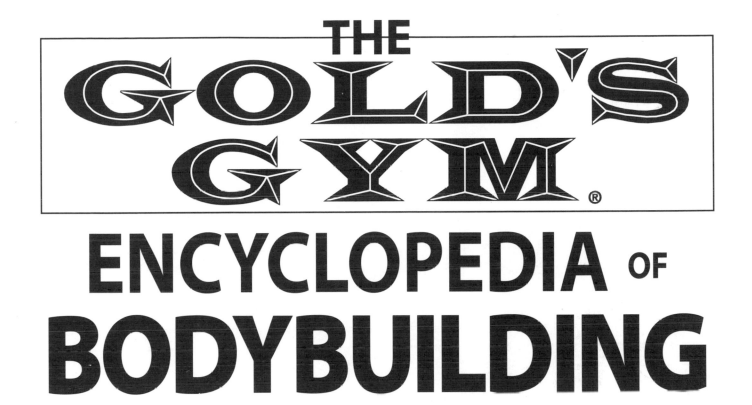

THE GOLD'S GYM
ENCYCLOPEDIA OF
BODYBUILDING

**Edward Connors, Michael J. B. McCormick,
Peter Grymkowski, and Tim Kimber**

CONTEMPORARY BOOKS

Library of Congress Cataloging-in-Publication Data

The Gold's Gym encyclopedia of bodybuilding / Edward Connors . . .
    [et al.].
            p.   cm.
        Includes bibliographical references (p.   ) and index
        ISBN 0-8092-3006-2
        1. Bodybuilding.   I. Connors, Ed.
    GV546.5.G636   1998
    646.7'5—dc21
                                                        97-42287
                                                        CIP

Cover design by Todd Petersen
Cover photo copyright © 1996 by Irvin J. Gelb
Interior photos copyright © by Irvin J. Gelb
Interior design by Hespenheide Design

Published by Contemporary Books
An imprint of NTC/Contemporary Publishing Company
4255 West Touhy Avenue, Lincolnwood (Chicago), Illinois 60646-1975 U.S.A.
Copyright © 1998 by Michael J. McCormick and Gold's Gym International, Inc.
Printed in the United States of America
International Standard Book Number: 0-8092-3006-2
18   17   16   15   14   13   12   11   10   9   8   7   6   5   4   3   2   1

Contents

Acknowledgments

To Michael and Carol McCormick.

Special thanks to Mom and Dad, Gloria and Bianca Watson, and Maxine T.D.

Thanks also to Tim, Pat, Mark, and Molly McCormick; Irv Gelb, John Wiedemann; Don MacLeod; Matt Dimmel; Dave Young; Chris Santiago-Adams; NOW Foods; Scott Prohaska; Christine Charles and Eastman Kodak; Anthony Clark; Pete Gisondi; Chris Noone, Esq.; James Hendricks, Esq.; Jim and Lee Rockell; Chuck and John MacAllister; Gerry Welcher; Ali' Helvacioglu; Tony Fitton; Linda Metz; George Martin; Harry Otto; Webster Frances, III; Don Stulpin; Donny Williams; Gunnar Sikk; Greg Zulak; Dr. Pcrisamy Sammikanu; Dr. Mauro DiPasquale; Dr. Michael Weintraub; Dr. Gilbert Forbes; Dr. Pierre Tariot; Dr. Allen Cuseo; Dr. Joseph Kelly; Dr. Lou Fussilli; Steve Healy; Brad Silvers; Bruce Lista; Don Ross; Mike Lambert; Chris Liotta; Melvin Arnone; Tony Civilletti; Jan Taraszkiewicz; Bob Reilich; Rick Bilitiere; Dave Futor; Mark Glickman; Jeff Logan; Johnny Johnson; Gerry Boga; Doug Majors; Tom Vaccarrella; Ned Lowe; Lloyd Kennerson; James Kennerson; Dave Maxwell; Bill Hess; Al Parker; Wolfgang Foque; Joe Vazzana; Terry Wester; and Russ Testo.

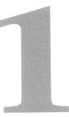

Gold's Gym: First Venice, Then the World

A Brief History

GOLD'S GYM VENICE, 1965

1965 was the year the first workout occurred inside the walls of Gold's Gym in Venice, California.

    Opened as a no-frills, no-nonsense, best-atmosphere-for-training gym, Gold's soon replaced Muscle Beach as the bodybuilding capital of Southern California. Of course, Southern California was the

Gold's Gym, Venice, California—1965

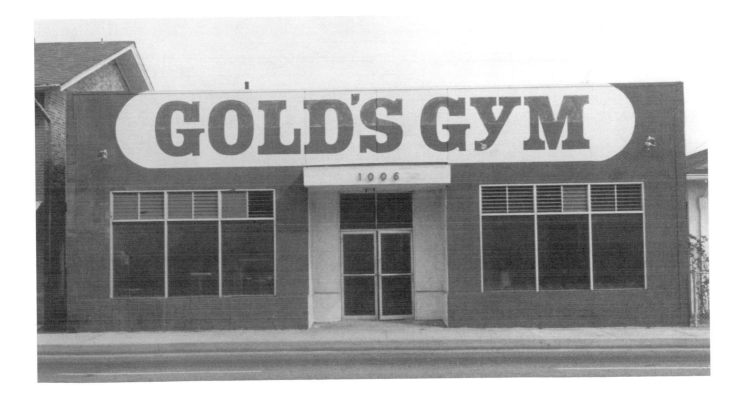

bodybuilding capital of the world. Soon Gold's Venice was able to qualify as the hot spot on the global map of bodybuilding.

The twentieth century's gold rush was not to *dig* for gold. Instead, thousands roared into Venice Beach to *pump* for gold—to pump for size at the real source of bodybuilding treasure: Gold's Venice.

In 1975, just a decade after the doors swung open, the famous muscle flick *Pumping Iron* featured Arnold Schwarzenegger in the midst of one of his Olympia contest preps. Gold's Venice was featured as Arnold's personal arena for his titanic battle preparations. Arnold's presence—with Gold's Venice as the backdrop—set the tone for the ensuing 20 years of bodybuilding.

1980

At the end of the 1970s, we realized bodybuilding's mainstream press was referring to Gold's as the "Mecca of bodybuilding." By 1980, people arriving from all over the world to train here were overwhelming the gym's daily use by top International Federation of Bodybuilders

Gold's Gym, Venice, California—1979

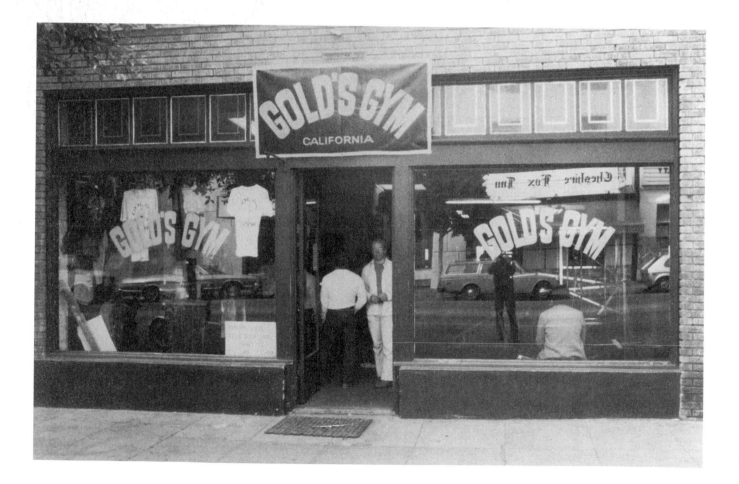

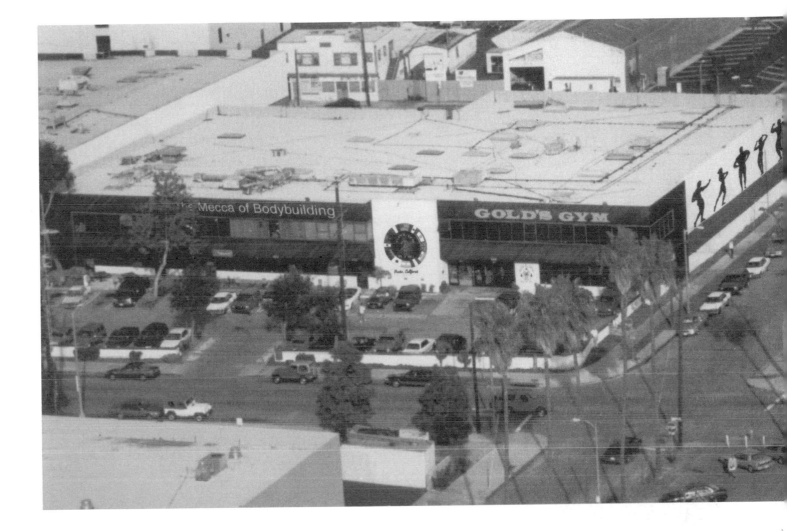

Gold's Gym, Venice, California—1997

pros and others. Gold's magnetic attraction was amazing. Of course, not everyone who wanted to train here could come to California, so the idea of bringing Gold's Venice to everyone was born.

The incredibly successful Gold's Gym licensee program allowed millions to train at Gold's Gyms. Highly motivated individuals who demonstrated a clear conception of the bodybuilding lifestyle were able to become members of the mushrooming Gold's family.

1997

Today, there are more than 500 Gold's Gym locations in 22 countries around the world, each bringing a "piece of Venice" to its members. Gold's is the largest international gym chain, and every year its reputation as the pinnacle of industry achievement grows stronger. On the domestic front, there are Gold's Gyms in 42 states and 376

American cities. There are more than 2 million Gold's Gym members worldwide.

Gold's is simply the best and most famous—and the most widely photographed—gym in the world.

The Gold's logo is among the world's most widely recognized, due in large part to the public's voracious appetite for officially licensed Gold's merchandise. Gold's logo items include the favorite bald-man T-shirts, men's and women's apparel for exercise and casual dress, fitness accessories, books, nutritional supplements, home-based training modules, VISA credit cards, customized leather jackets, and more.

GOLD'S VENICE—THE GYM

For more than three decades, bodybuilders have traveled distances both great and small to train at Gold's Venice. Some have been so magnetized by the atmosphere of Gold's that they have gone as far as to move to Venice. Gold's Venice is the gym of choice, not just for the world's best pro and amateur bodybuilders but for countless other professional athletes. An amazing number of celebrities train here in order to guarantee the highly productive workouts their stature demands. In fact, Gold's Venice has received an award for having the largest celebrity membership of any gym. The "mecca" is *the* place to train. No other gym in the world provides the exposure all bodybuilders want and need to succeed.

Gold's Venice is structured across 30,000 square feet in a sequence of activity-focused rooms. Literally every inch of available floor and loft space is covered in equipment. Only the 30-foot-high walls are off-limits for a productive bodybuilding encounter. No space is left unused in the quest for paramount physical prowess.

Industry Innovators

Equipment found nowhere else is used at Gold's every day year round. There is no dust here, baby. Some pieces are incredibly exotic, the experimental Lamborghini's of the weight world. More than a few of Gold's benches and machines have not been put into mass production because they are just too expensive to produce—incredible results or not.

Exercise equipment manufacturers use Gold's Venice as their test track. If the design is received with enthusiasm by our members, the light drops to green and it's a go. Gold's involvement in the process is somewhat altruistic but we also get to keep the machines no matter what! The real winners in this incredible, unique-to-the-industry relationship are the members of Gold's Gym.

Roland Cziurlok

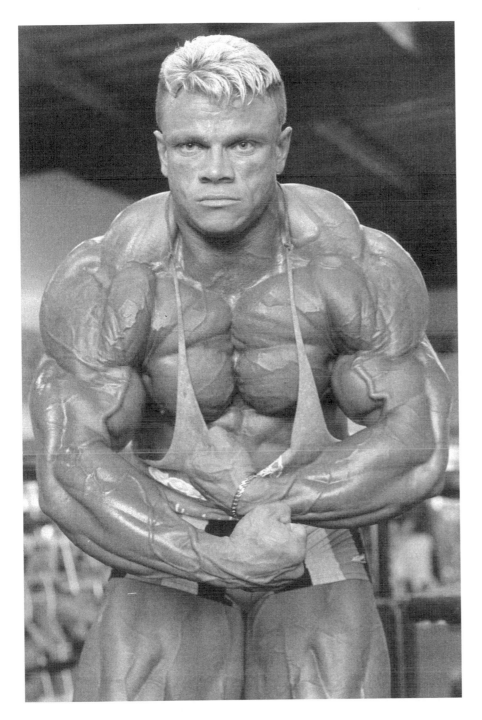

But Gold's offers far more than weight training. The aerobics room, featuring the innovative Cardio Theatre, has the most complete lineup of aerobics equipment available. A huge variety of heart-thumping, blood-pumping machines are ready to take you to the edge of cuts and separation.

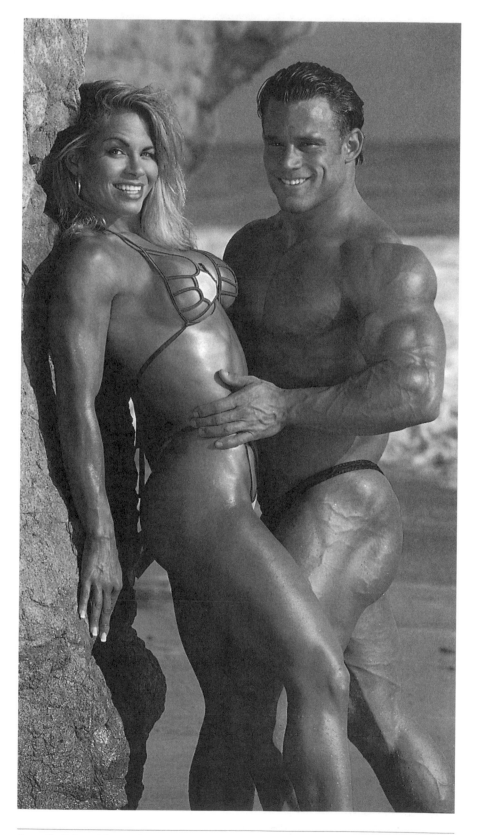

Amy Fadhli and Jason Arntz

Of course, there is also the world-famous Gold's Venice Pro Shop where you can purchase hundreds of officially licensed Gold's items, ranging from Gold's nutritional supplements to custom-designed Gold's Gym leather jackets.

Gold's Gym Web Site—The Electronic Mecca

If you are looking for a new hangout dedicated to the world of bodybuilding, all you need is a modem, computer, and access to the Internet.

Just as bodybuilding has been a force in the real world, the electronic world has recognized that delivering practical information on how to achieve your physical best is vital. Computer users once thought of as wimpy little geeks pounding away at their keyboards have shown the rest of the world they are like everyone else. Today people of every description use the Internet for information access and entertainment, and Gold's Gym has emerged as the Internet's bodybuilding leader by opening a web site that is the electronic twin of the Gold's Venice Pro Shop. The site also has up-to-date bodybuilding information you won't find in magazines. This electronic gym features training and diet areas, a clinic for seeking advice, contest results, and more. Even though you can't literally train in Gold's web site, think of it as our lobby. To get there simply set your web browser to http://www.goldsgym.com.

Bodybuilder's Paradise

If a survey were conducted asking the world's best bodybuilders where they would go to train for a pro card, the answer would surely be Gold's Venice. On a daily basis this gym features more bipedal beef than any magazine could. Why do you think all the big-muscle magazines send their photographers here? There is ZERO possibility of a bad or even mediocre workout. Far from being imposing or intimidating, the sheer thick-hulled presence of so many human battleships only draws forth the hidden energy and talent you are banking on to win as a bodybuilder. Gold's Venice is a think tank of innovative, reality-based bodybuilding technology.

TRUE BODYBUILDING EXPERIENCE

The following are excerpts from an interview with Gold's president Pete Grymkowski. Not only an innovative pioneer in the business of bodybuilding, Pete also enjoyed a long and successful career both as an amateur and IFBB professional.

What type of a child were you?
Serious on the inside while being nonchalant and casually relaxed on the outside.

How about activities or sports as a young man—were you involved with these?
I was too busy both working in terms of employment and with weights when I was young.

What type of neighborhood were you raised in?
[One with] hundreds of kids my age. I was one of the oldest, so being an Aries I developed leadership qualities. But I also learned to be synergistic, which also was a benefit [of] being from a large family.

Did you have any heroes as a child?
I had role models in bodybuilding like Steve Reeves, Dave Draper, Bill Pearl, and most of all Arnold, who I respected for his many accomplishments, not only in bodybuilding.

When did you start training and why?
I started training when I was 13. I had transferred from a small Catholic grammar school to a large public high school. There were lots of good-looking girls to impress as well as establishing a distinct identity for myself.

Were you gifted physically?
Yes. I was very lean and muscular with wide shoulders.

Was there any special type of training program at the start?
I trained very hard, but I never believed the magazines. They would preach dramatic results training only one hour a day. At 13 years I trained two and a half hours a day and by 15 only saw minor results. I didn't know anything about steroids at that time, so I could only assume that the magazines were not revealing the true training routines. Otherwise, why didn't I grow like they did? So I set my mind on going to Southern California some day to see for myself how the champions really train.

After high school you enlisted in the army. How was your enlistment?
I loved it! I volunteered for basic training two times and went through it completely twice—the discipline was very good.

Dennis Newman

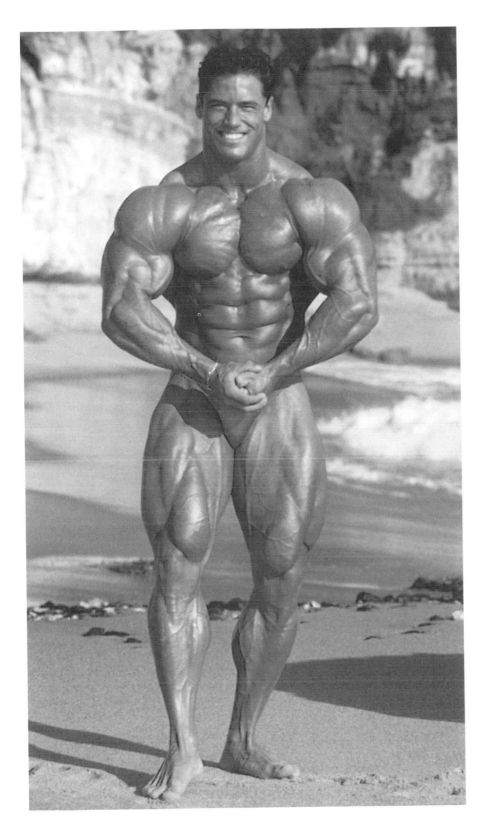

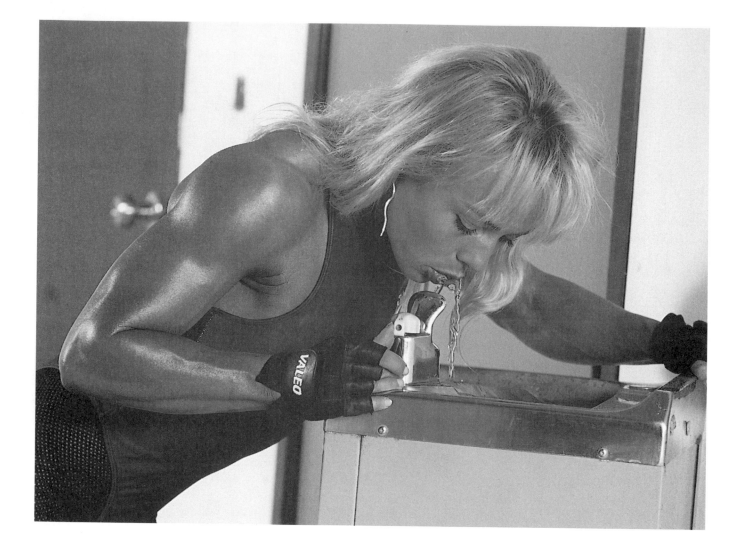

Gold's Venice—*The water fountain of bodybuilding!*

After your enlistment what came next as far as a career?
I worked for my father's building maintenance company. One of his customers was General Dynamics where I put a suggestion in the suggestion box and went to work as an expediter in engineering.

Where were you training and how was it at first?
I was training at the YMCA in Rochester, New York. I was 5 feet 10 inches, 179 pounds [with a] 48-inch chest and 17$\frac{1}{4}$-inch arms.

What led to your realization that there were more inside secrets [than] Bob Hoffman's Protein from the Sea available to help you grow?
I was training three hours a day and thought I was doing great. I entered the Junior USA. This was my second contest and the first time I had ever been around national competitors. I was amazed at

their incredible size. Ken Waller won at 232 pounds. When they said he only trained two hours a day, I said something doesn't make sense!

What were your next competitions and their results?
The next contest I entered was the 1971 Mr. America contest. I came in at 232 pounds and placed second to Casey Viator. I had a 60-inch chest and $20^7/8$-inch arms. Those five-hour workouts really paid off!

Can you provide an overview of your training methods?
Monday, Wednesday, and Friday: back, biceps, thigh biceps, abs, calves. Tuesday, Thursday, and Saturday: chest, triceps, quads, abs, calves. I trained like a determined lunatic, often five to seven hours per day. No one else would do it as a full-time job. I started at 11:00 A.M., brought my lunch, and went home for dinner at 8:00 P.M. It was totally radical!

What was your condition like at these major contests?
In 1973 I placed second to Jim Morris. I outweighed him 256 to 209 pounds.

What happened next in your life?
I moved to California with my training partner Tim Kimber. Together with Ed Connors, we purchased Gold's Gym and helped to start the NPC [National Physique Committee].

How about some info on your unique training experiences?
During 1971 and 1972 I did live in De Land, Florida, for a short time and trained with Arthur Jones and Casey Viator. I went back to Rochester, followed the Nautilus routine, and eventually fine-tuned it for the 1973 competitions.

Do you feel you would have been competitive in current pro events?
Yes, because I always seek out a better way to do things. There were many things that I did then that bodybuilders are just now understanding. Techniques such as proportionate levels of protein, carbs, and fats, which I found to be 100 [grams of] protein, 30 [grams of] carbs, and 15 [grams of] fat required to assimilate that 100 grams of protein! Further research will prove this combination to be best for muscular growth.

In 1977 you left Rochester, moved to Florida for a while, and eventually settled in California. Isn't this the start of the Gold's story as we now know it?

Yes. In Florida Tim and I trained at the Orange Avenue Gym with Kent Kuehn and Rocky Theresa. They were a tremendous asset to my 1977 Mr. America and Mr. World titles. On February 9, 1977, Tim and I met Ed Connors at the gym. Ed was in Orlando interviewing for a job at Disney World and had a crowd around him as he explained what life was like in Venice, California. Ed told me I had potential to win the IFBB Mr. America contest. I was broke and living in my 1965 Corvette behind the Orange Avenue Gym, so Ed sent me a plane ticket. I entered the Mr. America contest [June 9, 1977] and won. I stayed in California and talked Tim into coming here from Florida to help me train for the Mr. World, which I won.

What were the immediate events leading up to the purchase of Gold's Gym?
I was training at Gold's from midnight to 7:00 A.M. while the janitors were cleaning. In between sets, I would imagine what it would be like to own Gold's and the different things that it could be involved with. The previous owner's wife became ill with cancer and he decided to sell it. The rest is history. Together with the two people I trusted most as partners, Tim [and] Ed, [I] formed Gold's Gym Enterprises. We purchased Gold's in February 1979. I competed and did exhibitions until 1982. The NPC was formed in 1978 and I was already a pro doing exhibitions. I remember doing 26 exhibitions one year! I trained all over the world, made considerable money, and put it all back into Gold's Gym.

I remember the most commonly asked question was what life was like at Gold's Gym in Venice. I would answer just as Ed Connors had explained it to Tim and [me] in Orlando. Out of this [answer] came one of our mottos: If everyone can't come to Gold's Gym Venice, then we'll bring Gold's Gym Venice to everyone!

Gold's Gyms are now 500 strong and in some of the most exotic places—Qatar, Saipan, Russia, Japan, Korea, Israel, Indonesia, Hungary, Guam, French West Indies, Venezuela, Virgin Islands, Mexico, Italy, Cyprus, Portugal, Germany, England, Finland, Australia, Canada, Argentina, Bauhaus, Moscow, and the Netherlands Antilles.

Tell us about Pete Grymkowski now.
Physique-wise I'm 185 pounds—very muscular at 4 percent body fat. I feel like time has stood still for the past 25 years—I'm in better shape now than I was at 25. As far as how old I am—I never think about that. I have a personal motto: age is not a number—it's a condition! I also have other hobbies such as Gracie jujitsu and auto drag racing. I own and drive two dragsters and two funny

cars. I'm building a new top-fuel dragster with over 6,000 horse-power with four tires on the back for better traction. At first we'll use it for exhibition only, with hopes of setting up a new division of top-fuel dragsters called monster fuelers. Grymko Motorsports, named by the late great writer Bill Reynolds, will build these special types of cars.

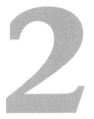

An Introduction to Bodybuilding

OUR SUGGESTION ON HOW TO BEST USE THIS BOOK

There is much more to bodybuilding than just training with weights. The workout only initiates the process of growth that we call bodybuilding, it does not complete it. In that context, there is much more to this book than phenomenal exercise photos. The expected chapters on nutrition, supplements, gaining weight, etc., are included. But unique to this book is quite a bit of material not found in a gym script but based on personal knowledge.

Twenty years ago successful books on bodybuilding only needed sound basic information and a lot of incredible photos. The impact that technology has had on the sport is unavoidable. Newly revised details become more numerous by the month. Diet, nutrition, and of

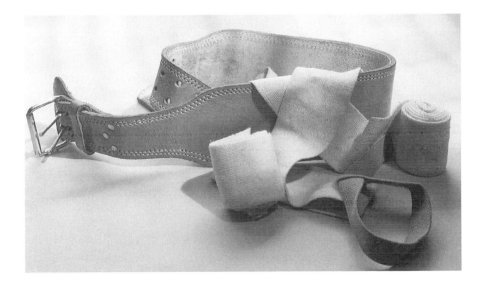

A bodybuilder's tools

Marika Johansson

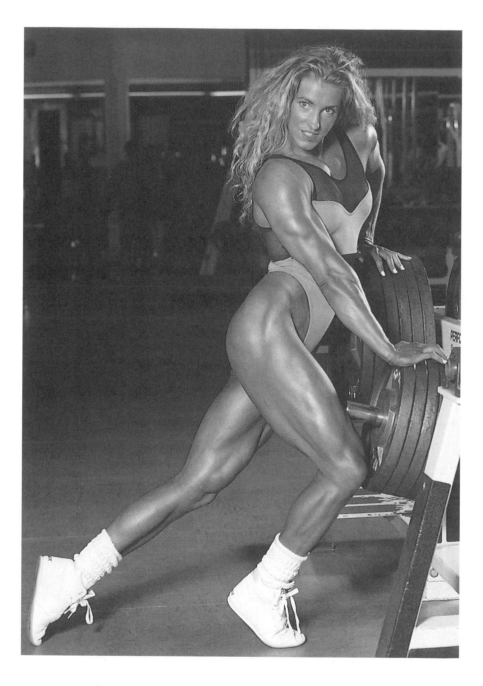

course, supplementation concepts pop up every month. Many bodybuilders find this much advanced information to be more confusing
than helpful. The scope and depth of bodybuilding knowledge is growing by leaps and bounds.

   The third chapter of this book was written specifically for the purpose of bridging some of the gap between what bodybuilders could
know and what they are able to learn and utilize in a practical sense.
Collectively there is enough material in this book to answer most of
your immediate questions. Additionally, we hope to address many
of your later bodybuilding concerns before they become dilemmas.

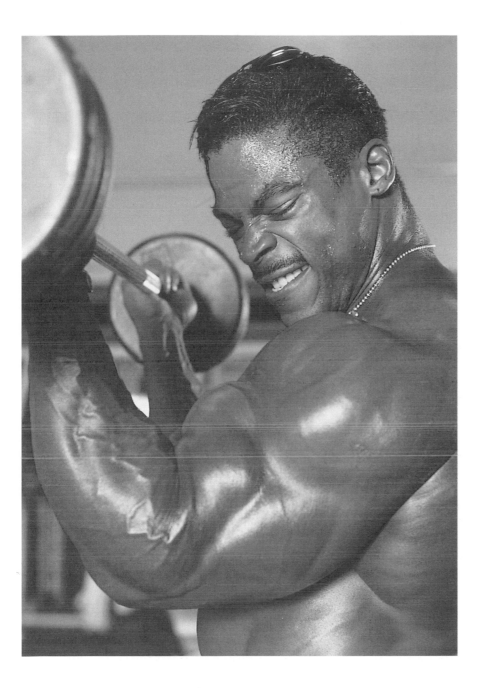

Aaron Baker

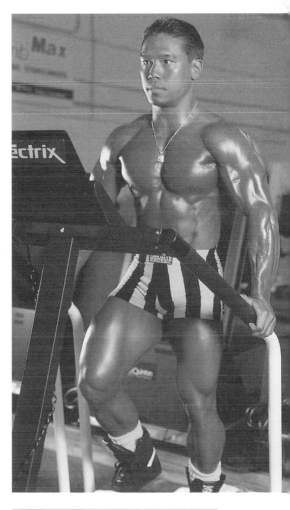

Here are some hints at how you can use this book to your best advantage:

- Read it.
- Keep it handy.
- Reread it.
- Study it.
- Consult it.
- Discuss it.
- Question it.

Chris Faildo

Craig Titus

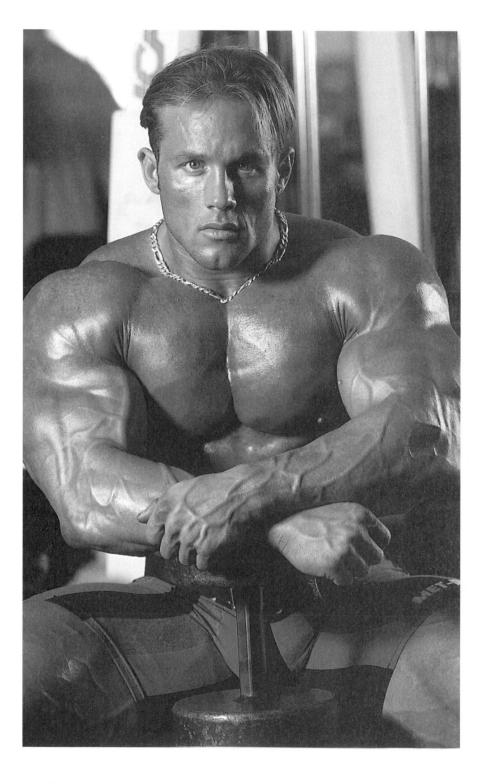

Note: most of the pictures that have appeared in the muscle magazines featuring bodybuilding champions were taken at Gold's Gym Venice. The atmosphere of success makes the Gold's presence felt—no matter how it is packaged. Whether it's via the Internet or a muscle magazine, you cannot escape the fact that Gold's Venice rules!

FOR THOSE OF YOU STARTING OUT

Who doesn't want a better body? Some of us, however, wanted more than simply better—we thought we could become one of the best. If this were not such a common thought, then why would there be a need for more than 500 Gold's Gyms worldwide? The large number of Gold's locations along with the magnetic attraction Gold's has for the best bodybuilders makes it likely that you followed thousands before you by starting your training in a Gold's Gym.

But if on the other hand this book is part of your first bodybuilding experience, congratulations! The best advice we could possibly convey is to keep your ears and eyes open when you go to the gym. Learn to look and listen. Not all those in the gym with tremendous muscle size actually figured it out for themselves. The fact is that some of them will know less about bodybuilding than you will after reading this book. But most of these massive bodybuilders have been doing something right. So it makes sense to watch what they do. Be attentive to the successful bodybuilders, then put a program together for yourself. Always watch and study—be an observer of human behavior.

If you're a little intimidated, it's no big deal. Try going to the gym when traffic is a little slower—at one of the gym's nonpeak times. Admittedly, a large gym at 5:00 P.M. Monday is going to be noisy and confusing to the novice.

If you think you might get in the way, go to the gym when there are fewer members training to get familiar with the gym's layout and equipment. Anytime before 3:00 P.M. and after 9:00 P.M. is likely to provide more room to roam. The hours of 3:00 P.M. to 9:00 P.M. are considered peak usage hours. It is not advisable to join as a member, then proceed to immediately begin training for the first time. The first few workouts are always excitedly confusing, if not slightly overwhelming.

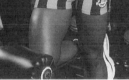

Carol Ann Hensley

COMMON-SENSE RULES

Believe it or not, we actually must tell some less socialized bodybuilders that you:

- do not spit in water fountains or sinks
- should put the weights away after your set
- should strip down the bar after your sets; don't leave it loaded
- never pull a plate off a barbell one side at a time; always get someone to help you pull the plates off simultaneously or the bar will flip upward

Remember that at one time we all were new to bodybuilding, so if you don't become a nuisance, there is a good chance your questions

Aaron Baker

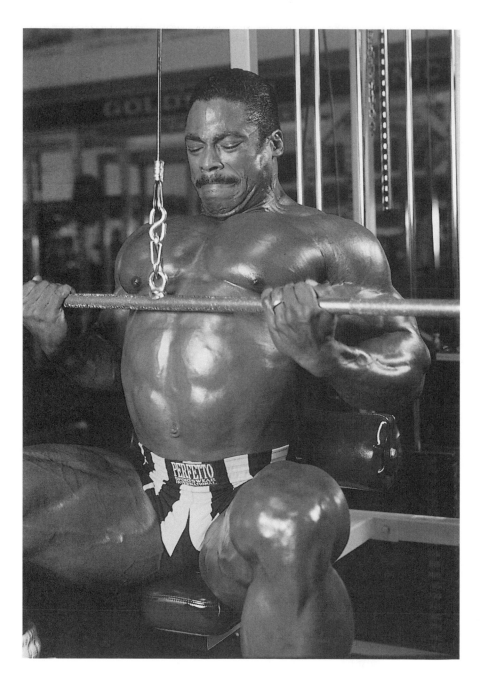

will be answered. And forget about impressing anybody, regardless of what you think or your little brother says.

BENEFITS OF BODYBUILDING

The benefits of bodybuilding include:

- increased muscle mass
- increased bone-mineral density

Mike Francois

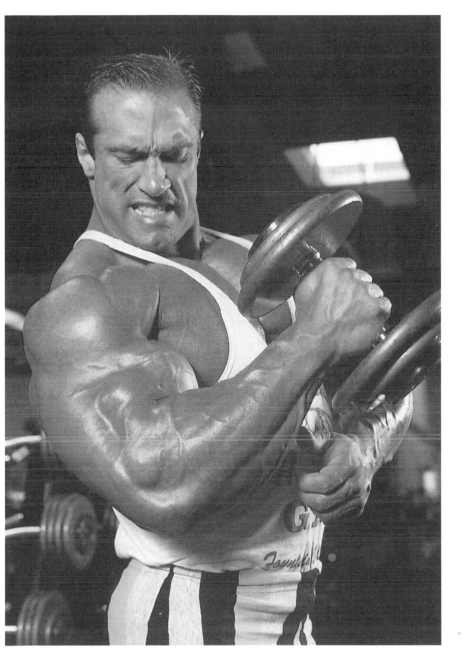

- increased metabolic rate
- reduced body fat
- improved glucose and carbohydrate metabolism
- reduced resting blood pressure
- improved self-image
- improved physical appearance
- improved awareness of eating habits
- improved self-discipline
- improved goal-setting skills

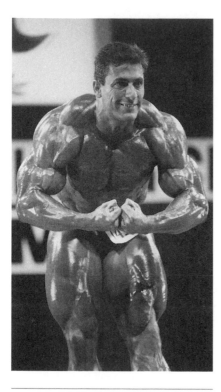

Agathoklis Agathockeous

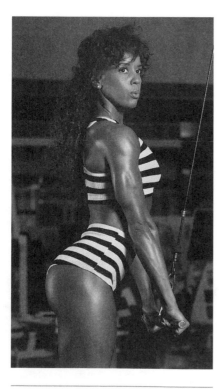

Saryn Muldrow

BASICS

For new bodybuilders, here are some ideas to incorporate into your bodybuilding planning.

Clothes

The most important comment here is to make certain your workout clothes are washed and clean; still some don't get this concept. Styles change and vary, but in general, wear loose or elastic fabrics that allow sufficient freedom of movement. Some facilities require members to wear gym clothing while training. This varies from gym to gym, so ask before you join.

Gyms

If you live in an area that offers a Gold's Gym, then say no more—join today. The other gym owners didn't write a 400-page bodybuilding textbook did they? If you aren't lucky enough to be in a Gold's territory, then the choice is yours. Many great former bodybuilding champions have accomplished much in their garages. For example, Bernard Sealy from Barbados won the middleweight pro-qualifying contest of the IFBB World Amateur Championship after training in his backyard under a coconut tree. When it rained, the training stopped. There was no indoor gym where he lived.

Outside the United States, well-equipped gyms can be few and far between. European bodybuilders are known to hold high esteem for Gold's Gym. Hakan Helvacioglu, a bright, talented bodybuilder from Turkey, says it all: "Here In Turkey when it is 110 degrees Fahrenheit, we all dream of traveling to Venice and training at Gold's. Then we will go to cool off in the Pacific Ocean after our workouts!"

Hakan's gym has limited equipment, only a few fans, and no air conditioning. Yet he continues to make gains in spite of these challenges. So take full advantage of the gym you join.

Gym Behavior

Two rules to remember at the gym are:

- Never interrupt someone performing a set.
- Never walk directly in front of someone performing a set; stay at least four or five feet in front of them.

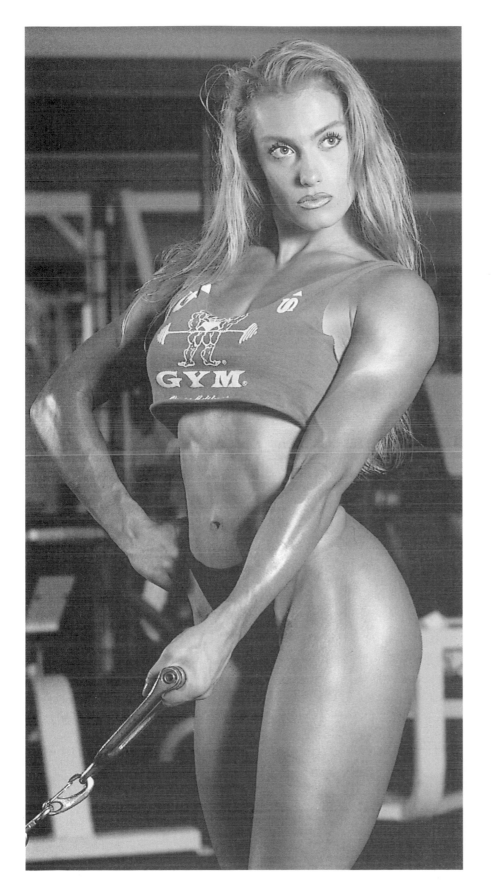

April Moore

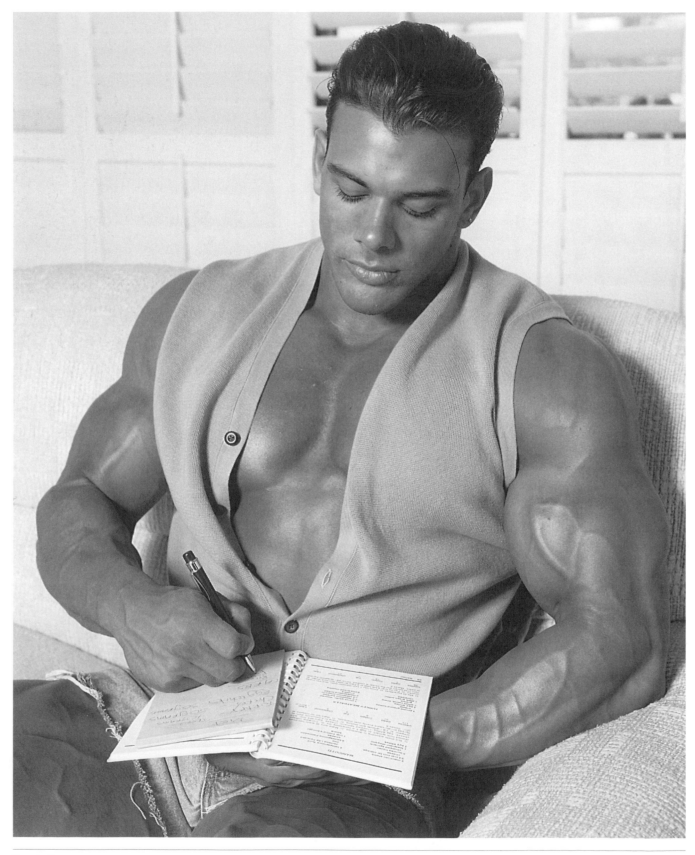

Frank Sepe

Lifting Belts

You will need a lifting belt, so take care of this as soon as possible. There are a couple of styles available. Bodybuilders generally use a leather belt with a four-inch rear width that tapers to a two-and-a-half-inch front and has a buckle adjustment. Wide belts that are four inches around and up to double thickness are used for powerlifting. These can also be used for bodybuilding but tend to be very uncomfortable because they are heavy and extremely stiff.

Newer types of belts are constructed from various synthetic materials. Most bodybuilders still prefer strapping on the familiar leather belt. It is a matter of personal taste. For your first belt, go with a buckled, leather two-and-a-half-inch by four-inch lifting belt.

Accessories

Knee Wraps. Training with knee or wrist wraps is not recommended unless you are directed to do so by a medical professional. Newer generation wraps are extremely tight when correctly employed and will send you to the floor in a second. They take a lot of getting used to—see chapter 7.

Fanny Packs. Although it's hard to wear a lifting belt correctly while wearing a fanny pack, this is a personal choice.

Personal Stereos. Again, using personal stereos is a personal choice.

Cell Phones. Give the cell phone a rest; be considerate of other bodybuilders while in the gym.

Notebooks. See the section on training diaries.

Workout Gloves. In all honesty workout gloves are a little overdone. If you plan to be big, you'll have to use heavy weights sooner or later, so why bother with gloves? You cannot use them safely when training with near maximum weights. If anything, gloves hurt your grip by becoming slippery from sweat. Bodybuilders must endure some things and the tough skin on your palms identifies you as a bodybuilder!

FIRST WORKOUTS

One word covers first workouts for a while—*sore*. Soreness does go away and is something we all have experienced. Now as to the gains you hope will occur during the first part of your training career, do not expect a steady line of growth. Some very gifted individuals are able to

Ms. Olympia—Kim Chizevsky

Jason Arntz undergoing a skin caliper body composition assessment

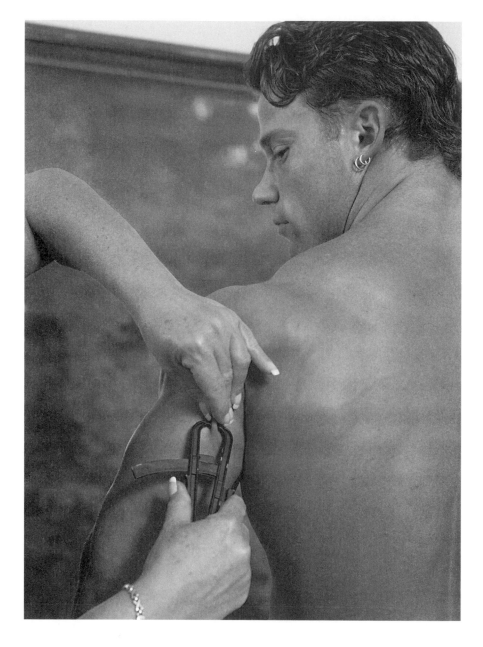

accomplish this, but the majority of us simply have to roll up our sleeves and get to work. Patience is essential to successful bodybuilding.

The first year of training is a tremendously exciting time. Never forget these early memories. They may be just the thing that keeps you on target during a tough precontest diet.

TRAINING PARTNERS

Young guys are virtually guaranteed to ignore the following advice: in general, males train better with male training partners and likewise with females. The strength required for spotting and assisting with heavy weights is important. Most men train with weights a female partner can't help with.

It has long been generally accepted that training with a partner is beneficial. You have a greater degree of commitment if you know someone is waiting at the gym and depending on you.

Whether you wish to train with someone of greater or lesser bodybuilding accomplishment is a matter of circumstance and personal choice. Take some time when you first get to the gym and look for someone physically similar to you to consider as a training partner.

PERSONAL TRAINERS

Rest assured, a personal trainer directly associated with a Gold's Gym will meet the highest standards. Personal training services are somewhat costly in most parts of the country. If you are a student or just starting out in a career, then personal training may have to wait until a later time. If, however, you are not greatly concerned with funding, by all means go ahead and employ a trainer. First look around to determine what your area has to offer. Many different certifications are available for personal trainers. It is not our position to recommend one over another. Just be certain your trainer has some *verifiable* type of certification, current CPR card, and insurance coverage.

Using a personal trainer is almost expected for a middle-aged, out-of-condition business executive who may not have the same motivation and goal structure as a bodybuilder. And it goes without saying that the middle-aged executive will need a different type of trainer than a bodybuilder. The amount of time a nonbodybuilder will expend on physical conditioning is likely to be minimal beyond going to the gym. In contrast, a bodybuilder assumes a lifestyle of near total immersion in the sport. Your responsibilities to yourself as a bodybuilder dictate that you accomplish on your own much of what a personal trainer does for a client. For example, regardless of your background or knowledge, you are the best judge of how your body reacts to specific nutrient combinations and diets.

Remember the rule on using personal trainers: *character over charisma!*

TRAINING DIARIES AND FOOD RECORDS

Although not required to train successfully, training diaries and food records are two additional steps that, when continuously maintained as valuable habits, become part of a healthy day-to-day lifestyle.

Shawn Ray

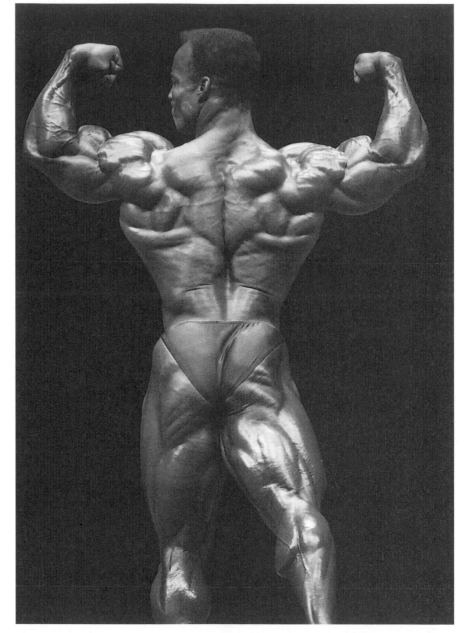

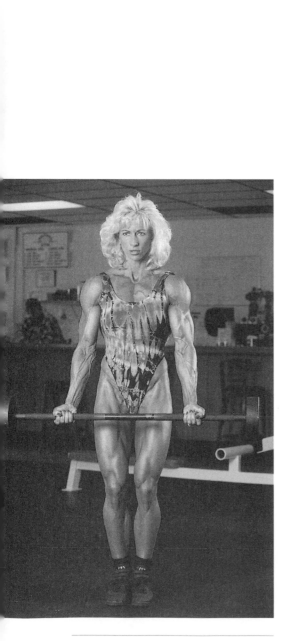

Betty Pariso

It is next to impossible to remember each of three or four weekly workouts and 30 to 35 meals with all the details intact. As you will see later in the book, much of what is done to increase muscular size revolves around specific diets and workout details. If you intend to tuck a first-place trophy under your arm, this is one bodybuilding habit you must start. These are important tools to capture and record the details about the most important bodybuilder you know—yourself.

Your ability to look back and monitor the preparation for a contest is incredibly important regardless of the contest's outcome. The same

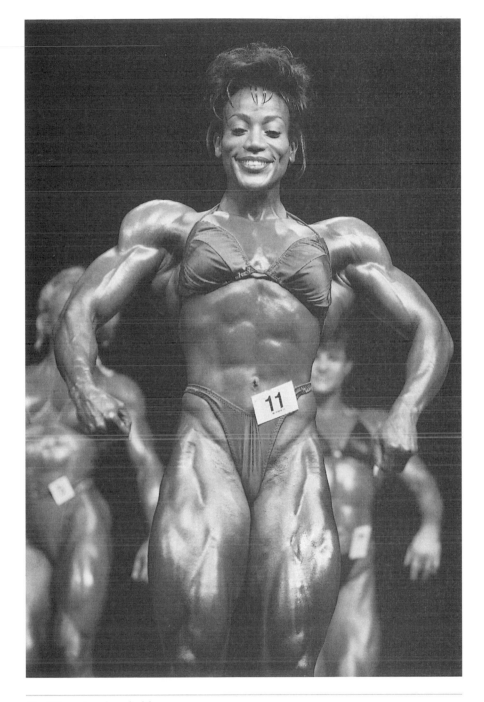

Ms. Olympia—Lenda Murray

holds true for your efforts in packing on extra pounds. You need to be sure what works and what does not. Too many times needless mistakes are repeated year to year, not due to laziness but as the result of overlooking small details. Rest assured that the people winning the competitions keep notes and review what they did to get in shape.

Carol Ann Hensley

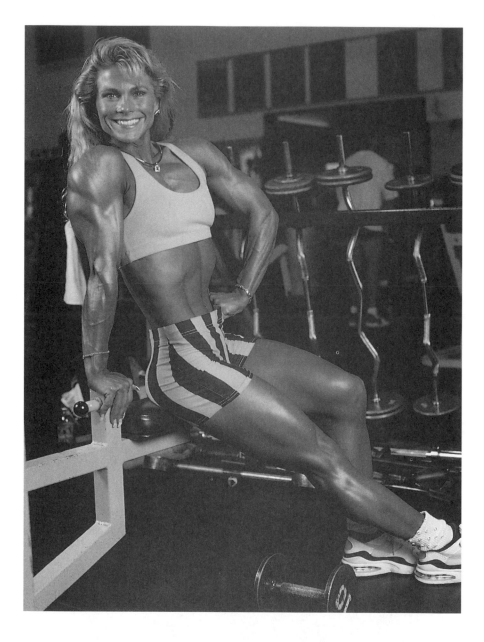

The competitor who is able to go back and check the record from the last contest is in a better position to spot mistakes and avoid them. A simple small notebook is fine for training diaries and food records. Generally you will want to use one which opens flat when folded back to the day's page. A stenographer's pad is often used by bodybuilders. Of course, the notebook's size depends on how much detail you want to record.

BODY FAT AND BODY COMPOSITION TESTING

Testing body fat and composition is an area of some controversy. For decades bodybuilders have simply hopped up on the scale to weigh.

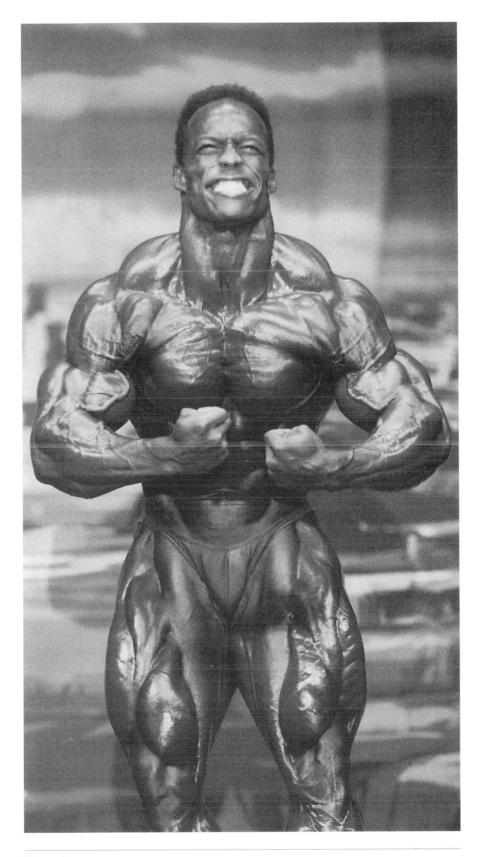

Shawn Ray

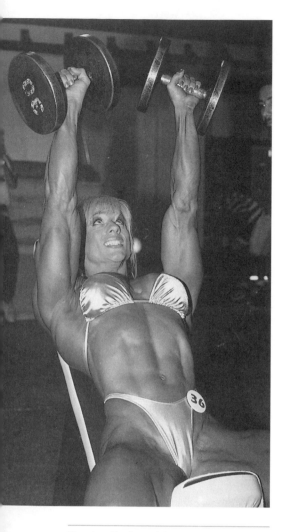

Denise Rutkowski

However, science now allows for more refined assessments. Body weight is made up of muscle, fat, water, and bone. The bathroom scale only tells you the grand total, not what percentage of each you have. The following methods are used to find these percentages. (Keep in mind that the most accurate methods are generally found in hospitals):

- DEXA body-scan dual-energy x-ray absorptiometry
- K-40 potassium isotope measurement
- whole-body immersion—water displacement
- electrical impedance
- skin-fold caliper assessment

In that some of these body-composition assessment tools are not FDA-approved, they cannot and should not be used to diagnose or treat a disease.

MUSCLE SORENESS

Sore, aching muscles are part and parcel of a bodybuilder's life. To the knowing bodybuilder, the sensation of slight soreness is a good indicator that the last training load was just right. At present, there are two schools of thought about why exercise-induced muscle soreness occurs. The first is mechanical and the second is metabolic. Some of the soreness is a result of changes in your muscle cell's chemistry. Soreness also arises from muscle cell structural disruption or damage.

The novice is not yet training with maximum weights. Yet because the novice's body has not yet fully adapted, the unaccustomed stress of even moderate training produces soreness as a muscle response. After some period of time, the body acclimates itself to the stress of training with an overall weight gain and strength increase.

If you are new to bodybuilding, don't despair. The to-be-expected soreness does mellow out. Before you know it you'll be looking for that sensation as a gauge of a good workout. Additionally, these first few months of soreness can produce tremendous bursts of size. The roles of diet, rest, and supplementation become primary after finishing each workout. Too little of any of these three supporting players and you might miss out on some of the gains.

Why?

The process of muscle metabolism that eventually produces muscle soreness likely occurs in one of two ways:

1. disruption of the cellular membrane (this is more pronounced during the eccentric or lowering portion of the exercise; see chapter 3)

2. increased internal temperature especially during eccentric motion—likely due to increased friction.

These two scenarios involve less than maximum intensity workouts. Hard-core, high-end pain training takes you beyond mere discomfort. In the case of the experienced bodybuilder who is using near maximum weights in high-intensity workouts, the damage to the muscle is due to severe microtraumas. The degree of discomfort felt after low-intensity exercise is different from that of more extreme training attacks. With the more intensive approaches, the disruption and metabolic alteration may take up to seven days to fully resolve. In instances where training has generated a major muscle trauma, the time frame required to regenerate damaged muscle tissue can be up to 20 days.

How?

Specifically, the mechanisms leading to soreness are:

- elevated internal muscle temperature, especially from the lowering or downward (eccentric) portion of an exercise
- influx of calcium ions into the muscle fibers; calcium is the cation responsible for muscle contractions and must be pumped back across the cell membrane into storage
- the calcium releasing a substance called *protease*, which is similar to a digestive enzyme but on a much smaller scale, at a specific point during the buildup within the muscle cell
- the released protease breaking down damaged muscle cells and transport from the muscle
- a protective response initiating within the cell to prevent any further damage as the protease degrades the damaged tissue

Unfortunately, once the damage has occurred to the muscle, it then exhibits a buildup of metabolites such as histamine, serotonin, and potassium. This accumulation of material inside the muscle is responsible for the post-exercise inflammation or injury. The inflammatory effect may take more than 24 hours to become apparent due to the time required for all this buildup.

This last point is important. If it takes at least 24 hours to accumulate enough of these waste products in the muscle, does it make good sense to train the same muscle again within three days or so? No—this would not provide recovery time.

At first it may appear we've given you too much information on just muscle soreness. However, as later chapters detail, there is no better way for a bodybuilder to estimate the degree of effort exerted during a workout. So self-awareness as it concerns muscle soreness cannot be overemphasized. The line between too much and too little in bodybuilding is small, so be cautious with the degree of soreness.

ESTIMATED EXERCISE RECOVERY TIMES	
Process of Recovery	Time Required
Restoration of ATP-CP	3–5 minutes
Muscle glycogen restoration after bodybuilding or strength workout	24 hours
Lactic acid clearance	1–2 hours
Recovery of nervous system and muscle tissues after max intensity bodybuilding	2.5–3 days

RECUPERATION GUIDELINES

Expect the following when recuperating after a workout:

- Female bodybuilders tend to recover at a slightly slower rate than their male counterparts.
- Younger bodybuilders recover from intense training at significantly faster rates than do older bodybuilders.
- Generally, the more experience you have as a bodybuilder the greater the ability of your body to recover.

The influence of your emotional state is no longer disputed. Negative emotions decrease performance and recovery, while the opposite holds true for a positive outlook. Food intake and your related nutrient profile are responsible for the biochemical mobilization of active recovery processes. Inadequate nutrition will doom your training to less than its best.

Methods of Accelerated Recovery

The following can help speed up muscle recovery:

- massage therapy
- heat therapy
- cold therapy
- intermittent temperature therapy
- water therapy
- magnetic therapy
- meditation
- visualization techniques

- biofeedback
- numerous types of drug therapies
- stretching techniques
- light aerobic exercise at less than 60 percent of your target heart rate (see chapter 15)
- use of specific nutrients (chemotherapeutics)

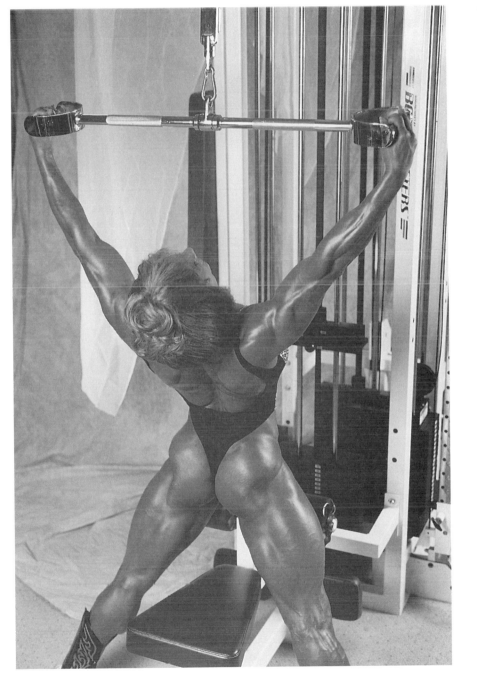

Laura Creavelle

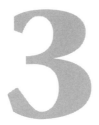

3

Essential Bodybuilding Knowledge

If you don't become Mr. Olympia it won't be because you had poor technique when performing barbell curls. It will be due to more cerebral factors.

In bodybuilding it can be said that what works for one generally works for all (with some adjustments of course). The tricky part is knowing what actually works. The people at Gold's Venice know what works—we've seen the best train for their biggest shows.

There are no unique problems in bodybuilding—only unique solutions!

As the best in the bodybuilding business, our goal in this chapter is to effectively train you to answer your own bodybuilding questions by providing information not presented in other bodybuilding books. The same practicality reflected in the success of Gold's is yours for the asking.

Our experience indicates that many new bodybuilders are overexposed and underinformed about bodybuilding's more intellectual aspects. Until 1992 or so, bodybuilders only needed to understand the basics of training about five days a week, using milk and egg protein supplements, and getting plenty of rest. Much has changed since then.

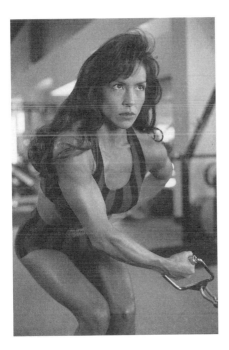

Kimiko Tanaka

TOPICS COVERED

Topics to be covered in this chapter include:

> *diet*
> *nutrition*
> *muscles and their structure*
> *hyperplasia versus hypertrophy?*
> *types of muscular contraction*

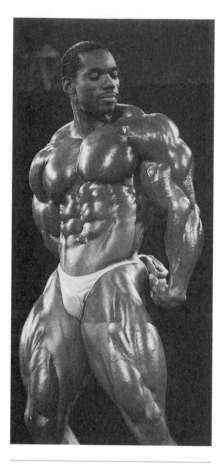

Flex Wheeler
Mike Matarazzo

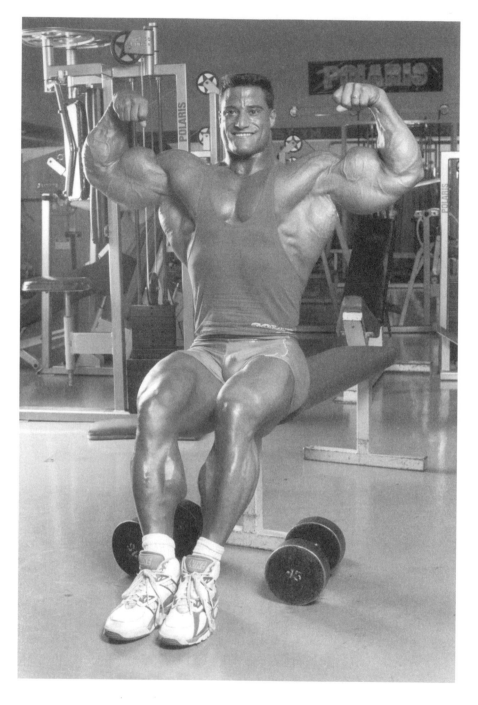

contraction fuel
energy systems
training
stress and stressors
intensity and recovery
manipulation of growth
gaining body weight
somatotypes
must-know terms

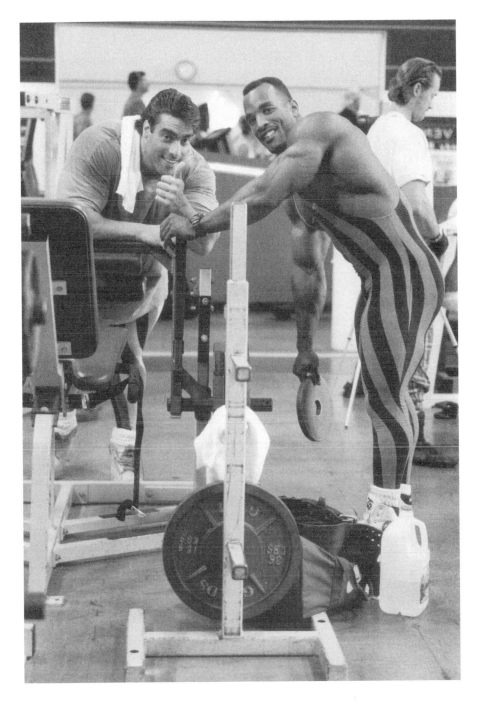

Jim Mentis and Darrem Charles

Several of these topics are also covered in other chapters because they are crucial areas on which bodybuilders should be clear.

EVERYBODY GETS CONFUSED

We begin with diet and nutrition as the two required templates for growth. They are followed by some aspects of muscle-structure form and function, training and recovery, and finally, growth.

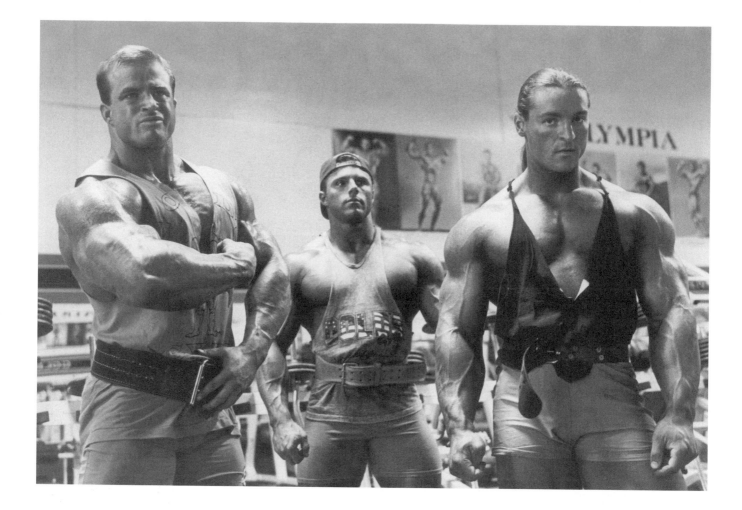

Andrew Dale, Kevin Christie, and
Gordon Lavelle

Your success as a bodybuilder requires great desire and knowledge—bodybuilding knowledge drawn from a number of different areas of science and research. The details we provide on how to train, diet, and condition for your ultimate physique are based on expert opinions. But the qualifications for becoming a successful bodybuilder do not include formal advanced education. So if you didn't earn a master's in biochemistry, you can still succeed.

Most bodybuilders get their information from monthly muscle magazines. There are 10 or so newsstand muscle magazines, each with a wide range of articles. What if you bought them all and attempted to read each cover to cover? Would this help your bodybuilding efforts? Would you be able to draw all that information together to develop a plan of attack for yourself? For many the answer is "no." This is not only due to the volume of material in the magazines but also the content and subject matter.

The muscle mags now have doctors and biochemists on their writing staffs. Until the mid-1990s this was unheard of. The accuracy of these highly trained writers has cleared away many misconceptions.

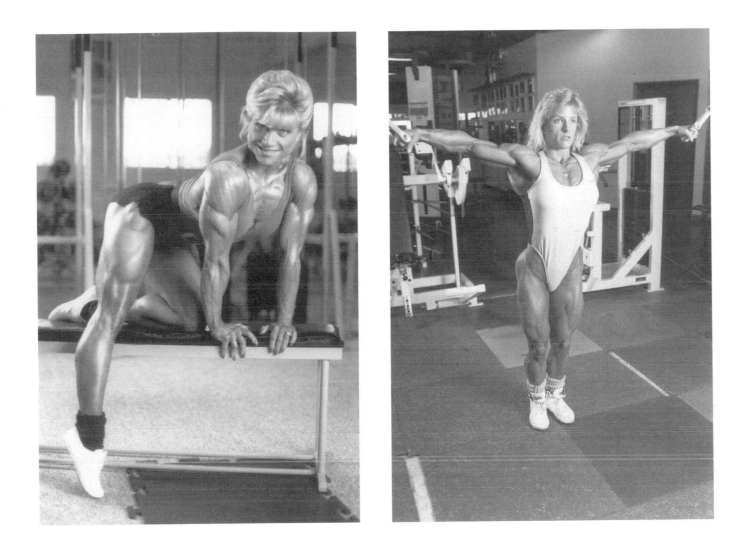

Drorit Kernes
Sue Price

The problem is whether or not you can use the articles for practical learning. Due to their educational backgrounds, many of these writers are not necessarily understood by their intended audience. All the info in the world won't do you any good if you don't understand how to use it. Even the terms used to explain something as basic as muscle contraction are enough to suck up all your available mental RAM.

What is the average Joe to do? The answers are hidden in the mags but how do you find them? By filling in some essential areas of bodybuilding knowledge, we hope in this chapter to provide you the tools to excavate the hidden gems of bodybuilding wealth.

DIET

Training accounts for only 4 percent of real-time bodybuilding. Once you've left the gym you're faced with approximately 96 percent of the week's hours left open for growth. Anything that takes up 96 percent

King Kamali

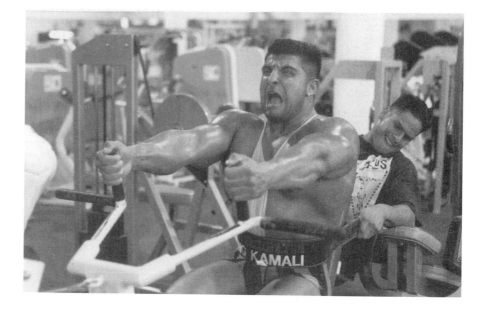

of our time merits our attention. It stands to reason that if you're getting 4 percent correct (the training) then making errors the other 96 percent of the time, you're compromising your success. Pay close attention to the chapters on nutrition and supplements. Diet is something bodybuilders must watch every day—not just during the period before a contest.

MUSCLE STRUCTURE

Muscle is tissue composed of fibers that are able to contract, causing and allowing movement of the parts and organs of the body. Muscle fibers are richly vascular, irritable and conductive, and elastic. Vascular refers to blood supply, irritable and conductive to electrical transference, and elastic to the contractile aspect.

There are two basic kinds of muscle: striated and smooth. Striated muscle, which comprises all skeletal muscles except for the myocardium, is long and voluntary. It responds very quickly to stimulation and is paralyzed by interruption of its innervation—the distribution or supply of nerve fibers or nerve impulses to a part of the body. Smooth muscle, which comprises all visceral muscles, is short and involuntary. It reacts slowly to stimuli and does not entirely lose its tone if innervation is interrupted.

The myocardium (heart muscle) is sometimes classified as a third kind of muscle. It is basically a striated muscle that does not contract as quickly as the other striated muscles. It is not completely paralyzed if it loses its neural stimuli.

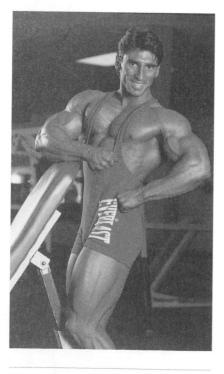

Todd Cummins

Paul DeMayo

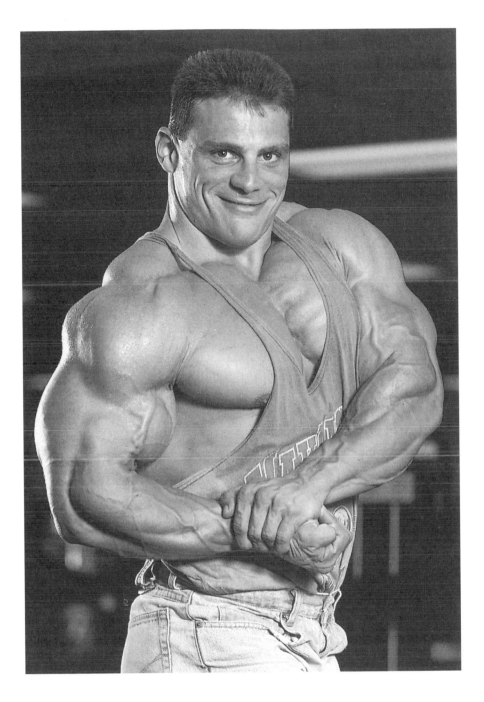

Striated muscle is muscle tissue consisting of myofibrils. Striated muscles are composed of bundles of parallel, striated fibers. Each striated muscle fiber is covered by a thin, connective epimysium and divided into bundles of sheathed fibers containing smaller myofibrils.

The muscle's contractile units, or sarcomeres, comprise the larger protein strands or myofibrils. A sarcomere is the smallest functional unit of a myofibril. Within each sarcomere are thick filaments of myosin and thinner filaments of actin.

Shawn Ray

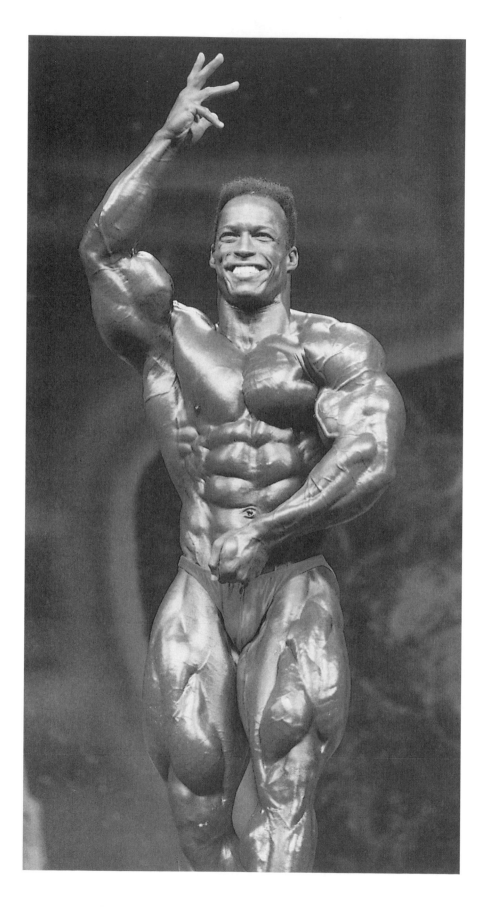

Cardiac muscle, or myocardium, is a special type of striated muscle. Cardiac muscle is the exception among involuntary muscles, which are characteristically smooth. Its contractile fibers resemble those of skeletal muscle but are not as large in diameter. The connective tissue of cardiac muscle is sparser than that of skeletal muscle.

Smooth muscle is composed of elongated, spindle-shaped cells found in muscles not under voluntary control, such as the muscles of the intestines, stomach, and other visceral organs.

Hyperplasia is an increase in the number of cells of a body part. This is where the idea of 100-repetition sets came from. It has been studied in experimental conditions using animals and chronic stretch overload. When considering the causal factor in muscle growth, hyperplasia likely becomes a player in some individuals at the point of extreme genetic threshold. Hypertrophy is probably responsible as the process behind your new lat spread. It is the increase in the size of an organ caused by an increase in the size of the cells rather than the number of cells.

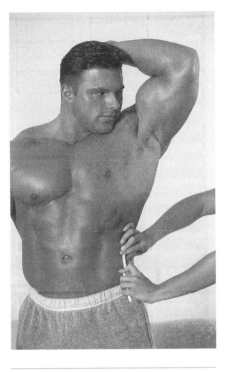

Kevin Christie

Muscular contraction occurs when an electrical pulse (caused by a chemical exchange) fires across the nerve's motor endplate. This electrical firing causes the muscle fiber's thin, threadlike filaments, actin and myosin, to become attracted to each other. Myosin is the skeletal muscle protein that makes up close to one half of the proteins in muscle tissue. Actin is a protein found in muscle fibers that acts with myosin to bring about contraction and relaxation. Taken together these two contractile proteins can be thought of as velcro caterpillars on velcro surfaces, easy going up but tough to pull down. The actual attraction is seen as a sliding toward one another, or inward movement. This sliding movement produces a shortening effect within the muscle's filaments. The shortened muscle is then said to be contracting. The contracted muscle produces internal muscular tension caused by cross-bridge activity between the actin and myosin filaments within the muscle fiber.

The force generated by these contractile elements is transmitted to the bones via tendons and connective tissue. The bones move and produce external tension. The nerve impulse leading to the actual contraction travels incredibly fast, about 16 feet per second. There are three forms of athletic muscular contraction: isotonic, isometric, and isokinetic.

ISOTONIC CONTRACTION

In an isotonic contraction the tension within the muscle remains the same throughout the movement, which is to say the force of the contraction remains constant. This is also called the positive portion of an

Ian Harrison

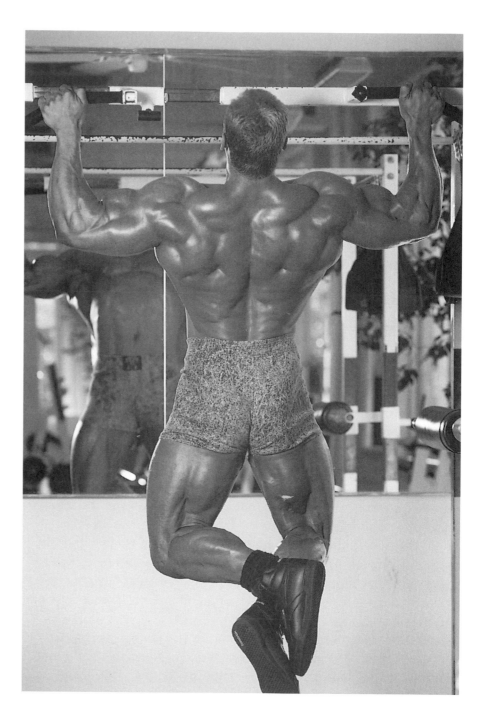

exercise movement. There are two aspects of isotonic contraction, concentric and eccentric. Concentric contraction occurs when the muscle fibers shorten as tension develops. At the onset of the movement, the actin and myosin filaments have tremendous pulling force. Thus you will be stronger in the initial phase of most movements. Toward the end or near the peak of contraction, the ability of the filaments to slide toward each other reaches a limit and strength weakens.

An eccentric contraction is the type of muscle contraction that involves lengthening the muscle fibers, such as when a weight is lowered through a range of motion. The muscle yields to the resistance, allowing itself to be stretched. Here the actin and myosin slide away from each other. The level of force generated is much higher in the eccentric phase as opposed to the concentric phase. This is due to the added friction in the eccentric portion.

Concentric aspect is a form of muscle contraction that occurs when muscle fibers shorten as tension develops. Eccentric aspect is a contraction that involves lengthening the muscle fibers, such as when a weight is lowered through a range of motion. The muscle yields to the resistance, allowing itself to be stretched. This is the age of the focused eccentric contraction. Too often bodybuilders focus their attention only on the positive motion (concentric) and pay little attention to the negative motion (eccentric). It is a matter of common sense to perform the lowering of resistance with at least as much focus and effort given to lifting the same weight.

ISOMETRIC CONTRACTION

Isometric contraction is a muscular contraction not accompanied by movement of the joint. The muscle is neither lengthened nor shortened but tension changes can be measured. Due to the lack of visible muscle shortening, there is no movement of the actins. This is the exercise method Charles Atlas made famous many decades ago. Atlas called this "dynamic tension."

ISOKINETIC CONTRACTION

Finally, there is isokinetic contraction, which pertains to a concentric or eccentric contraction that occurs at a set speed against a force of maximal resistance produced at all points in the range of motion. This contraction type is performed under controlled same-speed conditions.

MUSCLE FUEL

Your ultimate success as a bodybuilder may be due to more than the effectiveness of your training. As much or perhaps more than training, your gains will be contingent on your ability to eat enough food to provide the energy to support your existing level of muscle size, fuel your training, and support the process of recovery and growth. This adds up to more food than nonbodybuilders can imagine. This section

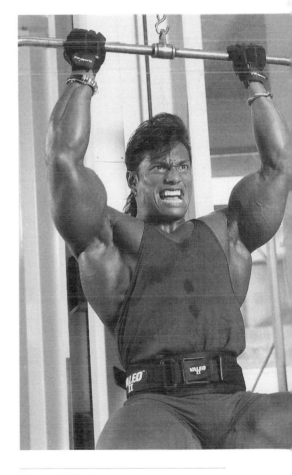

Romeo Villarino

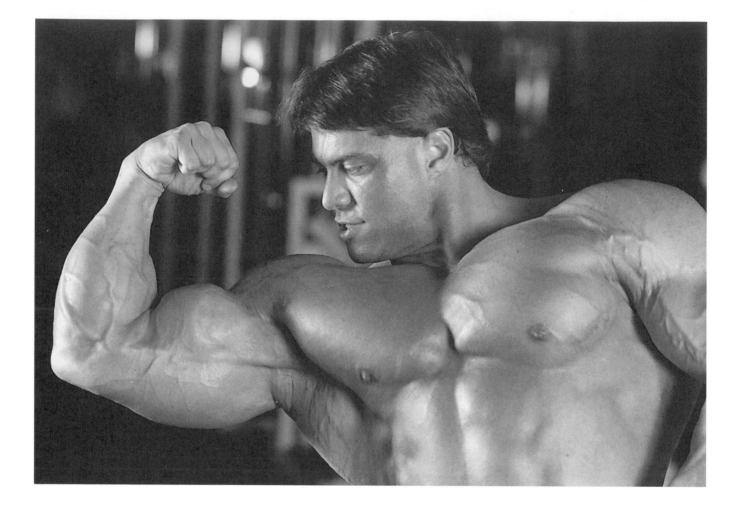

Phil Hernon

on muscle fuel is intended to provide an overall glance at the three stages of fuel utilization by the human body. Specific details on energy balance during growth or body-fat reduction are provided in later chapters.

Ultimately the energy used by the body must come from calories. Calories come from foods or fat stores in the body. Of course, many intermediate steps are involved before your muscles use that bowl of rice for the big pump.

ANAEROBIC ENERGY

ATP–CP System

The body's ATP–CP system supplies 8 to 10 seconds of energy employed in quick, explosive movements. After the store of adenosine triphosphate in the muscle tissue is depleted, phosphocreatine or creatine

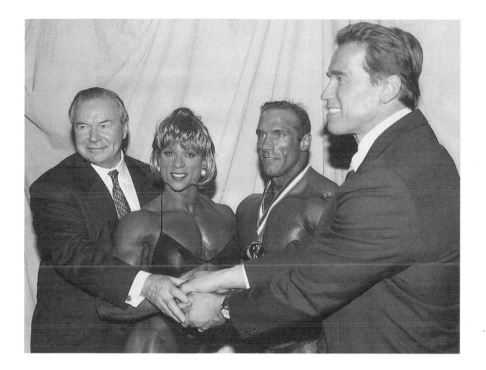

Arnold Schwarzenegger and Jim Lorimer (left) with Laura Creavelle and Mike Francois

phosphate is split into creatine and phosphate. The energy produced by splitting the CP molecule provides energy for the resynthesis of ATP from CP.

Lactic Acid or Phosphagen System

Characterized by the incomplete utilization of glucose with lactic acid as the residual metabolite, the lactic acid or phosphagen system is co-active with the ATP–CP system but in a secondary role. It takes over as the muscle's store of ATP is exhausted. After about one and a half to two minutes, the excess by-product of energy production accumulates and the internal environment becomes unable to further engage in sufficient glycolysis. For activity of less than two minutes in duration, the system by which fuel is metabolized into a consumable form is called anaerobic glycolysis or the lactic acid cycle.

Lactic acid is a three-carbon organic acid produced by anaerobic respiration. D-lactic acid is produced by the fermentation of dextrose. L-lactic acid, a product of glucose and glycogen metabolism, is involved in muscular contractions. L-lactic acid is a racemic mixture found in the stomach, in sour milk, and in certain other foods.

Anaerobic energy is created without the presence of oxygen. Olympic-caliber 100-meter sprinters never take a breath—the entire race is powered through the anaerobic system!

Saryn Muldrow

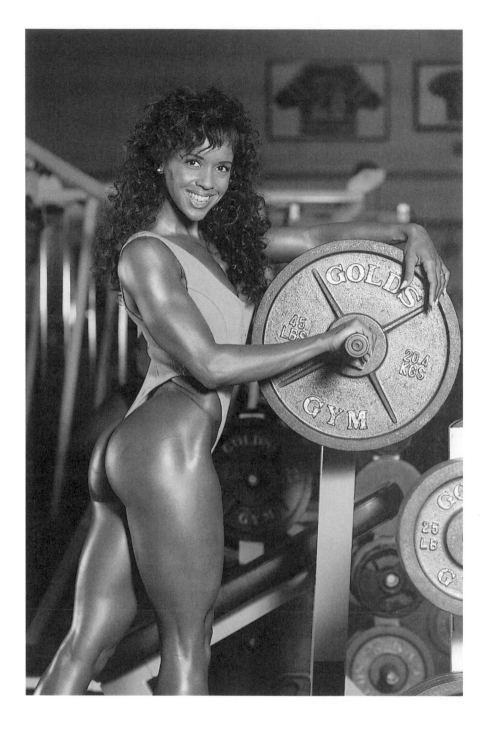

When you train you use energy—think of it as a drop in battery power. The full battery charge is similar to adenosine triphosphate (one unit adenosine and three units phosphates). When used by the muscle, a single unit of phosphate is lost resulting in adenosine diphosphate (one unit of adenosine and two units of phosphate). For the purposes of exercise, you can either store a limited amount of ATP, or alternatively, you can recharge the lost phosphate unit from ADP.

AEROBIC ENERGY

Aerobic indicates the presence of oxygen. Aerobic exercise is any physical activity that requires additional effort by the heart and lungs to meet the increased demand by the skeletal muscles for oxygen. The exercise generally requires heavier breathing than passive muscular activity and results in increased heart and lung efficiency with a minimum of wasted energy.

Glycolysis is a series of enzymatically catalyzed reactions, occurring within cells, by which glucose and other sugars are broken down to yield lactic acid or pyruvic acid, releasing energy in the form of adenosine triphosphate. Aerobic glycolysis yields pyruvic acid in the presence of adequate oxygen. Anaerobic glycolysis yields lactic acid.

Aerobic Glycolysis

The aerobic system is more efficient than either the ATP–CP or lactic acid cycle. The aerobic system can burn more than just glucose for energy. In contrast, the other systems cannot. Specifically, the aerobic system can use glycogen along with amino acids and fatty acids. It is a series of enzymatically catalyzed reactions, which occur in the presence of sufficient oxygen, by which glucose and other sugars are broken down to yield pyruvic acid. Energy is then released from the pyruvic acid, in the form of ATP. Aerobic glycolysis yields pyruvic acid in the presence of adequate oxygen.

Succinic acid, resulting from the oxidative decarboxylation of alpha-ketoglutaric acid, is oxidized to fumaric acid, and its oxidation regenerates oxaloacetic acid, which condenses with acetyl-CoA, closing the cycle.

The process, also called the Krebs cycle, is a sequence of enzymatic reactions involving the metabolism of sugars, fatty acids, and amino acids to yield carbon dioxide, water, and high-energy phosphate bonds. The cycle is initiated when pyruvate combines with coenzyme A (CoA) to form acetyl-CoA, which enters the cycle in subsequent steps to form alpha-ketoglutaric acid, and subsequently, succinic acid. After a few more steps, end-cycle metabolites combine with acetyl-CoA, closing the cycle. The Krebs cycle provides a major source of ATP. These various transformational sequences also produce intermediate molecules that are starting points for other vital metabolic cycles, including amino acid synthesis.

Acetylcoenzyme A is a two-carbon molecule that is formed in the course of several important metabolic processes. The formation of acetylcoenzyme A is the critical intermediate step between anaerobic glycolysis and the citric acid cycle. A coenzyme is a nonprotein substance that combines with an apoenzyme to form a complete enzyme

Dinah Anderson

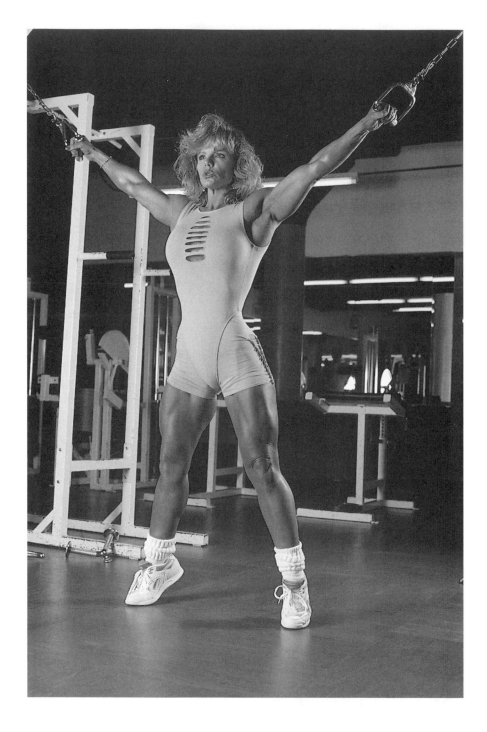

or holoenzyme. Coenzymes include some of the vitamins, such as B_1 and B_2, and have smaller molecules than enzymes.

Aerobic glycolysis provides a major source of ATP energy and also produces intermediate molecules that are starting points for a number of vital metabolic pathways, including amino acid synthesis.

FATIGUE AND EXHAUSTION

Fatigue is the loss of strength or endurance that occurs when muscle tissue is unable to respond to stimuli that normally evoke muscular contraction or other activity. Exhaustion is indicated by extreme loss of physical or mental abilities caused by fatigue or illness.

As exercise increases in duration, the body transitions through a sequence of energy systems, each contributing to fatigue, and ultimately, to exhaustion. In order of depletion, your energy systems are:

- activation and depletion of ATP–CP
- anaerobic glycolysis with increasing acidosis and calcium influx in the muscle
- aerobic glycolysis with depletion of glycogen stores leading to increased access to fat stores and release and increased oxidation of free fatty acids

TRAINING

Without a doubt bodybuilding brings to mind training. The reality is that only a small percentage of the time you spend every week as a bodybuilder is devoted to training.

In the course of the seven-day week there are 16 waking hours per day if you get eight or so hours of sleep at night. That equals 116 waking hours per week. If you train one and a half hours three days a week, that is four and a half hours spent training. This is 4 percent of the total waking hours available to you each week. The other 96 percent of the time is yours to use for maximizing the time you spend in the gym. Training is vital, but, as we now know, there are other pieces of the bodybuilding puzzle.

Intensity Levels

In general, intensity of training effort falls into three separate areas. They are:

1. positive or concentric full-rep momentary failure

2. positive or concentric full- and partial-rep momentary failure

3. positive or concentric full-rep momentary failure plus additional negative or eccentric-only reps

These are ranked from top down in order of increasing stress or intensity. Accordingly, the body's ability to recover (grow) from training decreases as you increase the level of intensity. Always remember that the bigger you become or more intensely you train, the amount of time required for total recovery also increases.

Spotters

Using a spotter is a great idea that can be overused, especially by young, inexperienced bodybuilders. A spotter takes whatever position is required to safely perform one of two responsibilities:

1. assist you in the completion of a stalled or missed repetition

2. assist you in stopping the exercise and replacing the weights in their starting position

Far too often overly enthusiastic lifters attempt to lift too much weight and the spotter (best friend and buddy) kicks in. Instead of racking the weight and reducing it by a few pounds, this spotter helps his buddy blindly grind out 4 to 6 two-man repetitions. Then, amazingly enough, these two switch positions and repeat the same sequence, sometimes through the majority of the workout. This overuse of the spotting concept is not inherently bad, but it certainly can hold back your gains if your spotting partner is performing part of your sets.

In the case of forced reps, drop sets, assisted reps, or eccentric exercises, the advantages to having a spotter become clear. When using heavy weights, use of a spotter is mandatory. However, if you are new to the gym and a more accomplished bodybuilder asks you to spot, *do not* grab the bar until that bodybuilder tells you to take it. Make this mistake and you'll know what a bad temper looks like! Generally spotters should be hands off.

STRESS

A stressor is anything that causes stress (wear and tear) on the body's physical or mental resources. Working out is a great way to reduce your perceived level of stress. You always feel better after a good workout. Training is simply another form of stress in your body. Lifting weights is the type of stress you want to be able to master—not the other way around.

Stress often involves negative connotations. Yet stress itself is not bad. Bodybuilding success, for example, is centered around control of the stress input and the resulting stress response. Time spent in the gym is one form of active bodybuilding stress. Other factors involved in bodybuilding, such as your emotional state and social and economic conditions, add to the cumulative stress incurred. These secondary

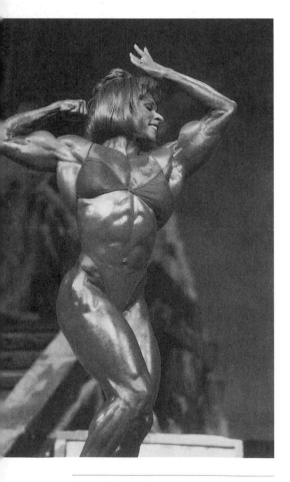

Laura Creavelle

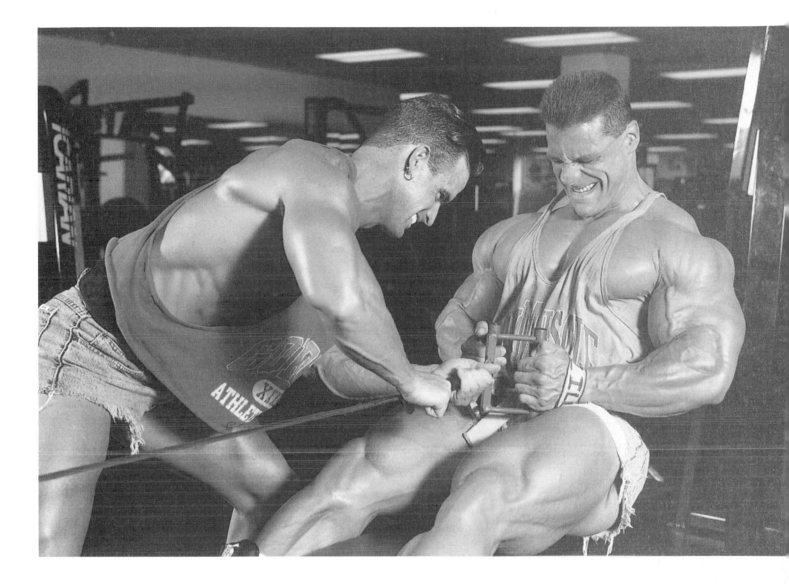

Paul DeMayo (right) and
Ted Hanley (left)

stressors should ideally be a distant second to your training. The period of recovery outside the gym is the period during which you hope your body's stress response is greater than the amount of stress incurred. If all factors are in place, muscle growth will occur.

Manipulation of Growth

General Adaptation Syndrome (GAS) is the defense response of the body or mind to injury or prolonged stress, as described by Hans Selye (1907–1982). It consists of the following three stages:

1. an initial shock reaction

2. an increasing resistance or adaptation, using the various defense mechanisms of the body or mind

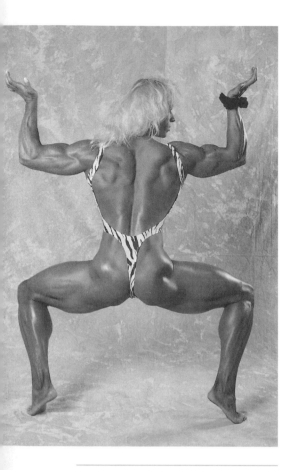

Ms. Olympia—Kim Chizevsky

3. final stage of either adjustment and healing or exhaustion and disintegration

Bodybuilding is first physical stress, and second, mental and emotional stress. It is the delicate balance between GAS from your body and the continued onslaught of training that yields pounds of hard-won muscle. Train less, eat and sleep more is the generalized prescription for taking advantage of your body's GAS. Remember that steroids only speed the recovery side of the GAS equation; they do not specifically produce new muscle growth. There must always be the initial source of stress—the training.

MUSCLE TISSUE DAMAGE

Muscle tissue damage is an area of bodybuilding debate that will outlast this book. Some experts in the field of muscle physiology are of the opinion that the upper limit of human muscular growth can be accomplished only through hyperplasia, or the creation of new muscle fibers. Even more interesting is the idea of how hyperplasia may occur. It centers around the damage or trauma to the contractile elements within the muscle itself.

Upon reaching peak contraction in a repetition, the downward eccentric portion begins. With a sufficiently heavy weight, measurable microtrauma, or small tears, appear inside the contractile proteins. The exact sequence of the intracellular cascade of growth factors this trauma initiates is presently unknown.

How Much Is Needed

Very little of this type of research has been conducted. You are largely on your own and best advised to employ intense self-awareness as the assessment tool. The sensation of muscle tissue being injured on this microscale has been described as a phantom tickle deep inside the muscle. You can actually become attuned to this sensation during a properly executed eccentric repetition.

When pumping out fast reps, you produce an incredible feeling of a deep, tight, and full pump. The pump is an unmistakable feeling and is never forgotten. The pump goes away after five hours or so and does not strongly correlate with eventual and permanent size increases. In comparison, the feeling from eccentrically induced microtrauma is less of an immediate pumping. Here minor tissue damage appears to be related to a unique form of the pump. It is more along the lines of less-than-maximum volume but produces a very tight sensation centered in the deeper muscle tissue.

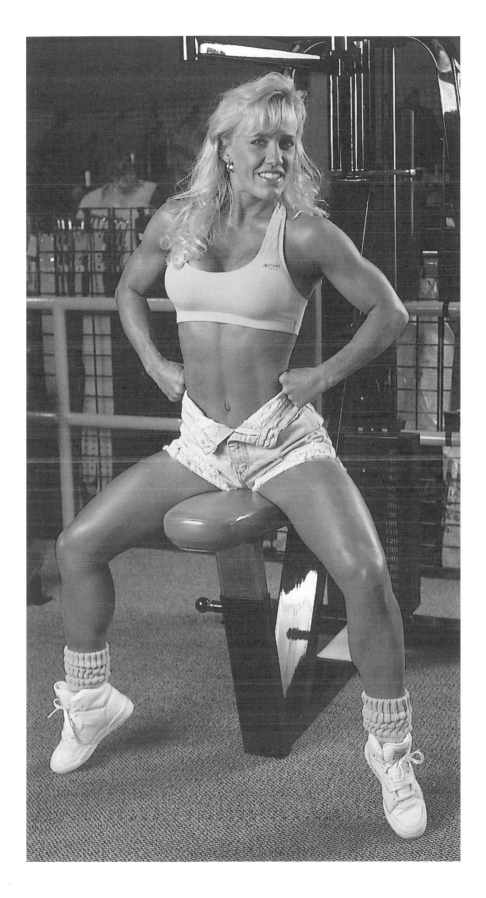

Suzy Duby

Jason Arntz

Learning to recognize this feeling is an area in which self-experimentation is required. Give the training some time and you'll soon be able to tell the pump from miniscule tissue damage patterns.

POST-TRAINING GROWTH

The intricate balance between overtraining and undertraining is vague. One way to assess the growth patterns is to weigh yourself on a schedule, recording each observation. After accounting for fat accumulation, this is pretty much how bodybuilders gauge their growth gains.

The ideal condition for training-induced growth is moderate to intense fatigue. If you are able to hold off on training until the fatigue is ameliorated through recovery, then the pounds will stack up. Growth and recovery are energy-expensive and energy-dependent metabolic activities. If you take in too few calories, you will not grow.

Muscle cells generally require a refractory or recovery period after activity, during which time cells restore their energy supplies and excrete metabolic waste products. Exhaustion is indicated by a decreased capacity for physical and mental work regardless of adequate sleep, loss of appetite and body weight, increased incidents of infection, fatigue, or lack of energy, and inability to maintain usual routines.

To take all precautionary steps to make certain you are recovering well enough to avoid exhaustion and to continue to grow:

- consistently eat the required amount of food (this is not as easy as it sounds, so beware)
- consume proper quantities of water
- use the appropriate supplements
- be consistent in sleep and training

Other aids to recovery include meditation techniques, hydrotherapy, massage therapy, heat therapy, and stretching.

ABOUT GAINING WEIGHT

Gains in body weight almost never come in a steady stream. They seem to come in bursts of significant weight increase followed by a refractory period of no increase. When you begin to grow beyond your initial burst, you'll notice how the scale responds by jumping offside on intervals of anywhere from 10 to 18 days. Here are some rough guidelines as to how much weight you might expect to pack on. (These figures are collected from anecdotal evidence—knowledge based on isolated observations and not yet verified by controlled scientific studies):

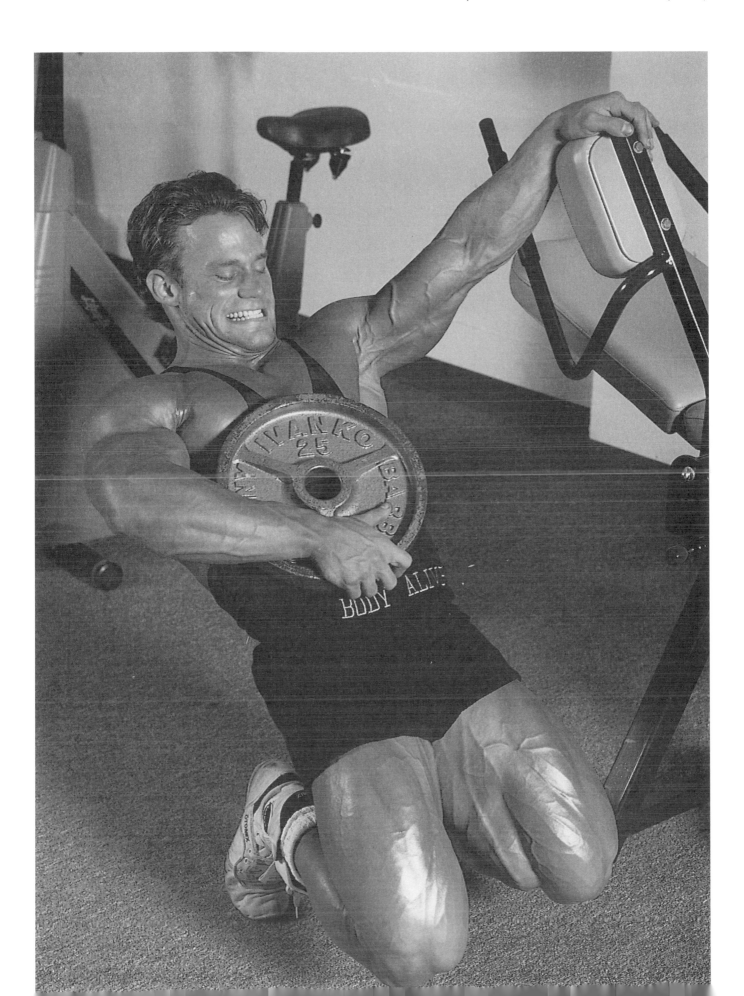

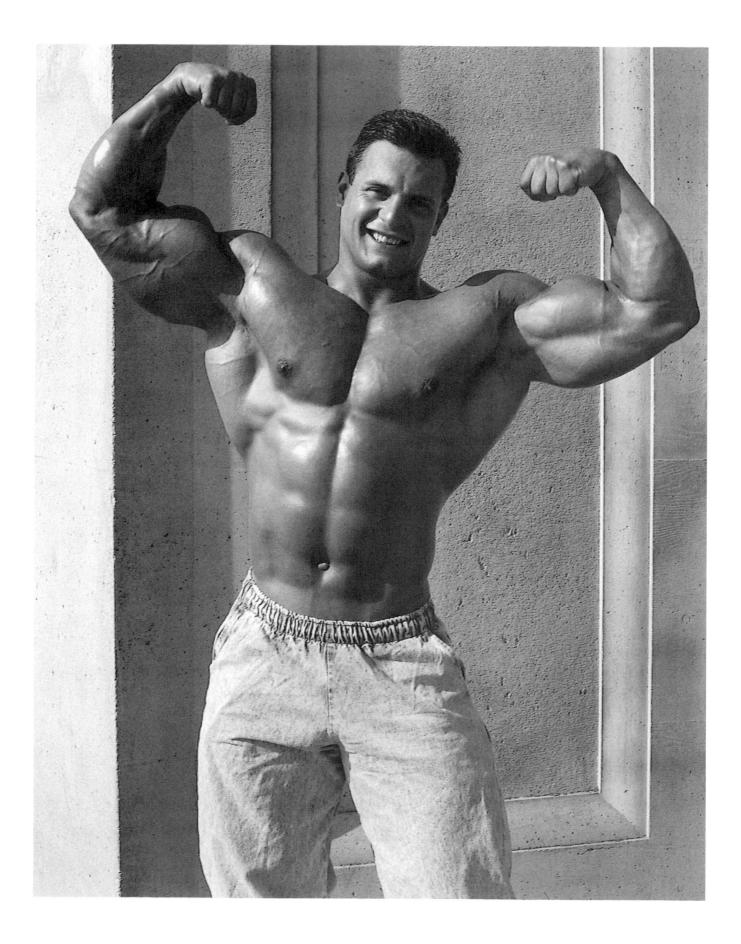

- Five to 10 pounds per year is normal.
- Ten pounds or more is good reason to be happy.
- More than 15 pounds per year is phenomenal.

A Textbook Example of How to Gain Weight

To illustrate, we will use an anonymous bodybuilder. He does exist; we will provide only the details of his training and diet.

He's less than 35 years of age, stands six feet tall, and for more than seven years, never weighed more than 243 pounds in the off-season. His best-conditioned competition weight was around 227 pounds. Year after year he heard the same national judges tell him, "It's all there; you just need to pack on more beef to take advantage of your structure." And year after year he showed up in about the same condition.

Reviewing his past competitive seasons indicated he had trained the same way with the same people, eaten the same food, and in spite of what outwardly appeared to be alterations in his workout structure, never moved any distance from the high-volume, pumping-up style still unknowingly imitated by so many bodybuilders. His lifting form and technique were lousy, sloppy, and loose. He became a victim of the big-fish–little-pond complex. He was bigger than everyone in his neighborhood, but not than his competitors at the nationals.

A few years back, Mr. Anonymous went to a training engineer for some help. The consultant maintained that any lack of continued size gains or progress was due 95 percent of the time to too little food, especially protein, and too much training. It was his firm conviction that he could help our anonymous subject by reducing his training volume and dramatically increasing his protein.

Prior to the onset of the first 28-day period with this consultant, Mr. Anonymous had trained six days per week, each session lasting one and a half to two hours. Each body part was trained twice per seven-day period, with 12 to 14 sets per part. Specifically, before restructuring his training, he completed two workouts per week at 13 sets per workout, or 26 sets per body part every seven days.

After restructuring each body part, Mr. Anonymous completed one workout per week at five sets per workout, or five sets per body part every seven days. That's an 80 percent reduction in volume! His training method and exercise form also were considered a problem area due to a lack of emphasis on the eccentric portion, the most important for growth.

His results were as follows: after a 28-day period consisting of 12 training sessions of approximately 75 minutes each, he gained an amazing 33 pounds of muscle and chopped his body fat by 2.8 pounds. That registers on the Detecto as 30 extra pounds, or in his case, 265 total pounds. Simply put, he slapped on more muscle in 28 days than he had in the previous five years.

The biggest factors in these amazing gains were the protein increase along with the correction of his loose form. By vastly boosting his protein consumption to about 400 grams per day, sleeping more, and decreasing the amount of training, he accomplished in 28 days what had eluded him for more than half a decade.

TERMS TO KNOW

Lastly, we have some commonly misunderstood bodybuilding terms. Give these a good review and check back every now and then. Some areas of biomedical bodybuilding do not lend themselves to a quick read. It's not a good idea to proceed through information guessing here and there what words mean. You need precision to be sure the idea in your head matches the facts. The following terms give bodybuilders trouble year after year.

Somatotypes. Body classifications based on physique are called somatotypes. The three somatotype classifications are ectomorph, endomorph, and mesomorph.

An ectomorph or asthenic habitus is a person whose physique is characterized by a slender build with long limbs, an angular profile, and prominent muscles or bones. A mesomorph or athletic habitus is a person whose physique is characterized by a predominance of muscle, bone, and connective-tissue structures, a well-proportioned, muscular body with broad shoulders, thick neck, deep chest, and flat abdomen. An endomorph or pyknic is a person whose body build is characterized by a soft, round physique with a large trunk and thighs, tapering extremities, an accumulation of fat throughout the body, short, round limbs, a full face, a short neck, stockiness, and a tendency toward obesity.

Lateral. The term *lateral* is most often used to describe exercises such as dumbbell laterals or cable laterals that move to the side of the body in a lateral plane of travel.

Supine versus Prone. There are decades of confusion between the terms *supine* and *prone* due to different writers indicating the same concept with different words. The word *supine* indicates a person lying horizontally (flat) on the back. In contrast, *prone* indicates a person lying horizontally facedown.

Hormone. Hormones are complex chemical substances produced in one part or organ of the body but initiating or regulating the activity of an organ or group of cells in another part of the body. Hormones are secreted by the endocrine glands and carried through the bloodstream

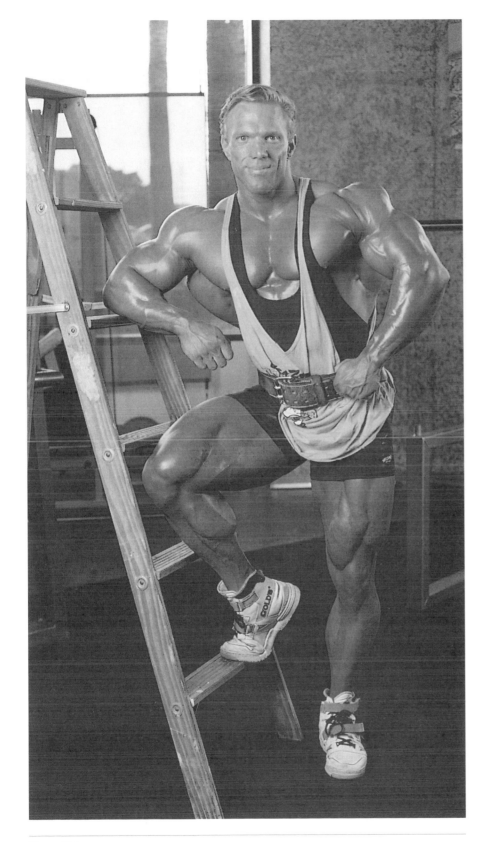

Dave Fisher

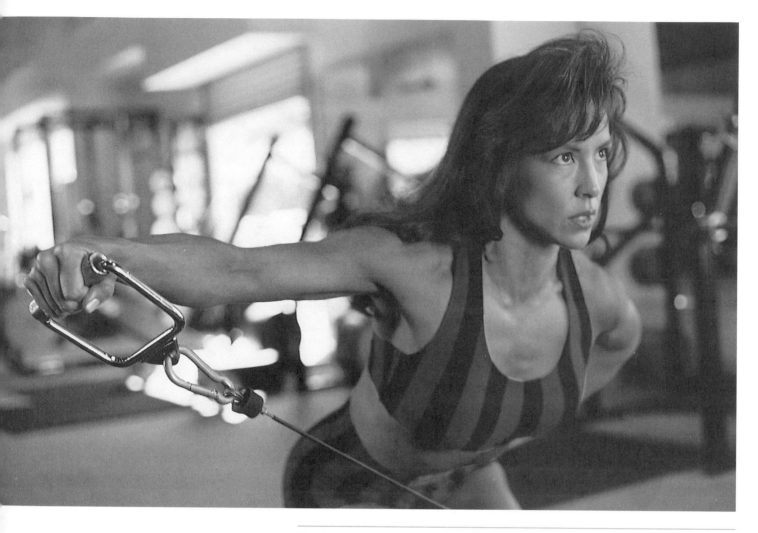

Kimiko Tanaka

to the target organ. Secretion of hormones is regulated by other hormones, neurotransmitters, and a negative-feedback system in which an excess of target-organ activity signals a decreased need for the stimulating hormone.

Steroid. Steroids are hormonal substances with a similar basic chemical structure, produced mainly in the adrenal cortex and gonads.

Steroid Hormones. Ductless gland secretions that contain the basic steroid nucleus in their chemical formula are steroid hormones. The natural steroid hormones include the androgens, estrogens, and adrenal cortex secretions.

Anabolism. Anabolism is the constructive metabolism characterized by the conversion of simple substances into the more complex compounds of living matter.

Anabolic Steroid. Compounds derived from testosterone or prepared synthetically to promote general body growth, oppose the effects of endogenous estrogen, or promote masculinizing effects are called anabolic steroids. All such compounds cause a mixed androgenic-anabolic effect.

Anabolic steroids are sometimes prescribed in the treatment of cachexia or anorexia, aplastic anemia, red-cell aplasia, and hemolytic anemia, and in anemias associated with renal failure, myeloid metaplasia, and leukemia. Some common compounds used in such therapies are oxymetholone, oxandrolone, methenolone, and nandrolone esters. Anabolic steroids used in the treatment of breast cancer in women carry the risk of causing masculinization. The symptoms of such undesirable effects are acne, growth of facial hair, and hoarsening or deepening of the voice.

Catabolism. Catabolism is a complex, metabolic process in which energy is liberated for use in work, energy storage, or heat production by the destruction of complex substances by living cells to form simple compounds. Carbon dioxide and water are produced, as well as energy.

Proteins. Any of a large group of naturally occurring, complex, organic nitrogenous compounds, proteins are composed of large combinations of amino acids containing the elements carbon, hydrogen, nitrogen, oxygen, usually sulfur, and occasionally phosphorus, iron, iodine, or other essential constituents of living cells.

Protein is the major source of building material for muscles, blood, skin, hair, nails, and the internal organs. It is necessary for the formation of hormones, enzymes, and antibodies. Protein may also act as a source of heat and energy, and it functions as an essential element in proper elimination of waste materials.

Rich dietary sources are meat, poultry, fish, eggs, milk, and cheese, which are classified as complete proteins because they contain the eight essential amino acids. Nuts and legumes, including navy beans, chick-peas, soybeans, and split peas, are also good sources but are incomplete proteins because they do not contain all the essential amino acids. Protein deficiency in adults results in a lack of energy and endurance, physical weakness, depression, lowered resistance to infection, and impaired healing of wounds.

Polypeptides. Chains of amino acids joined by peptide bonds are called polypeptides. A polypeptide has a larger molecular weight than a peptide but a smaller molecular weight than a protein. Polypeptides are formed by partial hydrolysis of proteins or by synthesis of amino acids into chains. Peptides are chains of molecules composed of two or more amino acids joined by peptide bonds.

Amino Acids. Organic chemical compounds composed of one or more basic amino groups and one or more acidic carboxyl groups are called amino acids. Twenty of the more than 100 amino acids that occur in nature are the building blocks of peptides, polypeptides, and proteins. Twenty-two amino acids have been identified as vital for proper growth, development, and maintenance of health. The body can synthesize 14 of these amino acids, called nonessential, whereas the remaining eight must be obtained from dietary sources and are termed essential.

The eight essential amino acids are isoleucine, leucine, lysine, methionine, phenylalanine, threonine, tryptophan, and valine. Arginine and histidine are essential in infants. Cysteine and tyrosine are quasi-essential because they may be synthesized from methionine and phenylalanine, respectively. The main nonessential amino acids are alanine, asparagine, aspartic acid, glutamine, glutamic acid, glycine, proline, and serine. From their structures, the amino acids can be classified as neutral, basic, or acidic. Each group is transported across cell membranes by different carrier mechanisms. Arginine, histidine, and lysine are basic amino acids, aspartic acid and glutamic acid are acidic, and the remainder are neutral.

Splanchnic and viscera. Splanchnic pertains to the internal organs or viscera. Viscera are the internal organs enclosed within a body cavity, primarily the abdominal organs.

Cachexia. A term referring to general ill health and malnutrition, cachexia is marked by weakness and emaciation, usually associated with serious disease such as tuberculosis or cancer. Many medical articles discuss cachexia. This process is the opposite of what a bodybuilder wants to do. We want to gain weight—not lose.

Anorexia. A lack or loss of appetite, resulting in the inability to eat, anorexia may result from poorly prepared or unattractive food or surroundings, unfavorable company, or various physical and psychological causes.

Anorexia Nervosa. A disorder characterized by a prolonged refusal to eat, anorexia nervosa results in emaciation, amenorrhea, emotional disturbance concerning body image, and an abnormal fear of becoming obese. The condition is seen primarily in adolescents, predominantly girls, and is usually associated with emotional stress or conflict, such as anxiety, irritation, anger, and fear, which may accompany a major change in the person's life. Treatment consists of measures to improve nourishment, followed by therapy to overcome the underlying emotional conflicts. This condition has been observed in the past histories

Nanna Bjone

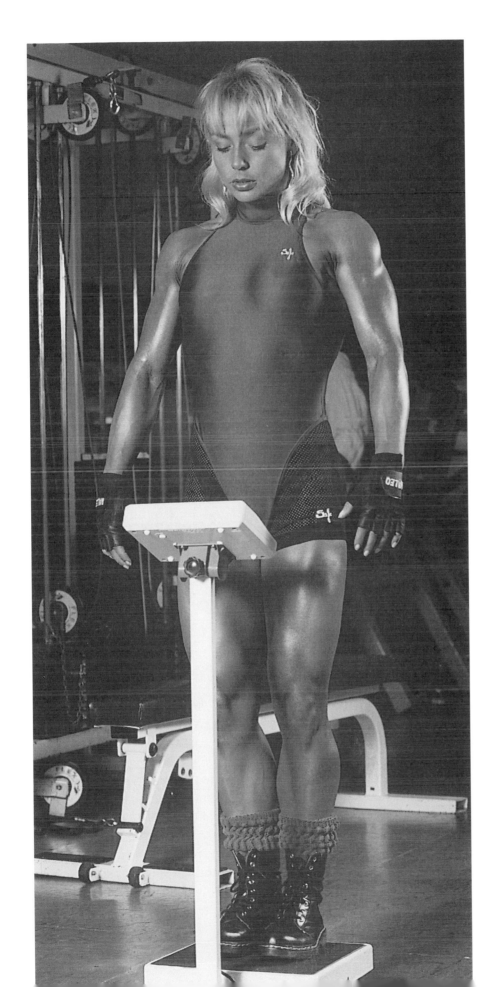

Lee Garoutte

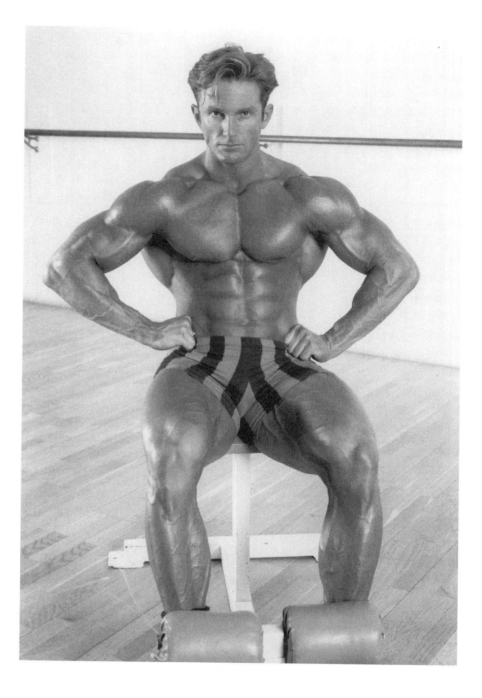

of some top female bodybuilders. These brave women have battled their disease through bodybuilding.

Reverse Anorexia Nervosa. A newly diagnosed "disorder," reverse anorexia nervosa is characterized by a prolonged period of near continuous eating, resulting in hypertrophy of the limbs and only interrupted by short intense bursts of weight-lifting. The body is seen as always too small, never big enough. The sufferer lives in a state of neverending fear of smallness. The condition is seen primarily in young males and is associated with emotional stress or conflict, such as anxiety, irritation, anger, and fear.

Thermoregulatory Centers. Thermoregulatory centers are areas located in the hypothalamus concerned mainly with the regulation of heat production, heat inhibition, and heat conservation to maintain a normal body temperature. Kinds of thermoregulatory centers include thermogenic center, thermoinhibitory center, and thermotactic center.

Thermogenesis. The production of heat, especially by the cells of the body, is called thermogenesis.

Thermoregulation. Thermoregulation is the control of heat production and heat loss, specifically the maintenance of body temperature through physiologic mechanisms activated by the hypothalamus.

Mitochondria. Mitochondria are small rodlike, threadlike, or granular organelles within the cytoplasm that function in cellular metabolism and respiration and occur in all living cells except bacteria, viruses, blue-green algae, and mature erythrocytes. They consist of two sets of membranes, a smooth outer one and a convoluted inner one, arranged in folds to form projections, or cristae, that extend into the matrix. Mitochondria provide the principal source of cellular energy through oxidative phosphorylation and adenosine triphosphate synthesis. They also contain the enzymes involved with electron transport and the citric and fatty acid cycles.

Oxidation. Any process in which the oxygen content of a compound is increased, oxidation also indicates any reaction in which the positive valence of a compound or a radical is increased because of a loss of electrons.

Oxidation-Reduction Reaction. Also called redox, oxidation-reduction reaction is a chemical change in which electrons are removed (oxidation) from an atom or molecule, accompanied by a simultaneous transfer of electrons (reduction) to another.

Oxidative Phosphorylation. An ATP-generating process in which oxygen serves as the final electron acceptor, oxidative phosphorylation occurs in mitochondria and is the major source of ATP generation in aerobic organisms.

Hypothalamic Hormones. Secreted by the hypothalamus, hypothalamic hormones include vasopressin, oxytocin, and the thyrotropin-releasing and gonadotropin-releasing hormones.

Hypothalamic-Pituitary-Adrenal Axis. The combined system of neuroendocrine units that in a negative-feedback network regulate the body's hormonal activities is called the hypothalamic-pituitary-adrenal axis.

Hypothalamus. The hypothalamus is the portion of the brain that activates, controls, and integrates the peripheral autonomic nervous system, endocrine processes, and many somatic functions, such as body temperature, sleep, and appetite.

Pituitary Gland. The endocrine gland suspended beneath the brain in the pituitary fossa of the sphenoid bone, the pituitary gland supplies numerous hormones that govern many vital processes. It is divided into an anterior adenohypophysis and a smaller posterior neurohypophysis. The anterior lobe of the gland is composed of polygonal cells related to the production of seven hormones. The hormones, controlled by hypothalamic releasing factors, include:

> *growth hormone (somatotropin)*
> *prolactin*
> *thyroid-stimulating hormone*
> *follicle-stimulating hormone*
> *luteinizing hormone*
> *adrenocorticotropic hormone*
> *melanocyte-stimulating hormone*

The posterior lobe is morphologically an extension of the hypothalamus and the source of vasopressin (antidiuretic hormone) and oxytocin. The pituitary gland is larger in a woman than in a man and becomes further enlarged during pregnancy.

Adrenal Gland. Either of two secretory organs perched atop the kidneys and surrounded by the protective fat capsule of the kidneys, each adrenal gland consists of two parts having independent functions: the cortex and the medulla. The adrenal cortex, in response to adrenocorticotropic hormone secreted by the anterior pituitary, secretes cortisol and androgens. Adrenal androgens serve as precursors that are converted by the liver to testosterone and estrogens. Renin from the kidneys controls adrenal cortical production of aldosterone. The adrenal medulla manufactures the catecholamines epinephrine and norepinephrine.

Adrenal Cortex. The outer and greater portion of the adrenal or suprarenal gland, the adrenal cortex is fused with the gland's medulla and produces mineralocorticoids, androgens, and glucocorticoids, hormones essential to homeostasis. The adrenal medulla is the inner portion of the adrenal gland. Adrenal medulla cells secrete epinephrine and norepinephrine. Epinephrine, or adrenaline, is an endogenous adrenal hormone and synthetic adrenergic vasoconstrictor.

CHAPTER 3 REFERENCES

Bompa, T. 1994. *Periodization of Strength: The New Wave in Strength Training.* Chandler, Arizona: Progenix.

Bucci, L., ed. 1993. *Nutrients as Ergogenic Aids for Sports and Exercise.* Boca Raton: CRC Press.

Ebbing, C., and P. Clarkson. 1989. "Exercise-Induced Muscle Damage and Adaptation." *Sports Medicine*: 7:207–234.

Ferrier, L. K., L. J. Caston, S. Leeson, J. Squires, B. J. Weaver, and B. J. Holub. 1995. "A-Linolcic Acid and Docosahexaenoic Acid–Enriched Eggs from Hens Fed Flaxseed: Influence on Blood Lipids and Platelet Phospholipid Fatty Acids in Humans." *American Journal of Clinical Nutrition*: 62:81–6.

Friedman, M., ed. 1989. *Absorption and Utilization of Amino Acids*, Vol. 1. Boca Raton: CRC Press.

Komi, P. V., and E. R. Buskirk. 1972. "Effect of Eccentric and Concentric Muscle Conditioning on Tension and Electrical Activity in Human Muscle." *Ergonomics*: 15:8.

Latifi, L., ed. 1994. *Amino Acids in Critical Care and Cancer.* Austin: R. G. Landes.

Talag, T. S. 1973. "Residual Muscular Soreness as Influenced by Concentric, Eccentric, and Static Contractions." *Research Quarterly*: 44:458–469.

Wolinsky, I., and J. F. Hickson, eds. 1994. *Nutrition in Exercise and Sport*, 2nd ed. Boca Raton: CRC Press.

4

Nutrition

This chapter on nutrition information is intended to provide the factual basis for your dietary choices as a bodybuilder. If nothing else, it should at least get the gray matter rumbling. Much of your success as a bodybuilder is determined by how well you are able to effectively apply sound nutritional knowledge. Nutrition is the intake, assimilation, and use of nutrients for proper body functioning.

Bodybuilding is far more than the discipline to go to your nearby Gold's Gym and train hard. The limiting factor to the ultimate success of your workouts is what happens after you leave the gym. The role of nutrition becomes primary during the other 23 nontraining hours in your day.

You can grow on too little training but you'll never grow eating too little food.

EFFECTIVE NUTRITION

Nutrition consists of both macronutrients and micronutrients. The macronutrients are proteins, carbohydrates, fats, and water. The prefix *macro* indicates a large nutrient. The micronutrients are vitamins, minerals, trace elements, and other minor but still vital metabolic substrates. *Micro,* of course, is a prefix meaning small.

The best source for effective nutrition is whole foods, not necessarily organically grown but unrefined and intact. It's not just the addition of other nonfood ingredients that adulterates processed food but the mechanical manipulation involved. Whole foods, especially in their natural state, contain many micronutrients not found in manufactured foods. For optimum nutrient effectiveness, never allow the use

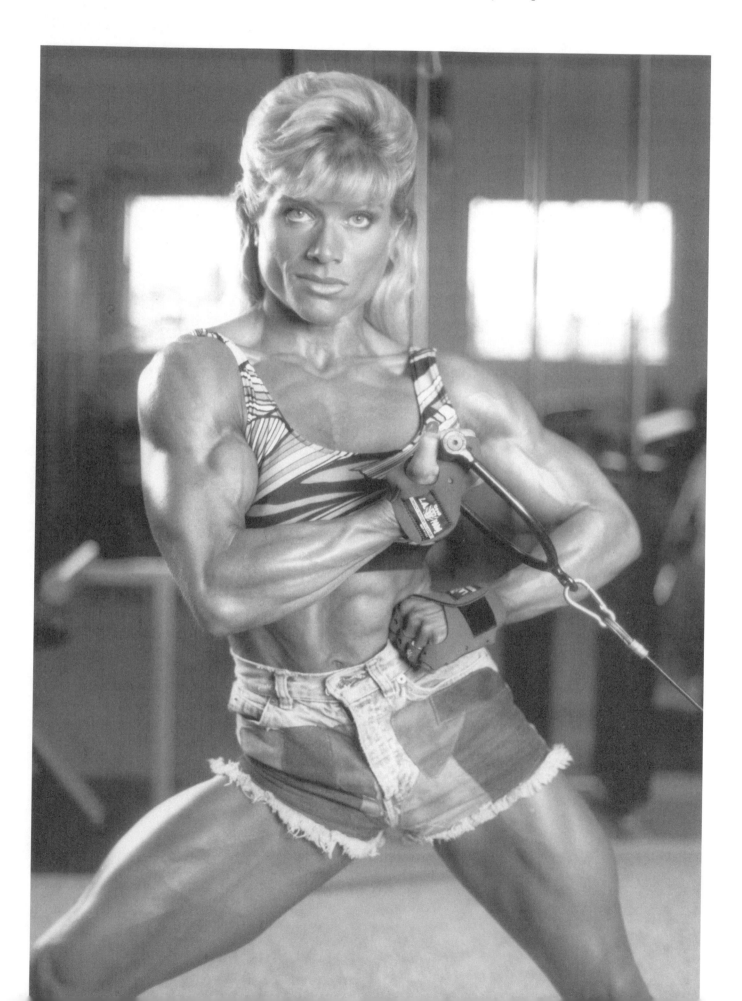

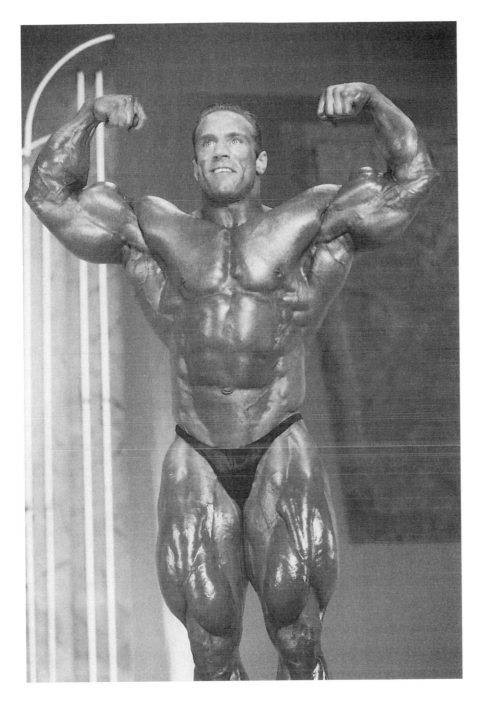

Drorit Kernes (opposite page)
Mike Francois

of supplements to overshadow the consumption of whole foods. These micronutrients have vital roles in optimal health and growth. Even though the modern supplement industry has the technology to produce well-balanced and structured products, the best source for nutrition will be nature itself.

Essentially the diet you follow from day to day is the total sum of your nutritional intake. You follow a specific bodybuilding diet because

Shawn Ray

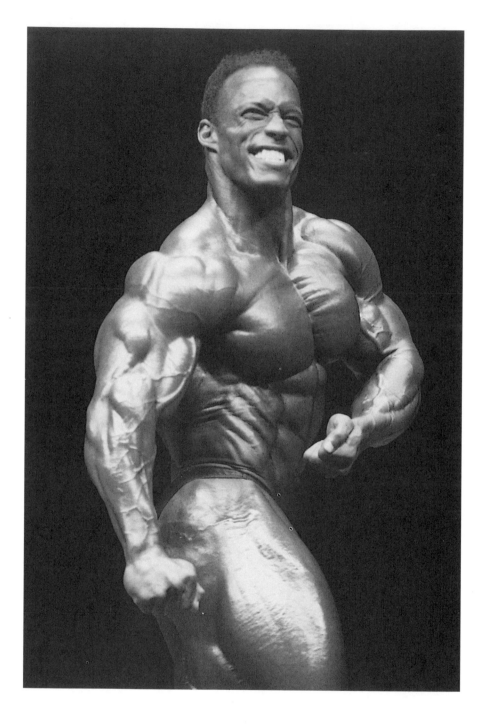

you believe it to be effective for your needs. There are almost as many ideas on correct diet as there are bodybuilders. By far, the most confusing aspects of obtaining your bodybuilding goals are nutrition and diet. First you must gain a workable understanding of what effective nutrition is, then your diet strategy will be much easier to create.

Approach your bodybuilding education with equal amounts logical reasoning and emotion. This balanced perspective is needed to give you the self-control to avoid fast diet fixes and nutritional fads.

A DIETARY SUGGESTION

Bodybuilding dictates that your goal is to maximize muscle mass with a minimum of body fat. To be up-front, the following possible dietary concepts are not carbohydrate-based but carbohydrate-balanced. You hear a lot about essential amino and fatty acids but not much about essential carbs!

In order to provide an optimum metabolic environment, the following suggestions are to serve as a strong template for the design of your vigorously customized nutrient attack plan. To roughly calculate your day-to-day caloric intake along the following guidelines, use the Worksheet for Estimating Daily Nutrient Proportions.

Cycle your carb intake along these lines:

- **from waking until four hours later:** 30 percent protein, 40 percent carb, 30 percent fat
- **from four hours to 10 hours:** 40 percent protein, 30 percent carb, 30 percent fat
- **from 10 hours to 16 hours awake:** 50 percent protein, 20 percent carb, 30 percent fat

The idea is to consume more carbs during the early part of your day.

WORKSHEET FOR ESTIMATING DAILY NUTRIENT PROPORTIONS

Calculate Your Daily Nutrient Levels As Follows:

Daily Protein Percentage as Grams of Protein per Meal
_____ calories per day × _____ % protein = _____ protein kcals
_____ protein kcals per 4 kcals per gr protein = _____ grams protein
_____ grams protein per # of daily meals = _____ protein grams per meal

Daily Carbohydrate Percentage as Grams of Carbohydrate per Meal
_____ calories per day × _____ % carbs = _____ carb kcals
_____ carb kcals per 4 kcals per gr carb = _____ grams carb
_____ grams carb per # of daily meals = _____ carb grams per meal

Daily Fat Percentage as Grams of Fat per Meal
_____ calories per day × _____ % fats = _____ fat kcals
_____ fat kcals per 4 kcals per gr fat = _____ grams fat
_____ grams fat per # of daily meals = _____ fat grams per meal

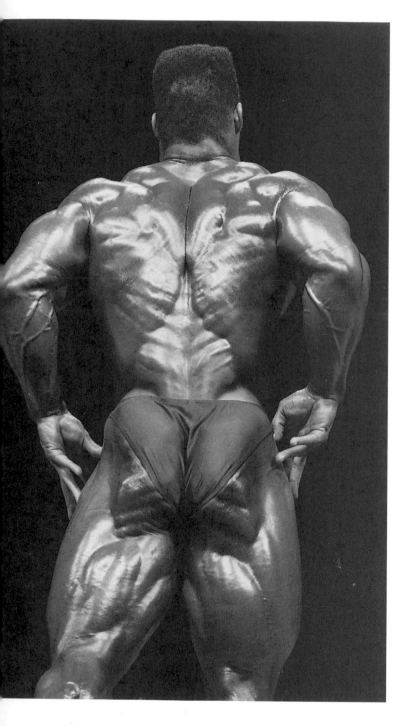

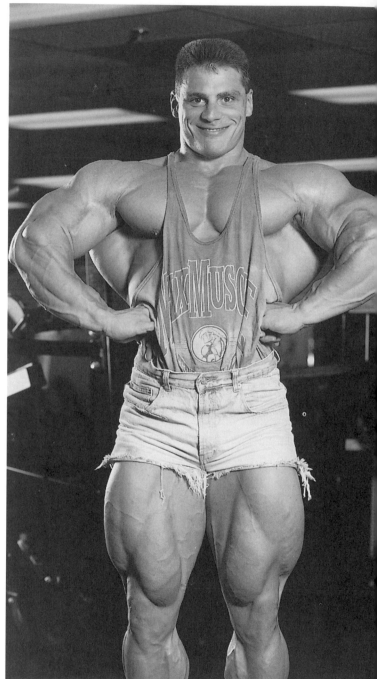

Shawn Ray (left)

Paul DeMayo (right)

PROTEIN

Drawing from scientific observations, it is acknowledged that man's tendency is to increase protein consumption in response to daily work expenditure. Increased total work equates with increased caloric expenditure. Simply put, the harder you work (effective bodybuilding is very hard work) the more your tendency is to increase protein in the diet. This tendency refers to both athletes and nonathletes. Let's first figure out exactly what the facts are when it comes to protein and bodybuilding.

From the largest member of this family of related organic structures to the smallest, you have in order: protein, peptides, amino acids, nitrogen. The end products of protein digestion are amino acids, along with di- and tripeptides. In direct circulation, amino acids are found almost exclusively, although some small peptides are also found.

Note: please remember as you read this section that your body uses previously consumed proteins, in the form of amino acids (enzymes, etc.), in order to use the protein you eat today. So in other words, you lose protein as you use protein. All in all, you likely should be eating more protein than you think.

Aminos and Peptides

A protein is formed from a long polypeptide, which itself consists of amino acids held together in peptide bonds. More than 100 different amino acids have been identified in nature but only 20 of these are incorporated into your body's structure. All human tissue protein is formed from these 20 primary amino acids through the process of anabolic synthesis.

Numerous derived amino acids are also formed from these 20 primary aminos. Some derived aminos are cystine, carboxyglutamate, and hydroxyproline. Each of the 20 primary amino acids is a unique structure with specific metabolic roles to perform well beyond the synthesis of larger protein structures.

Amino acids are further classified according to their respective dietary requirements. Those aminos that can be synthesized within the body in sufficient amounts are considered nonessential or dispensable. The essential aminos must be supplied through dietary sources and are considered to be indispensable. Remember: an indispensable amino acid is an essential amino acid; a dispensable amino acid is a nonessential amino acid.

In recent years, a third classification of amino acids has emerged, which is designated as "conditionally essential." This reflects the observation that under certain conditions of stress, the following aminos become essential: arginine, glycine, cystine, tyrosine, proline, glutamine, and taurine. Needless to say, if you're training hard, then the conditionally essential aminos may become essential due to the elevated metabolic stresses.

Protein Metabolism

Protein metabolism is the set of processes whereby whole proteins are used by the body. Dietary proteins are first broken down into amino

---

AMINO ACIDS CATEGORIES

Essential Amino Acids

1. arginine*
2. cystine*
3. glutamine*
4. glycine*
5. histidine
6. isoleucine
7. leucine
8. lysine
9. methionine
10. phenylalanine
11. proline*
12. taurine*
13. threonine
14. tryptophan
15. tyrosine*
16. valine

Nonessential Amino Acids

1. alanine
2. asparagine
3. aspartate
4. cysteine
5. glutamate
6. serine

*under specific conditions

THE 20 PRIMARY AMINO ACIDS

1. alanine—Ala
2. arginine—Arg
3. asparagine—Asn
4. aspartic acid—Asp
5. cysteine—Cys
6. glutamic acid—Glu
7. glutamine—Gln
8. glycine—Gly
9. histidine—His
10. isoleucine—Ile
11. leucine—Leu
12. lysine—Lys
13. methionine—Met
14. phenylalanine—Phe
15. proline—Pro
16. serine—Ser
17. threonine—Thr
18. tryptophan—Trp
19. tyrosine—Tyr
20. valine—Val

acids, then absorbed into the bloodstream, and finally used in body cells to form new proteins.

Amino acids in excess of the body's needs may be converted by liver enzymes into keto acids and urea. The keto acids may be used as sources of energy via the Krebs citric acid cycle, or they may be converted into glucose or fat for storage. Urea is excreted in urine and sweat. Growth hormones and androgens stimulate protein formation, and adrenal cortical hormones tend to cause breakdown of body proteins.

Many aspects of bodybuilding are deliberate efforts to force the body to surpass its natural parameters. This is not a negative observation, but a very positive one in that much has been learned about how individuals can take total control of their bodies through disciplined effort.

So, as you attempt to expand your existing levels of muscular development, you are actually continually forcing your genetic framework beyond its original set of metabolic instructions. It is almost as

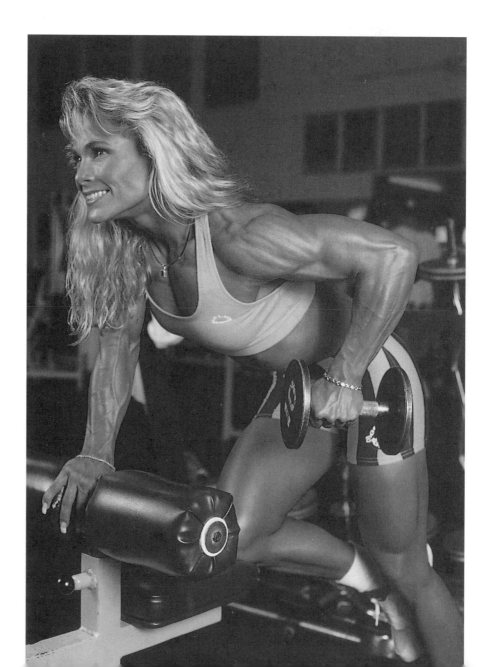

Carol Ann Hensley

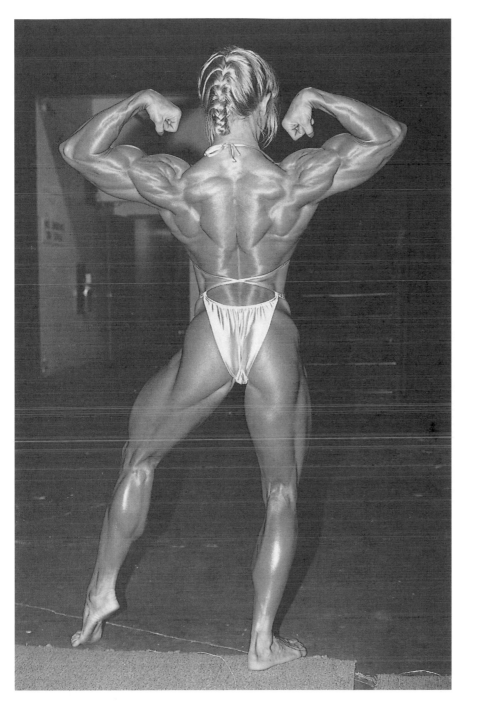

Denise Rutkowski

tough to accomplish as it sounds, but it is obtainable for those who want to grow badly enough!

Protein Uptake and Utilization

Once protein has entered the stomach, the major work of breaking whole proteins into smaller peptides, and eventually, free amino acids begins on a large scale. Upon leaving your stomach, many of the

MAJOR FUNCTIONS OF THE 20 PRIMARY AMINO ACIDS

ALANINE
- glycogenic precursor for energy
- maintains blood-glucose levels

ARGININE
- detoxification of ammonia
- supports immune system
- influences growth-hormone function

ASPARAGINE
- metabolic control of functions for brain and nervous system

ASPARTIC ACID
- used to form threonine
- aids in ammonia disposal
- involved in fatigue resistance

CYSTEINE
- protects against free radicals
- promotes the healing process
- stimulant to immune system
- membrane stabilizer

GLUTAMIC ACID
- 50% of amino acid content of brain structure
- fuel for the brain
- excitatory neurotransmitter

GLUTAMINE
- removal of ammonia from CNS
- rapid turnover as fuel for intestinal system

GLYCINE
- simplest amino acid
- role in GH release
- used as a sweetening agent

HISTIDINE
- used to treat allergic disorders
- therapy role in red and white blood cells

ISOLEUCINE
- found in high concentration in muscle tissue
- intermediate in Krebs cycle to be balanced in proportion to leucine and valine

LEUCINE
- lowers blood sugar
- to be balanced in proportion to leucine and valine found in high concentration in muscle tissue

LYSINE
- treatment of herpes simplex
- promotes bone metabolism role in collagen formation

METHIONINE
- antioxidant function
- contains sulphur
- lipotropic
- vital role in liver function

PHENYLALANINE
- substrate for norepinephrine
- precursor to tyrosine role in appetite control and pain control

PROLINE
- maintenance of tendons and joints
- major constituent of collagen

SERINE
- participates in synthesis of purine, pyrimadines, and porphyrin

THREONINE
- may be converted to intermediate in Krebs cycle
- helps prevent fatty accumulations in liver

TRYPTOPHAN
- precursor to serotonin
- role in migraine headaches
- used for insomnia
- dilates the blood vessels

TYROSINE
- precursor to adrenaline and thyroid hormones
- thermoregulation

VALINE
- found in high concentration in muscle tissue
- intermediate in production of succinate
- to be balanced in proportion to leucine and valine

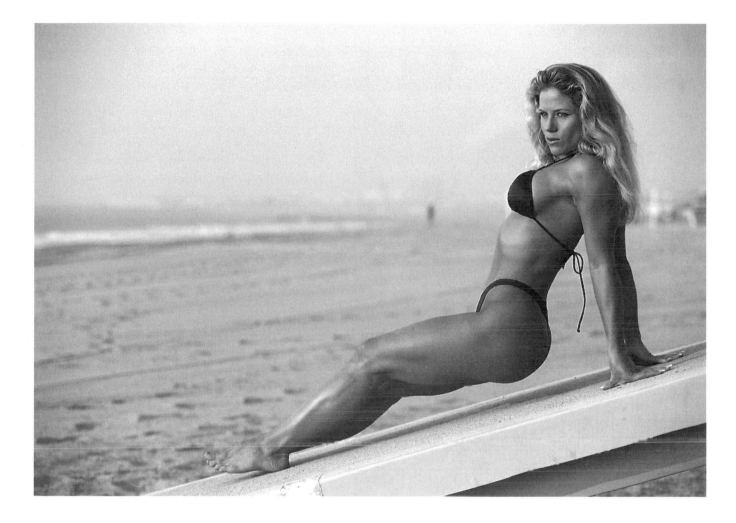

Monica Brandt

amino acids ingested may never reach general circulation due to their required role in the organs involved in the transport process. For example, after the stomach, the small intestine has first choice on the aminos. The liver then restores its amino needs and releases the remaining aminos and small peptides (dipeptides and tripeptides) into general circulation to tissues such as skeletal muscle.

Once the amino acid enters a cell, peptide structures are formed, which in turn create proteins. This ongoing process of repair and synthesis leaves relatively few amino acids for storage inside cells. However, the liver, kidneys, and intestinal mucosa do store large amounts of aminos for their respective needs. From a bodybuilder's point of view, this indicates the benefit of maintaining a steady supply of amino acids in your body throughout the day.

Proteins are also used to produce body tissue and synthesis of hormones and their agonists and antagonists, buffering compounds such as glutathione and carnosine. The enzymes utilized to break whole proteins into their smaller components are synthesized from amino acids.

Note: along with an increase in protein intake goes a simultaneous increase in the body's requirements for the B vitamin family. Among other things, the B-complex group is essential for proper protein metabolism.

Protein to Energy

Protein performs or provides the materials for more than muscle growth. Dietary protein is also used in the production of energy as in gluconeogenesis, the formation of glycogen from fatty acids and proteins rather than carbohydrates. An example of this protein-to-energy shuttle is known as the glutamine-alanine cycle. Glutamine, the most abundant free amino acid in skeletal muscle tissue, is mainly synthesized from other amino acids.

Roles of Protein: First Maintenance, Then Growth

We need to separate your daily protein needs into two distinct areas: maintenance and growth. Of the two aspects of protein requirements, growth is more often thought of as a bodybuilding role—you need protein to grow. After puberty, there is essentially a cessation of growth that leaves us with daily protein intake being shuttled through the body to take care of existing lean body mass.

Within your body, protein is broken down into its amino or peptide structure. It's then transported to the correct metabolic arena for final active absorption. Once actively absorbed, protein's constituents are responsible for the following areas:

- synthesis of hormones, neurotransmitters, enzymes, and other biochemicals
- energy consumption during periods of intense stress, injury, and caloric deficiency
- optimal functioning of your immune system
- repair of existing tissue levels
- synthesis of new tissue
- synthesis of other amino acids

Protein and the Immune System

The immune system's reliance on protein is total—not enough dietary protein and trouble ensues. As is so often the case, science turns to the lab mouse for a demonstration. Two groups of mice were exposed to the bacteria responsible for tuberculosis. Group One was provided with a diet adequate in both calories and protein, while the otherwise identical Group Two received a diet severely deficient in protein with the missing calories replaced with carbs and fats.

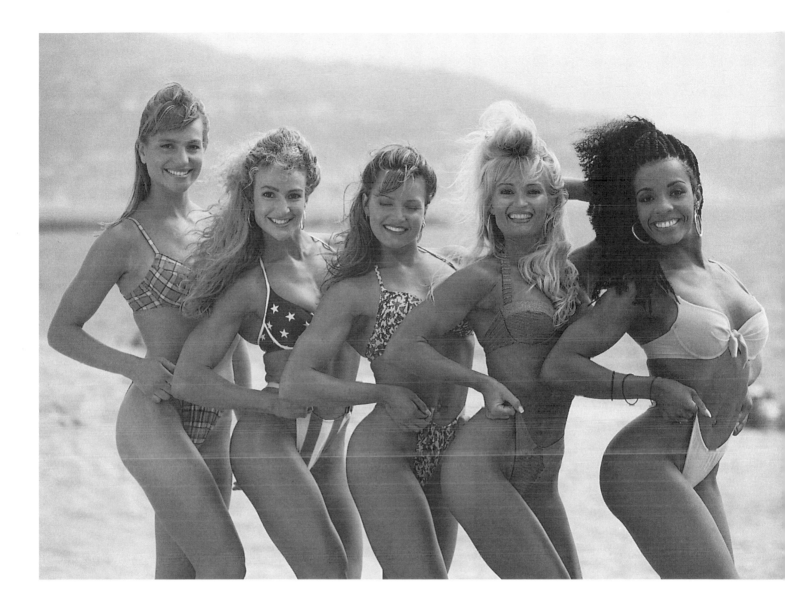

Fitness America contestants

Both groups were exposed to the same bacteria on the same day. Group One demonstrated a vigorously effective immune response. However, Group Two was unable to initiate the needed immune response, and therefore, did not survive as long as Group One. Interestingly, a second related investigation showed that when dying protein-deficient mice were returned to a normal protein diet, their immune responses normalized.

This research was presented in the December 10, 1996, proceedings of the National Academy of Sciences. The investigator's conclusion was that the age of immune system manipulation through diet has arrived. With infectious disease now the largest threat to life on earth, immuno-modification through specific alterations in diet, hence nutrient intake, is becoming the penicillin for the next century.

ESTIMATED DAILY PROTEIN INTAKE BY BODY WEIGHT

USRDA is 0.8 grams protein/kilo/day

100 lb. (45 kilos)
1.5 g protein/k/day = 68 grams
2.5 g protein/k/day = 113 grams
3.5 g protein/k/day = 158 grams
5.0 g protein/k/day = 225 grams

125 lb. (57 kilos)
1.5 g protein/k/day = 86 grams
2.5 g protein/k/day = 143 grams
3.5 g protein/k/day = 200 grams
5.0 g protein/k/day = 285 grams

150 lb. (68 kilos)
1.5 g protein/k/day = 102 grams
2.5 g protein/k/day = 170 grams
3.5 g protein/k/day = 238 grams
5.0 g protein/k/day = 340 grams

175 lb. (80 kilos)
1.5 g protein/k/day = 120 grams
2.5 g protein/k/day = 200 grams
3.5 g protein/k/day = 280 grams
5.0 g protein/k/day = 400 grams

200 lb. (91 kilos)
1.5 g protein/k/day = 137 grams
2.5 g protein/k/day = 228 grams
3.5 g protein/k/day = 319 grams
5.0 g protein/k/day = 455 grams

225 lb. (102 kilos)
1.5 g protein/k/day = 153 grams
2.5 g protein/k/day = 255 grams
3.5 g protein/k/day = 357 grams
5.0 g protein/k/day = 510 grams

250 lb. (114 kilos)
1.5 g protein/k/day = 171 grams
2.5 g protein/k/day = 285 grams
3.5 g protein/k/day = 399 grams
5.0 g protein/k/day = 570 grams

275 lb. (125 kilos)
1.5 g protein/k/day = 188 grams
2.5 g protein/k/day = 313 grams
3.5 g protein/k/day = 438 grams
5.0 g protein/k/day = 625 grams

Protein Requirements

Granted, the biggest bodybuilders are generously gifted, not only physically but in the incredible amounts of proteins and carbs they are able to eat. For those beyond 220 pounds, bodybuilding also becomes a race for the refrigerator. It takes very little hard lifting to cause a jump in the need for both maintenance protein and additional protein for the growth-inducing recuperation process.

Note: 1 kilogram (kilo or K) = 2.201 pounds.

Keep in mind that the government's Recommended Daily Allowance is based on a very broad population, including young and old who by comparison to athletes are relatively sedentary individuals. Active people need more protein—the more active, the more protein.

Shawn Ray

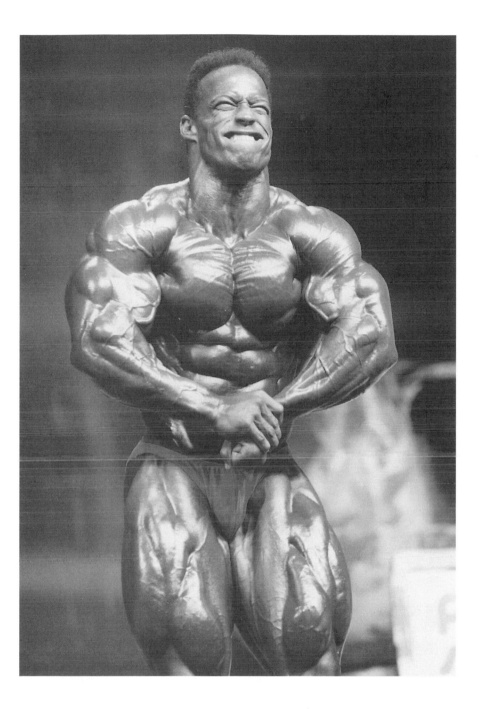

Precautions

Even if you are able to force yourself to consume 80 percent of your total daily calories in the form of protein, there will likely be minimal negative side effects if you are a normal, healthy individual. This proportion of protein in the diet has produced only minor alterations in the biochemistry of experimental subjects.

The idea that too much protein will hurt your kidneys is a common fallacy. This incorrect association of higher levels of protein intake with kidney distress is the second line of the average guy's defense, the first being that there is no reason for extra protein—it'll only go to waste. The defenders of the average guy are wrong on both counts. There is no evidence that indicates any detriment to a healthy individual eating as much protein as desired.

However, there are some individuals who must restrict intake of specific amino acids, and hence, their overall protein consumption. The most widely known are those with phenylketonuria or PKU. This is an inborn metabolic disorder caused by the absence or a deficiency of phenylalanine hydroxylase, the enzyme responsible for the conversion of the amino acid phenylalanine into tyrosine. Accumulation of phenylalanine is toxic to brain tissue. You may be familiar with the warning found on cans of diet soda or other sugar-free foods indicating that the product contains phenylalanine (one of the amino acids contained in aspartame).

Sources of Protein

It doesn't matter whether you are starting out as a bodybuilder or well into your bodybuilding career, the simplest and most underutilized sources of protein are whole foods: lean meats, eggs, poultry, milk, fish, nuts, and so on. Supplements should be secondary to food. Dietary needs for those striving to be truly huge, say 230-plus pounds, are the exception. Due to the amount of protein required to expand their existing mass, a supplemental protein program is equally as important as whole foods. Let there be no doubt that a lot of protein can be packed into a blender and swigged down in four or five gulps. One particular type of whey protein, CFM, is incredibly soluble for protein drinks.

Cost is generally a limiting factor when it comes to using a protein supplement. Over the years many different forms of supplemental protein have become available through intensive marketing by countless supplement manufacturers. These include free-form amino acid crystals and capsules, protein powders (whey protein is the top of the line), pre-digested liquid proteins, protein tablets (amino acid tablets), and chewable protein wafers. The question of exactly what type of whey protein or egg powder to use is dependent on many different factors. Product quality is far more vital than the subjective differences between brands and types. Before you buy, do some comparing—strain the brain and push past the biggest advertising budget. When compared to whole food, supplements are generally more convenient but may cost more. However, whole-food proteins are often high in fat.

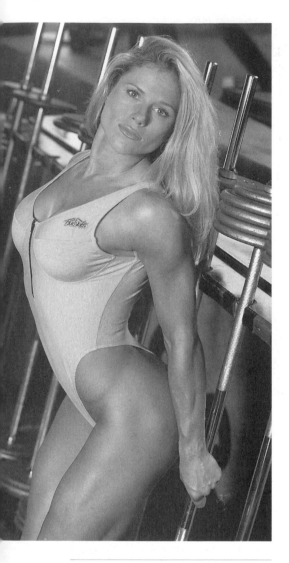
Monica Brandt

Ronnie Coleman (opposite page)

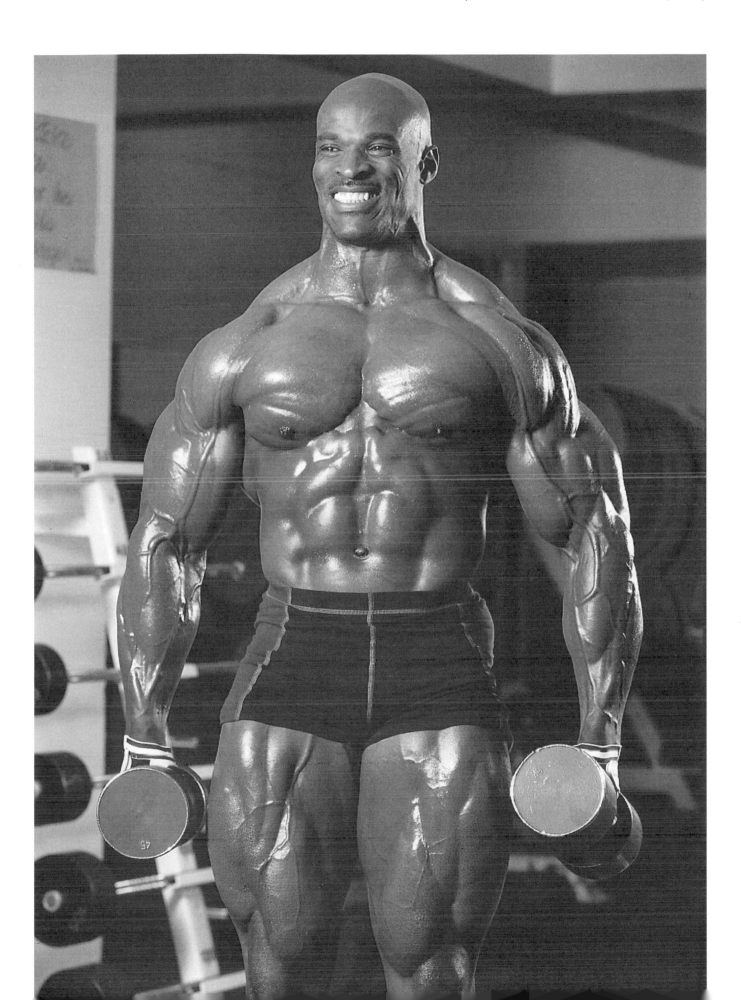

Maximize Your Protein Intake

Eating more than 150 to 200 grams of protein every day of the week is not an easy task to accomplish. But look at it this way: the bigger the dog, the bigger the bowl! To be big, you must eat big.

It is vital to understand one aspect of a bodybuilder's protein consumption: it will be effectively impossible for you to make the optimal degree of progress without the steady use of a quality protein supplement. Very few individuals can set aside the time to purchase, prepare, and have available throughout the day adequate dietary protein from whole foods.

Phil Hernon

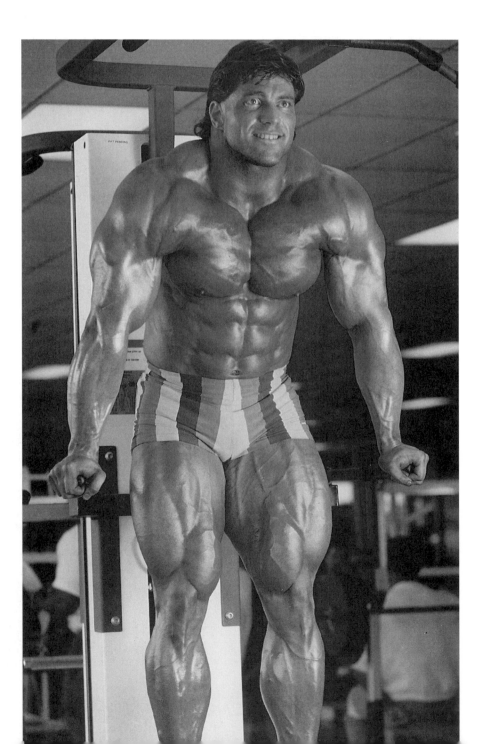

The following are suggestions as to how to best maximize your protein intake:

- Consume smaller and more frequent meals.
- If there is any doubt whether you are digesting protein correctly, use a supplement containing protein-digesting enzymes.
- Keep the extra stuff to a minimum and shoot for lots of protein.

CARBOHYDRATES

Remember, there is no such thing as an essential carbohydrate! Along with fats and proteins, carbohydrates are an important source of fuel for your body. In terms of first-line availability, carbohydrates supply the most accessible and utilized energy source. Though the major player in terms of hourly provision of energy substrates, carbohydrates supply at best 2 percent of the total available human fuel reserves. Fats contain the vast majority of the body's reserve energy platform at 80 percent, with skeletal muscle filling in the 18-percent gap.

You store far less carbohydrate energy than fat, but fats are in second place when it comes to stoking the furnace within. The explanation

Ronnie Coleman

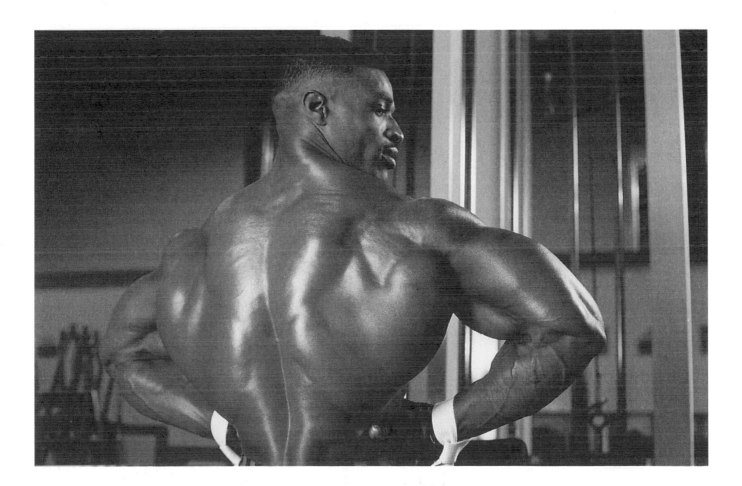

Ian Harrison

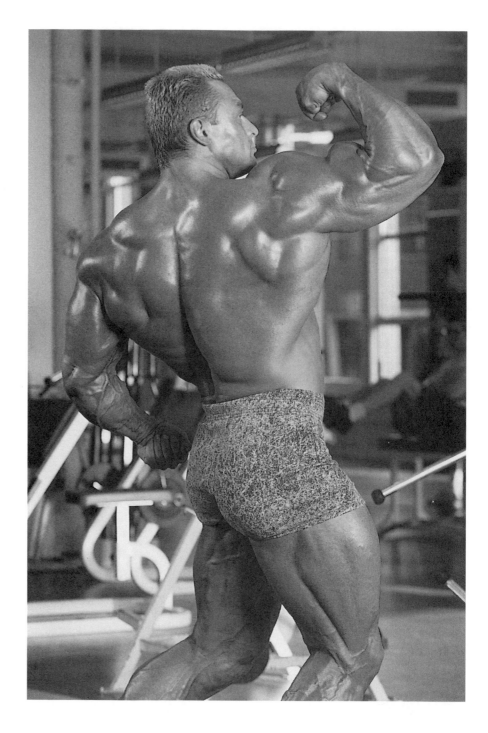

for so little carbohydrate being stored involves the manner with which the body holds carbs. A single gram of stored carbohydrate muscle glycogen is maintained along with perhaps four grams of water. In terms of evolution, it is better to carry your fuel reserves in as dense a form as possible. Fats provide just this needed form of compact energy reserve. Each gram of fat yields nine calories, while carbs and proteins provide four calories per gram.

So for every gram of carb, you have to drag around five grams of material. In the case of fats, they have a one-to-one ratio, with no excess water associated with the scenario. Additionally carbs burn at four calories per gram and fats at a little over nine calories per gram, so it becomes clear which storage strategy will allow greater range of functional mobility for the evolving human. It is a matter of evolution that our bodies use fats over carbs for survival. Nondietary carbohydrate sources of energy include skeletal muscle stores in the form of glycogen and blood glucose derived from the liver (more exactly, synthesized from amino acids in the liver).

Description of Carbohydrates

In human nutrition, carbohydrates are any of a group of organic compounds, the most important being saccharides, starch, cellulose, and gum. According to their particular molecular structure, carbs are classified as mono-, di-, tri-, poly-, or heterosaccharides.

Digestible carbs are classified as dietary carbohydrates, and indigestible are classified as dietary fiber or fibrous carbs. (The terms bodybuilders so often use are *starchy* and *fibrous* carbs.) Dietary carbohydrates fall under one of two categories: sugars or complex.

Simple Sugars

The two principal categories of sugars are monosaccharides and disaccharides. A monosaccharide is a single sugar, such as glucose, fructose, or galactose. A disaccharide is a double sugar, such as sucrose (table sugar) or lactose.

Complex Carbs

Complex carbs, or polysaccharides, are carbohydrates that contain three or more molecules of simple carbohydrates. Some examples of polysaccharides are dextrins, starches, glycogens, celluloses, gums, inulin, and pentose. Common sources for polysaccharides are grain products, legumes, potatoes, and other vegetables.

Carbohydrate Metabolism

Your carbohydrate metabolism is the sum of the anabolic and catabolic processes of the body involved in the synthesis and breakdown of carbohydrates. These metabolic carb processes are: glycogenesis—the synthesis of glycogen from glucose, glyconeogenesis—the formation of glycogen from fatty acids and proteins rather than carbohydrates, and glycolysis—the breakdown of glucose and other sugars.

TYPES OF CARBOHYDRATES

Starchy Carbs

barley	lima beans
red beans	black-eyed peas
corn	whole-wheat flour
lentils	pasta
oatmeal	peas
popcorn	rice
tomatoes	shredded wheat
yams	

Fibrous Carbs

asparagus	green beans
broccoli	brussels sprouts
cabbage	carrots
cauliflower	cucumbers
celery	eggplant
mushrooms	lettuce
green peppers	spinach
squash	zucchini

The status of your carbohydrate metabolism is based largely on the level of blood glucose or circulating carbohydrates. This is, in turn, dictated by the timing and frequency, along with the nutrient composition, of your last meal. The time of day that finds most of our blood sugars at their lowest level is early morning. Generally, upon awakening you have undergone essentially a seven-to-nine-hour fast without any new supply of ingested substrate for the needed maintenance of your blood glucose levels. (A blood sugar range of 40 to more than 400 milligrams/deciliter is acceptable.)

The source of the fuel in this postabsorptive or fasting state is 75 percent glycogenolysis and 25 percent gluconeogenesis. The process of blood sugar balance is a dynamic one, with the brain and functioning of the red blood cells (or erythrocytes), for example, using glucose as a preferred fuel source. The metabolites of incomplete utilization of fatty acids, ketones are able to serve as substitute fuels in the absence of sufficient glucose, but only after a period of great metabolic adjustment.

Note: understanding the subtle differences between medical terms that begin with the same set of letters is very important for an effective bodybuilding mind. Another very confusing aspect of this refined terminology is the different word forms that, though spelled differently, apply equally to the same concept. An example is *gluco* and *glyco*, which are equally correct forms for words such as the following:

- *Glycogenesis* is the synthesis of glycogen from glucose.
- *Glycolysis* is the process whereby glucose and other sugars are broken down to produce fuel for energy.
- *Glyconeogenesis* is the formation of glucose from noncarbohydrate sources such as amino acids and fatty acids.

Muscle and Insulin—Moving Carbs Where You Need Them Most

To understand insulin, we'll start with the pancreas. The pancreas is a gland that secretes various substances, such as digestive enzymes, insulin, and glucagon. It is a compound gland composed of exocrine and endocrine tissue. About 1 million endocrine cellular islets or islands of Langerhans are embedded between the exocrine units of the pancreas. Beta cells of the islands secrete insulin, which helps control carbohydrate metabolism.

There are two aspects to defining insulin. First is the internally synthesized or naturally occurring hormone secreted by the beta cells of the islands of Langerhans in the pancreas. The release of insulin is mandated by increased levels of glucose and amino acids in the blood. Insulin serves to maintain the metabolism of glucose along with intermediary metabolism of fats, carbohydrates, and proteins. Insulin low-

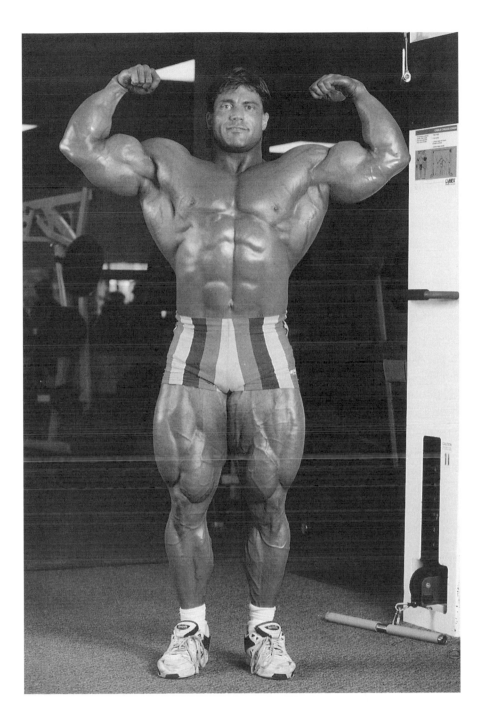

Phil Hernon

ers blood glucose levels and promotes transport and entry of glucose and amino acids into the muscle cells and other tissues. Too little secretion of insulin results in hyperglycemia (elevated blood sugar), hyperlipemia (elevated blood lipids or fats), and ketonemia (elevated blood ketones). Left uncorrected, severe insulin deficiency is fatal.

Second is the commercially prepared pharmacologic product used by diabetics. Several preparations of insulin are available, varying in rapidity of onset, intensity, and duration of action. They are termed rapid acting, intermediate acting, and long acting. Insulin is largely given by subcutaneous injection.

The alpha cells of the islets secrete glucagon that balances the action of insulin, and the acinar units of the pancreas secrete digestive enzymes. The beta cells of the pancreas are insulin-producing cells. The insulin-producing function of the beta cells accelerates the movement of glucose, amino acids, and fatty acids out of the blood and into the cellular arena, countering the glucagon function of alpha cells.

Glucagon is the countermeasure opposing insulin. Produced in the pancreas by alpha cells, glucagon functions to stimulate the conversion of glycogen to glucose in the liver. This system of energy conversion is built upon stored glycogen within the liver. Secretion of glucagon is stimulated by hypoglycemia and by growth hormone. A pharmaceutical preparation of purified, crystallized glucagon is used in the treatment of certain hypoglycemic states.

The Balancing Act

Hyperglycemia is a greater than normal amount of glucose in the blood. This abnormal profile of insulin production and utilization is one pattern of biochemistry that potentially leads to diabetes. The effect of elevated blood sugar is damaging and eventually fatal if left unchecked.

Not only are the undisposed carbs efficiently stored away as increased body fat levels, the elevated blood glucose levels are a contributing factor in the development of unhealthy blood fat levels. Ideally, carbs can be oxidized as fuel directly, but in less than ideal situations, high levels produce their peripheral storage as adipose tissue. Cases of uncontrolled severe diabetes are strongly associated with obesity. When diabetes is brought under control through diet and drug therapy, there is often dramatic fat loss in the patient.

At the other end of the blood sugar spectrum is hypoglycemia or low blood sugar. Hypoglycemia is a less-than-normal amount of glucose in the blood, usually caused by administration of too much insulin, excessive secretion of insulin by the islet cells of the pancreas, or dietary deficiency. Often hypoglycemia results in weakness, headache, hunger, visual disturbances, ataxia, anxiety, and personality changes. If severe and untreated, hypoglycemia may lead to delirium, coma, and death.

Alternative Carbohydrates

The body has a high priority set on maintaining blood glucose levels within a specific range. Although they are not termed essential, carbs do serve as the first line of energy provision for the entire body on a rhythmic pattern of ingestion and usage. Carbs are a fast and readily available fuel for oxidation. By contrast, the body must transition through numerous additional steps to access the available energy within both fats and proteins.

In only a few hours after your last meal, the body reverses from the state of predominately storing energy to one of energy consumption. There are three different alternative sources of carbohydrates: lactate, amino acids, and glycerol from fats. More than mere bananas and bread, carbs can actually be created when needed from materials or substrates within the body. The creation of glucose from secondary sources takes place within the liver or hepatic sink. As the liver's store of glycogen is depleted, a shift is initiated whereby the process of glucolysis and gluconeogenesis occurs. As the blood sugar level is lowered through the effect of insulin, the liver responds by releasing glucose into circulation, after it has metabolized stored glycogen into glucose.

Lactate

In addition to amino acids and fatty acids, a product of glucose oxidation—lactate—is able to serve as substrate for gluconeogenesis. When calculated by volume, the largest metabolic producer of lactate is skeletal muscle, though almost all body tissues contain lactate. The produced lactate is then shuttled back to the liver where it is able to produce liver glycogen.

Free Fatty Acids

Next we have free fatty acids (either from dietary sources or the liberation of body fat) and their ability to be metabolized into substitute glucose. The specific form of fat that is metabolized into glucose is glycerol.

Amino Acids to Glucose

In fasting states, where less protein is being maintained through synthesis and the degree of normal protein breakdown is held steady, the body will respond by shifting to utilizing ingested protein for a fuel source.

The amino acid transported from skeletal muscle tissue to the liver for conversion to glucose is alanine. A metabolic pathway for synthesizing glucose that is similar to the Cori cycle–lactic acid cycle is known specifically as the glucose-alanine cycle. Alanine is a nonessential amino acid produced in muscle tissue from other amino acids, especially leucine. Along with glutamine, alanine representatively

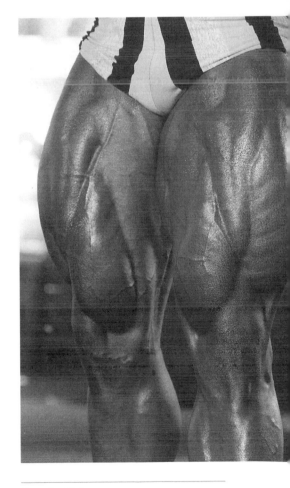

Ronnie Coleman

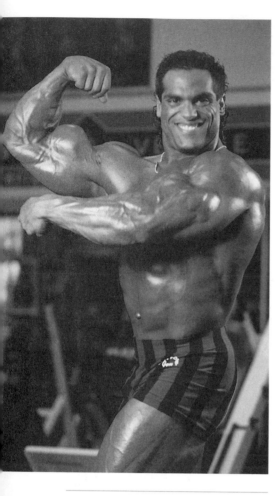

Dave Hughes

contributes 75 percent of the amino acids released from muscle tissue, although together they account for only about 18 percent of the amino acids founds in muscle protein.

Glutamine, is discussed here even though it does not supply a major source of synthetic glucose, due to the fact that it is associated with the movement or outward flow of alanine. Simultaneously we see a release of the BCAA (branched chain amino acids) from the liver. The BCAA are degraded into the alanine. Not directly utilized as material for the production of glucose, the BCAA (isoleucine, leucine, and valine) are pivotal to the process. The liver stores BCAA and is responsible for releasing them as required for transport to the major site of BCAA breakdown, the skeletal muscle system. Leucine is the predominate BCAA member utilized during gluconeogenesis. The breakdown of BCAA produces alanine. The BCAA are broken down from actual muscle tissue and used for energy in the muscle tissue itself. Large quantities of BCAA are available from storage in the liver and released into circulation for use as energy by the skeletal muscles.

The following is the sequence of events leading to the production of glucose from proteins as a secondary source:

1. depletion of glucose from the blood

2. release of glucose from stored glycogen in the liver

3. movement of BCAA from the liver to muscle tissue, with subsequent release of glutamine and alanine from muscle tissue to the liver

In terms of total amino acid loss by skeletal muscle tissue, by far glutamine and alanine suffer the biggest hits. Additionally, the source of the material for muscle tissue glutamine and alanine synthesis are the BCAA.

Note: excessive stress from either overtraining or undernutrition leads to a subtle state of chronic stress in your metabolic platform. Science has been able to measure the effects of metabolic stress by administering a triple hormone cocktail of adrenaline, cortisol, and glucagon. There was a clear shift in the subjects' protein metabolism from predominately anabolic (synthesizing new or maintaining old protein tissues) to catabolism of body proteins (a natural mechanism for renewal). These three hormones are also those released under conditions of emotional stress. So once again we have a situation where mental state and emotional attitude are either your friend or foe.

Fibrous Carbohydrates

We have focused on the digestible carbs that are eventually oxidized as energy. The other type of carbohydrate, fibrous, is not to be overlooked. A diet chronically lacking in fibrous carbs (cellulose, hemicellu-

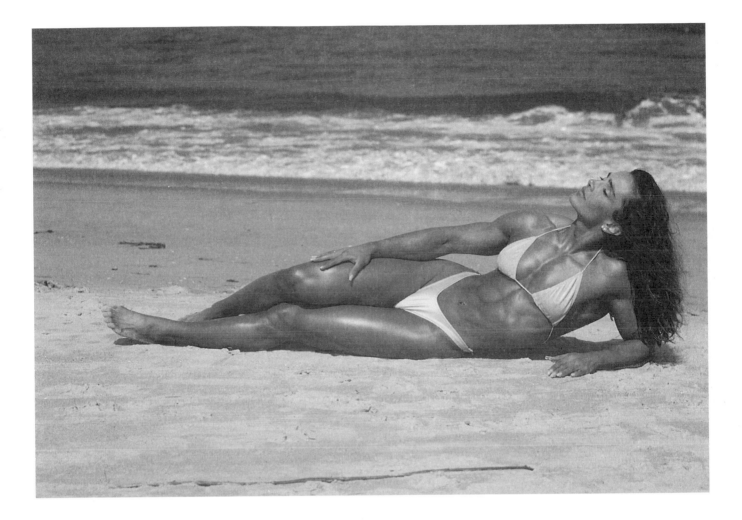

lose, and the pectins) is related to an increased occurrence of diseases such as certain cancers, heart disease, and diabetes. The digestible carbs are, of course, the in-and-out rechargeable fuel that the largest organ system in our body—skeletal muscle—utilizes on a primary basis.

Maximizing Carb Calories

To be a great or even good bodybuilder, you must pay attention to the types and amounts of foods consumed. Simply counting fat grams and considering carbs to be a safe food works for only 1 or 2 percent of bodybuilders. The rest of us have learned the hard way that nutrition is about balance. The following guidelines can help you to maximize the benefits from carbs.

Nutrient Structured and Timed Meals

Most adults demonstrate increased storage of ingested carbs in the form of muscle glycogen when the carbs are consumed four to six

GLYCEMIC INDEX

peanuts	13
soybeans	15
fructose	20
cherries	23
plums	25
grapefruit	26
peaches	26
sausages	28
lentils	29
kidney beans	29
skim milk	32
pears	34
whole milk	34
yogurt	36
lima beans	36
chick-peas	36
ice cream	36
tomatoes	38
apples	39
whole-wheat spaghetti	42
whole-grain rye bread	42
grapes	45
oatmeal	49
white spaghetti	50
sweet potato	51
potato chips	51
green peas	51
bran	59
pastry	59
sweet corn	59
sucrose	59
bananas	62
beets	64
raisins	64
swiss muesli	66
shredded wheat	67
Mars bar	68
white bread	69
white rice	70
white potato	70
whole-wheat bread	72
cornflakes	80
instant potato	80
honey	87
carrots	92
parsnips	98
russet potato	98
glucose	100
maltose	110

hours after waking. As the day progresses, the ability or tendency to store those carbs decreases. For most, a general rule is to consume more carbs early in the day with a shift to increased protein as the day progresses.

Glycemic Index Tables

The glycemic index for several foods is included to allow you to accurately structure the carbs you consume. It is designed around the principle of higher-numbered foods producing the largest release of insulin and the rapid lowering of the initially increased blood glucose level.

For best control over your blood sugar level, shoot for the foods with the lower GI number. The exception to this guideline is the two-to-three-hour post-exercise recovery period. During this time, the goal is to pump both carbs and proteins into the muscles which are in a state of increased sensitivity to the effects of insulin.

Combining Foods with Different GI Numbers

Along with timing the consumption of carbs, it is also a good idea to balance each meal in terms of the ratio of carbs to proteins to fats. (Refer to formula at the beginning of Chapter 4.) The goal here is to keep a steady balance between the release of insulin and its antagonist, glucagon. In strict terms, insulin is anabolic while glucagon is catabolic. The difficulty is that too far on the end of insulin anabolism is its anabolic effect on fat cells. Just like muscle cells, more and bigger fat cells are the end result of too many carbs at the wrong time. *Carbs increase insulin and inhibit glucagon; Protein and fats increase glucagon while inhibiting insulin.*

FATS

For more than 30 years, much has been said about dietary fats and health. Most of these comments or observations have been negative. Statements such as "if you don't eat fat, you won't get fat" have clouded the true picture of the effect of dietary fats and your health. Unfortunately, as the statistics demonstrate, the percentage of overly fat adults continues to grow year after year. So it would appear that even with the educational effort to date, there is something missing from the puzzle.

In the bodybuilding world, this overgeneralized anti-fat hype has served to confuse many athletes. In some cases, there may have been more negative impact than positive. There is far more to achieving a lean, chiseled physique than trying to remove as much dietary fat as possible. But first let's take a look at what roles nature has designed for fats.

Melissa Coates

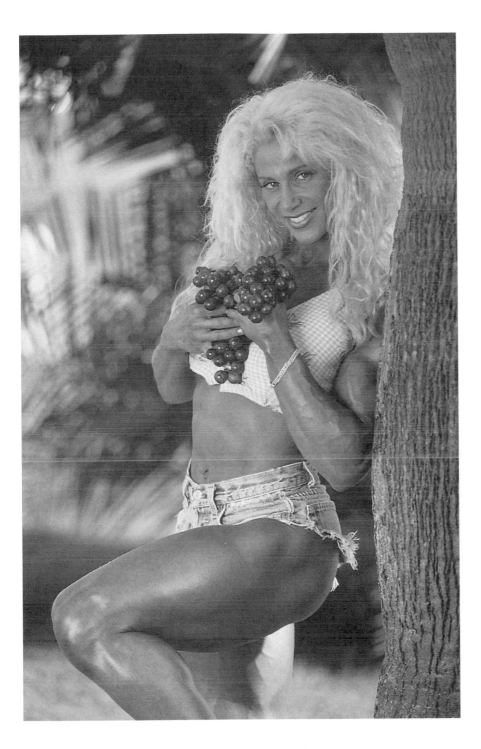

A fatty acid is any of several organic acids produced by the hydrolysis of neutral fats. In a living cell, a fatty acid usually occurs in combination with another molecule rather than in a free state. Essential
fatty acids are unsaturated molecules that cannot be produced by the
body and must therefore be included in the diet.

Free fatty acids are nonesterified fatty acids released by the hydrolysis of triglycerides within adipose tissue. Free fatty acids can be used

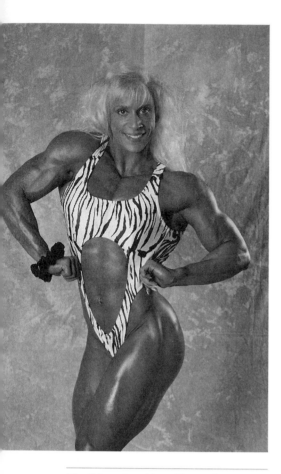

Ms. Olympia—Kim Chizevsky

as an immediate source of energy by many organs and can be converted by the liver into ketone bodies. Fatty acids are also broken down or catabolized, yielding the required glycerol component for conversion to glucose.

Types of Fats

Monosaturated Fatty Acids. An unsaturated fatty acid is any of a number of glyceryl esters of certain organic acids in which some of the atoms are joined by double or triple bonds. Monosaturated fatty acids have only one double or triple bond per molecule and are found in such foods as fowl, almonds, pecans, cashew nuts, peanuts, and olive oil.

Polyunsaturated Fatty Acids. Polyunsaturated fatty acids have more than one double or triple bond per molecule and are found in fish, corn, walnuts, sunflower seeds, soybeans, cottonseeds, and safflower oil. Diets high in polyunsaturated fatty acids and low in saturated fatty acids have been correlated with low serum cholesterol levels in some study populations.

Saturated Fatty Acids. Saturated fatty acids are any of a number of glyceryl esters of certain organic acids in which all the atoms are joined by single bonds. These fats are chiefly of animal origin and include beef, lamb, pork, veal, whole-milk products, butter, most cheeses, and a few plant fats such as cocoa butter, coconut oil, and palm oil. A diet high in saturated fatty acids may contribute to a high serum cholesterol level, and in some studies, is associated with an increased incidence of coronary heart disease.

Medium-Chain Triglycerides. A medium-chain triglyceride is a glycerine ester combined with an acid and distinguished from other triglycerides by having eight to 10 carbon atoms; MCTs can be absorbed directly into the portal system. MCTs are more readily used as energy than other types of fats, and in fact, burn in much the same way as carbs. They are also less prone to storage as body fat.

Essential Fatty Acids. Essential fatty acids are polyunsaturated fatty acids, such as linoleic acid, alpha-linolenic acid, and arachidonic acid. They are essential in the diet for the proper growth, maintenance, and functioning of the body. They are the building blocks or precursors of the prostaglandins. EFAs are vital to many important roles in fat transport, metabolism, and maintaining the function and integrity of cellular membranes. The essential fatty acids are also necessary for the normal functioning of the reproductive and endocrine systems and for breaking up cholesterol deposits on arterial walls.

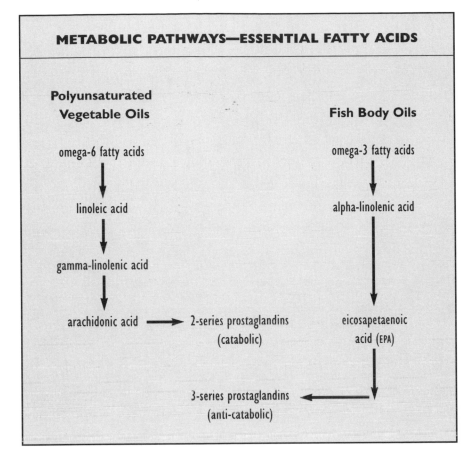

Prostaglandins are numerous potent, hormonelike unsaturated fatty acids that act in exceedingly low concentrations on local target organs. They are produced in small amounts and have a large array of significant effects. They effect changes in capillary permeability, smooth muscle tone, aggregation of platelets, endocrine and exocrine functions, and the autonomic and central nervous systems. A deficiency of essential fatty acids causes changes in cell structure and enzyme function resulting in decreased growth and other disorders.

Linoleic acid is an essential fatty acid with two unsaturated bonds, occurring in linseed and safflower oils. Linolenic acid is an unsaturated fatty acid essential for normal human nutrition. It occurs in glycerides of linseed and other vegetable oils. Arachidonic acid is an essential fatty acid that is a component of lecithin and a basic material for the biosynthesis of some prostaglandins.

As an aside, Canadian researchers have managed to increase the omega-3 fatty acid profile of human volunteers by having the subjects eat eggs from chickens for which diets had been altered to include flaxseed. The inclusion of the flaxseed yielded eggs with substantial levels of DHA (docosahexaenoic acid) and alpha-linolenic acid.

Ms. Olympia—Kim Chizevsky

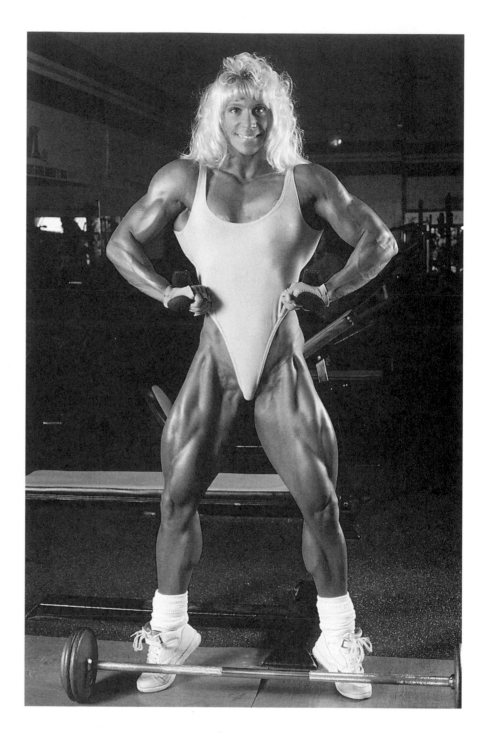

The test subjects ate four eggs a day for two weeks. Then their blood was analyzed for levels of the essential fatty acids and showed significant elevations in both DHA and a-LNA. Their cholesterol parameters were not significantly altered. The changes in the human subjects' fatty acid profiles resembled those seen in diets supplemented with fish oils. The truly fascinating aspect of this study involves the cholesterol measure. Even after 14 days of four eggs every day, the test subjects' levels of total cholesterol, HDL cholesterol, and triglyceride were not altered. Of the two essential fatty acids DHA and a-LNA, DHA seems to be the subject of ever-increasing scientific scrutiny. Keep an eye out for more information on nutritionally engineered eggs and DHA.

Role of Fats

Fats play numerous vital roles in optimal health and growth. In no particular order, fat functions to:

- insulate the body
- fuel the body
- pad vital organ structures
- provide essential fatty acids
- provide building blocks for other substances
- be a component of structures, especially cell membranes

These all-important aspects of human metabolism cannot be ignored without consequences. Remember, there are essential fatty acids and amino acids but there are no *essential* carbohydrates. Your body can manufacture the carbohydrates but not the fats and proteins it needs on a daily basis. The required fats and amino acids must be ingested in either whole foods or specific supplements.

Fat Metabolism

The biochemical process by which fats are broken down and elaborated by the cells of the body is called fat metabolism. Fats provide more food energy than carbohydrates; the catabolism of one gram of fat provides 9 calories of heat as compared with 4.1 calories yielded in the catabolism of one gram of carbohydrate.

Fat catabolism involves a series of chemical reactions, the last stages of which are similar to the final reactions of carbohydrate catabolism. Before the final reactions in fat catabolism can occur, fats must be hydrolyzed into fatty acids and glycerol. Conversion of glycerol provides a compound that can enter the citric acid cycle. Catabolism of fatty acids continues by beta oxidation to produce acetyl-CoA, which also enters the citric acid cycle.

The body synthesizes fats from fatty acids and glycerol, compounds derived from excess glucose, or amino acids, which is very difficult. Fat anabolism also includes the synthesis of complex compounds, such as phospholipids, an important component of cell membranes. The body can synthesize only saturated fatty acids. Essential unsaturated fatty acids must be supplied by the diet. Certain hormones, such as insulin, growth hormone, adrenocorticotropic hormone, and the glucocorticoids, control fat metabolism.

Note: fat catabolism is inversely related to the rate of carbohydrate catabolism.

Lipids are any of the free fatty acid fractions in the blood. They are stored in the body and serve as an energy reserve, but are elevated in various diseases such as atherosclerosis. Kinds of lipids are cholesterol, fatty acids, neutral fat, phospholipids, and triglycerides. Triglycerides are compounds consisting of a fatty acid (oleic, palmitic, or stearic) and glycerol. Triglycerides make up most animal and vegetable fats and are the principal lipids in the blood, where they circulate while bound to a protein, forming high- and low-density lipoproteins.

Chylomicrons are minute droplets of those lipoproteins measuring less than 0.5 mm in diameter. Chylomicrons consist of about 90 percent triglycerides with small amounts of cholesterol, phospholipids, and protein. They are synthesized in the gastrointestinal tract and carry dietary glycerides from the intestinal mucosa via the thoracic lymphatic duct into the plasma and ultimately to sites of utilization in the tissues.

VITAMINS

Vitamins are vital cofactors required for countless metabolic pathways within the body. In terms of dietary volume, vitamins are insignificant. In terms of value and requirements, vitamins are enormously important. Biochemically speaking, vitamins are organic compounds essential in small amounts for physiologic and metabolic functioning. Most vitamins cannot be synthesized by the body and must be obtained primarily from the diet, and secondarily, from dietary supplements. No one food contains all the vitamins.

Vitamins are classified according to their fat or water solubility, their physiologic effects, or their chemical structures, and they are designated by letters and chemical or other specific names.

Fat-soluble vitamins include:

- vitamin A (retinols and carotenes)
- vitamin D (calciferols)
- vitamin E (tocopherols)
- vitamin K (menadione and phylloquinone)

Water-soluble vitamins include:

- vitamin C (ascorbic acid)
- vitamin B_1 (thiamine)
- vitamin B_2 (riboflavin)
- vitamin B_3 (niacin)
- vitamin B_5 (pantothenic acid)
- vitamin B_6 (pyridoxine)
- vitamin B_{12} (cobalamin)
- folate
- vitamin H (biotin)

Edgar Fletcher

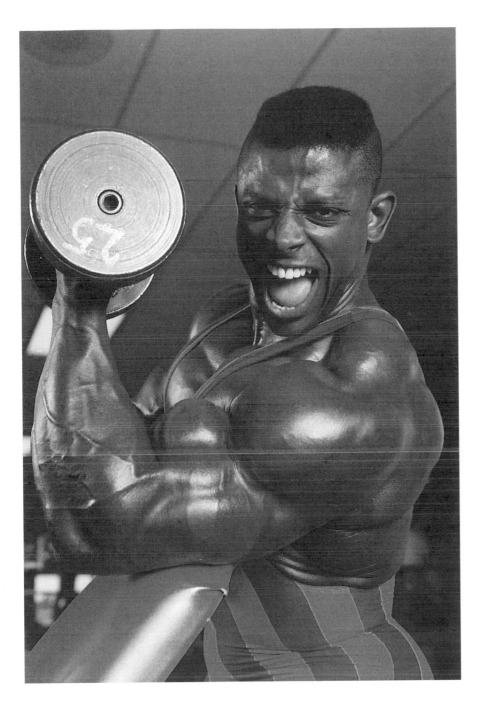

Sources of Vitamins

The best sources for meeting your vitamin requirements are fresh whole foods. Consistent intake of fresh foods in quantities sufficient for a growing bodybuilder is difficult even in an ideal setting. The challenge is to get the nutrients you need to grow, while maintaining a job, etc. This is where nutritional supplementation takes on the role of practical necessity.

Nutritional supplementation includes vitamins, minerals, and trace elements. Supplementation is a logical and convenient way to run your metabolism at peak efficiency. See chapter 5 for more information.

MINERALS

Minerals are inorganic structures required for proper metabolic functioning. They are usually referred to by the name of a metal, nonmetal, radical, or phosphate. A mineral is ingested as a compound, such as sodium chloride (table salt), rather than as a free element. Minerals play a vital role in regulating many body functions.

A chronic state of inadequate intake or absorption difficulty leads to a mineral deficiency. The deficiency may be caused by the inability to use one or more of the mineral elements (because of a genetic defect), malabsorption dysfunction, or lack of that mineral in the diet. The various symptoms resulting from a mineral deficiency depend on the functions of the element in maintenance and growth.

Roles of Minerals

Minerals are part of all body tissues and fluids. They are important factors in maintaining physiologic processes. As such, they act as catalysts in nerve response, muscle contraction, and nutrient metabolism. Minerals are also responsible for the regulation of your intricate electrolyte balance. Additionally, they influence optimum hormonal production.

Calcium and bone tissue are a good example of the relationship between a mineral and specific area of the body. Mineral deficiencies are treated by adding the specific element to the diet. The mineral may be added in supplementary form or derived from certain source foods. The following are the major essential minerals in human nutrition:

- calcium
- phosphorus
- magnesium
- iron
- zinc
- iodine
- selenium
- sodium
- chloride
- potassium
- copper
- manganese

- fluoride
- chromium
- molybdenum

WATER

Water is a molecule which contains one atom of oxygen and two atoms of hydrogen. Almost three quarters of the earth's surface is covered by water. Essential to life as it exists on this planet, water makes up more than 70 percent of all living things. At sea level, pure water freezes at zero degrees Celsius (32 degrees Fahrenheit) and boils at 100 degrees Celsius (212 degrees Fahrenheit). Human life is completely dependent on water for survival. Starvation might take months to kill you. Zero water intake will do the reaper's work after just a couple of days. Every aspect of your physiology and metabolism depends on water.

Water Functions

Water is required for most of the body's processes, from dissolving food to producing metabolic by-products. Upon the dissolution of these substances, the task of transportation is again dependent upon water for correct functioning. The thermoregulatory role of water cannot be overemphasized. For instance, in muscular contraction approximately 75 percent of the consumed energy is lost as heat. Too little water, and you'll overheat. Last, water acts as a shock absorber and lubricator for various joints and structures. So the list of water's functions in the human body includes:

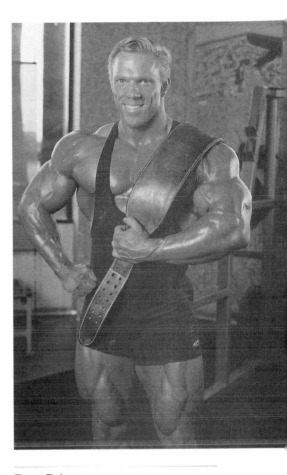

Dave Fisher

- regulation of cellular communication
- dissolution of substances within the body
- transport of dissolved materials within the body
- regulation of body temperature
- protective functions (shock absorption, etc.)

Where Is the Water?

There are three compartments of water within the human body:

Intracellular Water. Sixty-two percent of the body's water is located inside the cellular structure, surrounded by cell membranes.

Extracellular Water. Thirty-one percent of the body's water is located outside the cell membranes or in between tissues (interstitial) and in

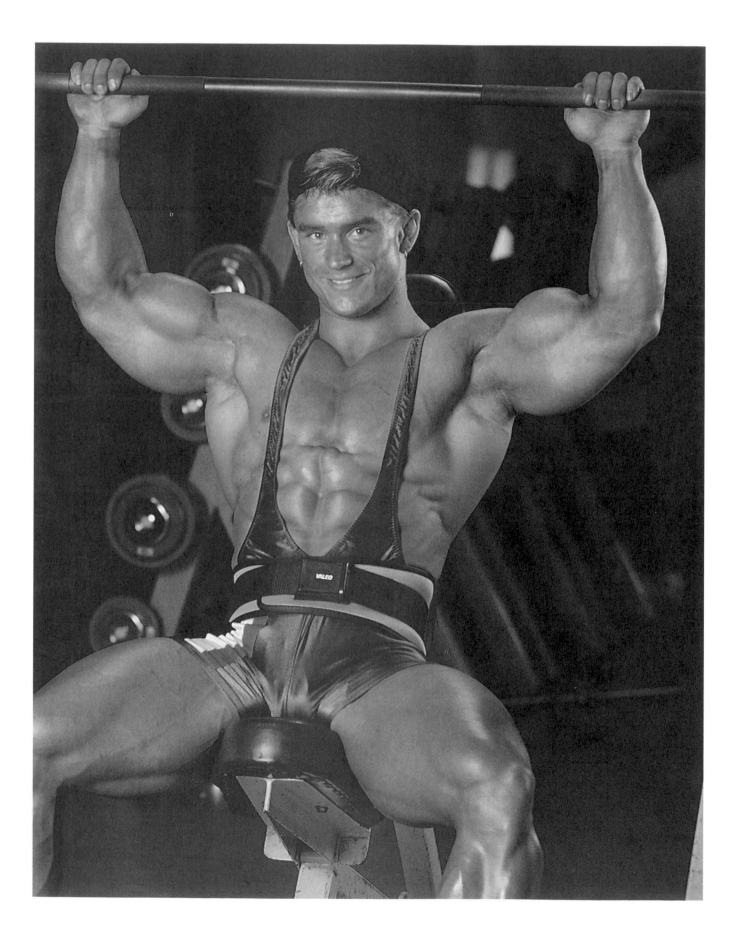

the plasma portion of blood (intravascular). One aspect of extracellular water is interstitial fluid. This is the extracellular fluid filling the spaces between most cells of the body, providing a percentage of the liquid within the body. Created by filtration through the blood capillaries, it drains away as lymph.

Transcellular Water. Seven percent of the body's water is in the often overlooked fluid found in the eye structure, joints, spinal cord, and digestive secretions.

Lee Priest

Not Only Water

Each of the three water compartments contains free water and the associated electrolyte molecules. Differences in the amounts of various electrolytes is one way in which the water compartments differ. The electrolyte levels of the extracellular fluids are approximately the same. Sodium and chloride contents are markedly higher in these fluids. Potassium, phosphate, and protein contents are markedly higher in intracellular fluid. The main electrolytes are: sodium, potassium, chloride, magnesium, and calcium.

How Much Water to Drink?

The average male of 175 pounds in a sedentary condition requires two liters of free water replacement every day. Sources of water loss are urine production, perspiration, respiration, and solid waste. Of course, as you increase both your physical size and muscle mass there is an associated increase in amount of water needed for simple physical activity. Accordingly, as you train harder this increased level of activity creates even more need for adequate water replacement. You need to strive for an optimum water balance.

Given that your muscles are constructed from relatively small amounts of protein and massive quantities of water, it is a sound idea to drink as much water as your body will hold, within reason. Essentially you should be training hard, using a high-quality protein supplement, and consuming optimal water levels daily. This is worth your attention.

There are additional sources of water beyond fluids. For example, the increased metabolic rate observed during intense exercise forms water from hydrogen and oxygen as a by-product of metabolic functioning. In the average-size man the hydrolysis of carbohydrates and fats also yields approximately 250 milliliters of water every day. For every gram of muscle glycogen, there are three to four grams of water stored along with the glycogen. This storage association between glycogen and water is one of the reasons for the dramatic weight loss seen during the initial period of a low-carb diet.

Marla Duncan

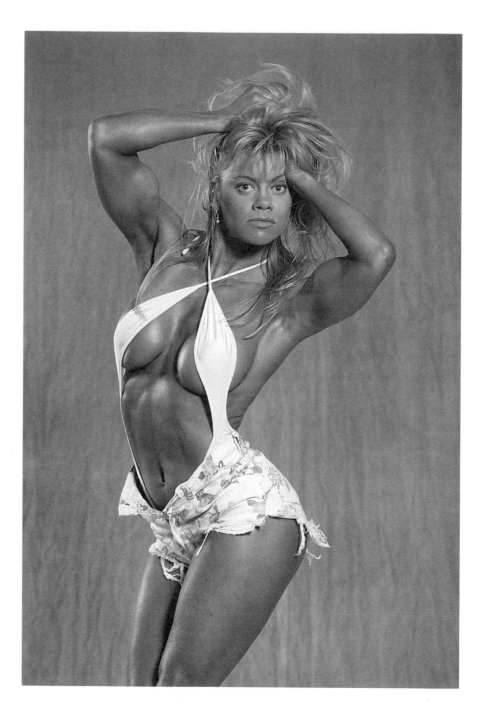

ELECTROLYTES

An electrolyte is an element or compound that, when melted or dissolved in water or other solvent, separates into ions and is able to conduct an electric current. Electrolytes differ in their concentrations in blood plasma, interstitial fluid, and cell fluid. Proper quantities of principal electrolytes and a balance among them are critical to normal metabolism and function. For example, calcium is necessary for the

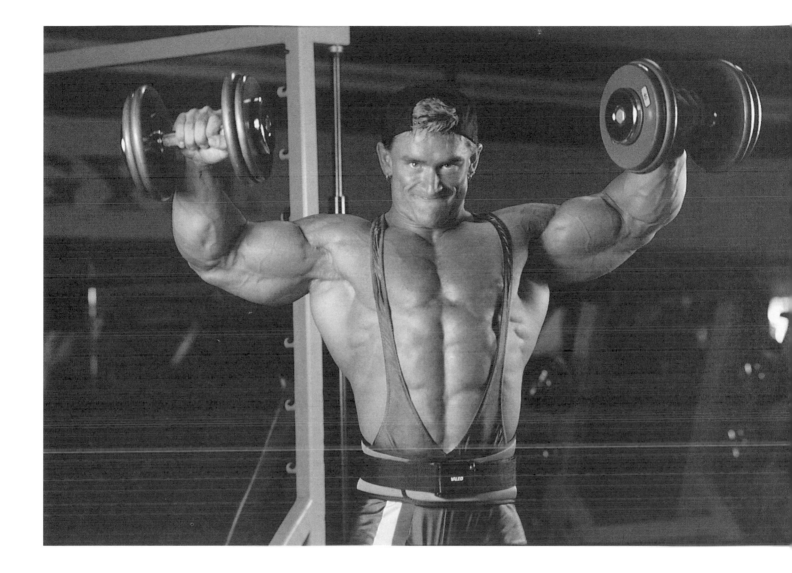

Lee Priest

relaxation of skeletal muscle and contraction of cardiac muscle; potassium is required for the contraction of skeletal muscle and relaxation of cardiac muscle; sodium is essential in maintaining fluid balance.

The electrical communication between cells resulting from the changes in electrical charges across cell membranes is accomplished through shifts in the balance between the charged electrolytes sodium, potassium, chloride, magnesium, and calcium.

THE IMMUNE SYSTEM AND NUTRITION

Your body is continually waging war against untold numbers of biological enemies such as viruses, bacteria, etc. The immune system is the biochemical mechanism that protects the body against pathogens, organisms capable of producing disease, and other foreign bodies. The immune system incorporates the humoral immune response, which produces antibodies to react with specific antigens, and the cell-mediated response, which uses T-cells to mobilize tissue macrophages in the presence of a foreign body.

The immune response is mobilized through the efforts of bone marrow, thymus, and lymphoid tissues. Also utilized by the system are the lymph nodes, the spleen, and the lymphatic vessels. Strategic aspects of the immune response are the immunoglobulins, lymphocytes, phagocytes, properdin, the migratory inhibitory factor, and interferon. Your diet must provide the necessary nutrients for your body's natural immunity to function as intended. The vitamins, minerals, fats, and especially, proteins that in one form or another are either eventually converted or play a supporting role in the conversion process, must be provided in sufficient amounts to allow the response process to occur.

USE A DAILY FOOD RECORD

There is little use for whining about not being able to grow if you haven't kept a thorough daily food record. This is an imperative step that must become a habit. Trying to remember what you eat in a day is less than ideal. Just jotting down the major details of every meal works to ensure you stay within the bounds of your dietary plan. The information gathered from your eating record provides the daily nutrient numbers critical for you to achieve your bodybuilding goals, especially in competition!

CHAPTER 4 REFERENCES

Bucci, L., ed. 1993. *Nutrients as Ergogenic Aids for Sports and Exercise*. Boca Raton: CRC Press.

Ferrier, L.K., L. J. Caston, S. Leeson, J. Squires, B. J. Weaver, and B. J. Holub. 1995. "A-Linolenic Acid and Docosahexaenoic Acid–Enriched Eggs from Hens Fed Flaxseed: Influence on Blood Lipids and Platelet Phospholipid Fatty Acids in Humans." *American Journal of Clinical Nutrition*: 62:81–6.

Friedman, M., ed. 1989. *Absorption and Utilization of Amino Acids*, Vol. 1. Boca Raton: CRC Press.

Latifi, L., ed. 1994. *Amino Acids in Critical Care and Cancer*. Austin: R. G. Landes.

Wolinsky, I., and J. F. Hickson, eds. 1994. *Nutrition in Exercise and Sport*, 2nd ed. Boca Raton: CRC Press.

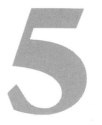

Supplements

Unfortunately, no matter how great fresh food is, you won't be able to eat enough to support continued growth past a certain point. You will need to use dietary supplements to become the best you can be. You can certainly accomplish much without using supplements. But bodybuilding without them would be like pole-vaulting in the Olympics with a bamboo pole while your competitors use carbon-fiber laminates.

The effective use of supplements has been called nature's genetic equalizer. Everyone can have a better body through nutritional technology. Millions haven't spent their money on useless nonsense—supplements work. (That's not to say there hasn't been some outrageous nonsense advertised over the years.)

Due to the ever-expanding genetic pool of bodybuilders, it makes sense to do your best to keep the field level by using supplements as effectively as your opponents. As you experience bodybuilding firsthand, it will soon become a matter of habit to budget for your supplement use. More muscle equals more strength equals more cuts, etc. The role of nutritional supplements in meeting this generic bodybuilding goal is beyond dispute. The loftier your bodybuilding goals, the more likely it is that supplements will play a strong supporting role.

WHAT IS A BODYBUILDING SUPPLEMENT?

We hear the term *food supplement* from different sources, but what qualifies as a supplement? In a broad sense, dietary supplements are compounds taken in the effort to achieve a specific bodily response. However, food does not qualify as a supplement nor do prescription medicines.

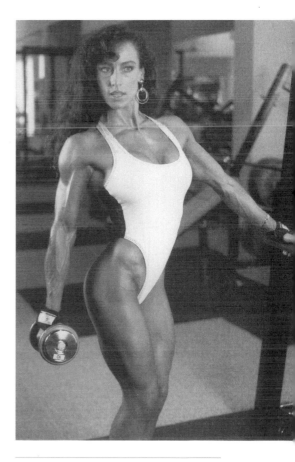

Sherilyn Godreau

Dave Fisher and Sue Price

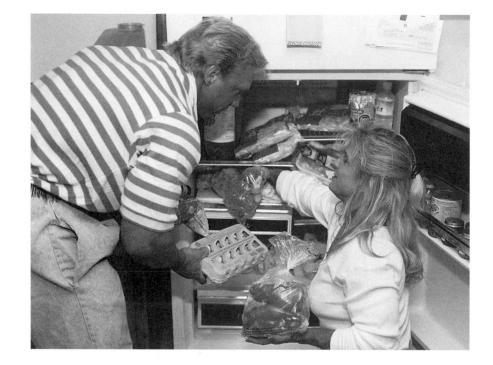

In today's competitive market, manufacturers can only stay strong by presenting on a consistent basis a wide range of tremendously powerful yet safe and innovative nutritional supplements. For the most part, flimsy fly-by-night scams don't last long in the world of bodybuilding supplements. Bodybuilders may get burned once by a company but they won't repurchase. They need real results others can see.

BACKGROUND

The relationship between bodybuilding as a specific activity and food fortified with dietary nutrients is more than 100 years old. Pioneers in the world of what was then known as physical culture, such as Bernard McFadden and Dr. Kellogg of Kellogg's cereal fame, prescribed exercise and healthy foods as well as specific substances to aid in the attainment of optimal health.

More recently, as muscle magazines have powered the amazing growth of bodybuilding, bodybuilding supplements have powered the phenomenal growth of the magazines. So we have a very close and mutually productive relationship between the needs of bodybuilders, the information provided in the muscle magazines, and the supplements sold through the magazines. It will likely stay this way for many years. The number of new, even better supplements will increase as alternatives to illegal and dangerous drugs. Approaching the goal of

NUTRITIONAL BODYBUILDING SUPPLEMENTS

Vitamins:
vitamin A
vitamin D
vitamin E
vitamin K
vitamin C
vitamin B_1 (thiamine)
vitamin B_2 (riboflavin)
vitamin B_3 (niacin)
vitamin B_5 (pantothenic acid)
vitamin B_6 (pyridoxine)
vitamin B_{12} (cobalamin complex)
folate
vitamin H (biotin)

Minerals:
iron
zinc
iodine
selenium
copper
manganese
fluoride
chromium
molybdenum
vanadium

Minerals and Electrolytes:
calcium
phosphorus
magnesium
sodium
chloride
potassium

creatine monohydrate (precursor for ATP)
orchic tissue
DHEA (dihydroepiandrostendione—hormonal precursor)
pregnenolone (hormonal precursor)
succinates (metabolic intermediary)
CLA (conjugated linolenic acid—fatty acid)

ALC (acetyl-L-carnitine—highly bioactive amino acid)
PHOS (phosphatidyl serine—highly bioactive fatty acid)
all amino acids (in any number of possible combinations)

Protein Powders:
whey isolates
caseinates
egg albumin
soya isolate
fish meal

weight-gain powders (calorie-dense extra meals)
weight-loss powders (calorie-sparse meal replacement)
orotic acid (metabolic intermediary)
glycerine gels (superhydration agent)
malto dextrins (highly soluble complex carbohydrates)
saw palmetto (active sterols—prostate)
pygeum extract (active sterols—prostate)
tribestan (plant extract)
guarana (plant extract—energy)
ephedra (plant extract—energy—thermogenic)
melatonin (active neurohormone—sleep response)
gingko biloba (plant extract—increased circulation)
enzymes
flavanoids
antioxidant cocktails (multiple antioxidants)
dessicated liver (cytochrome P-450)
ginseng (plant extract—energy)
bee pollen (extract—energy)
dimethylglycine (metabolic intermediary)
lecithin (source for phospholipids)
choline (precursor to acetylcholine)
MCT (medium-chain triglycerides)

Essential Fatty Acids:
omega-3 fatty acids
omega-6 fatty acids
GLA (gamma linoleic acid)
EPA (eicosapentaenoic acid)
DHA (docohexaenoic acid)
glucosamine sulfate

chrondotoin
NADH (nicotine adenine dinucleotide—metabolic intermediary)
caffeine (delay of fatigue)
water
electrolytes
sodium bicarbonate
aspartate salts (energy)
coenzyme Q_{10} (ubiquinone—metabolic intermediary)
inosine (metabolic intermediary)
adenosine (metabolic intermediary)
OKG (ornithine alpha ketoglutarate—anticatabolic)
AKG (alpha ketoglutarate—anticatabolic)
ferrulates (energy)
octacosanol (energy)
ATP (adenosine triphosphate—energy)
carnosine (metabolic intermediary)
GABA (gamma amino butyric acid—neurotransmitter)
GHB (gamma hydroxy butyric acid—neurotransmitter)
lipoic acid or thioctic acid (antioxidant)
sarcosine (metabolic intermediary)

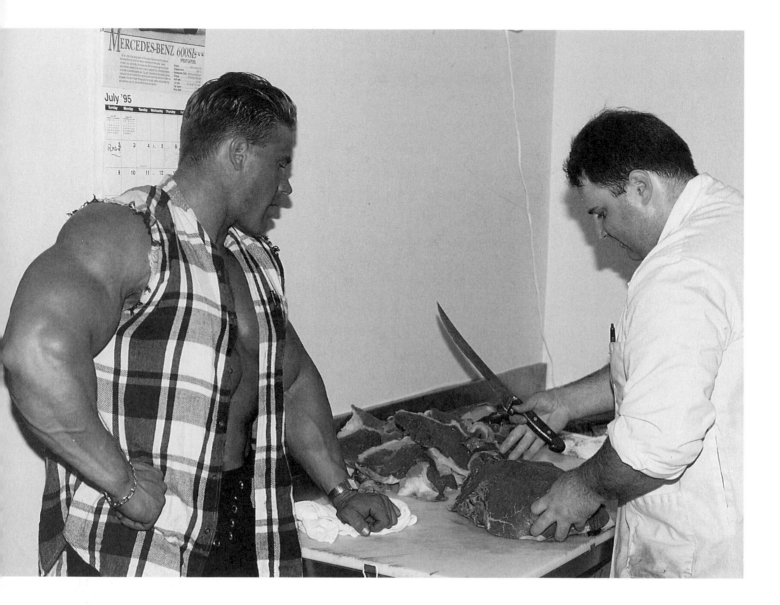

Jay Cutler

significantly increasing muscle tissue from purely a practical point removes the influence of marketing on choosing effective supplements.

While credit for the immense size of modern bodybuilders must surely be spread over many areas, the tremendous impact imparted by bodybuilding supplements cannot be minimized. Many of the other influences on today's competitors only function optimally as a result of the supernutrition provided through supplements. A likely first-generation supplement was powdered milk mixed in slightly stronger concentrations than normal. From there supplements progressed to the active ingredient in the powdered milk—the milk proteins. New technologies have empowered the supplement industry to expand its options for isolating many sought-after active nutrient groups. As this

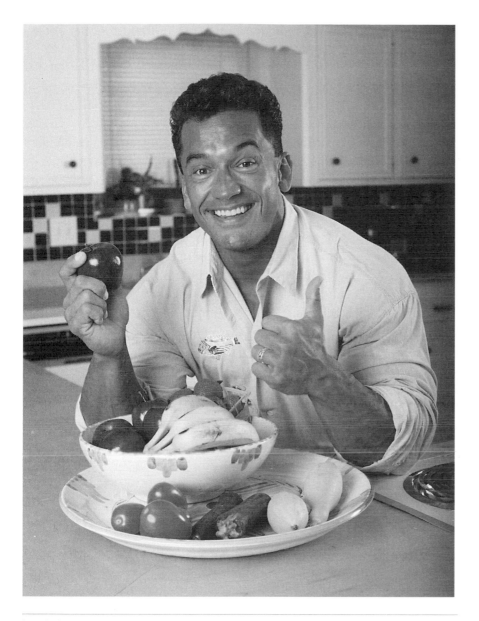

Lee Labrada

occurred, interestingly enough, the average size of bodybuilders increased simultaneously.

CONFUSED ABOUT SUPPLEMENTS?

It takes a brave person to enter the average U.S. health food store as a first-time shopper. Dietary supplement options number about 1,000; the bottles seem to multiply like rabbits from month to month. There

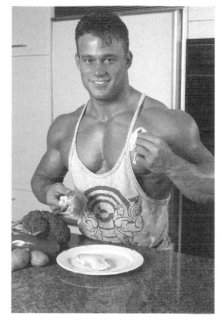

Jason Arntz

Dave Fisher and Sue Price

are so many different kinds of supplements to choose from, the aisles seem to get smaller as you try to get bigger.

Using the goal of controlling diabetes through the stabilization of blood sugar levels as the example, ponder how many different substances potentially fall under the supplement heading. These compounds are utilized by bodybuilders to achieve a higher rate of glucose disposal. Drawing from the plant world, in 1996 researchers catalogued more than 1,200 different species of plants exhibiting hypoglycemic or antidiabetic characteristics. Most were known only to the native populations in whatever part of the world they were found.

From these 1,200-plus possibilities, the same researchers have identified more than 200 chemical compounds responsible for the blood glucose lowering action. Time will tell how many of these 200 compounds will become indicated for the treatment or prevention of diabetes. Today we find the list of currently available hypoglycemic supplements consisting of: chromium, vanadium, hydroxycitric acid, cellulose gums, yohimbe, nicotinic acid, magnesium salts, quercetin, myircetin, and others.

With the field of nutrient research being driven by the heavy hand of need with just the right amount of greed, the question is not whether there will be more hypoglycemic nutritional supplements developed but how many. The first 25 years of the new century may see the number mushroom to upwards of 100. This imminent explosion of literally dozens of new types of bodybuilding supplements makes it difficult to accurately feature all soon-to-be-realized discoveries. It also produces the very strong possibility that more than one of today's supplements might undergo usage revisions or be replaced by safer and more effective compounds.

It is estimated that to bring a new drug to market in the United States costs more than $300 million of initial investment. Without the ability to produce exclusive prescription sales, and hence reap massive insurance payments, the drug companies have gone a different route of their own choosing. This prevents many possible natural compounds from being investigated due to less market protection as opposed to prescription drugs. This is the scenario for compounds that fall under tight FDA control and are sold as prescription medicines.

Compounds that qualify as food supplements fall under less-restrictive FDA control. This less-controlled regulatory and marketing environment sets the stage for supplement manufacturers to enter the research-and-development arena for the newest in effective supplementation. The trade-off is in the area of product labeling and claims. In the case of a prescription item, claims must be specific and given in great detail as in product specifications packaged with each medicine. For supplements to legally be labeled with specific claims, they must follow much the same approval process as prescription items. Labeling

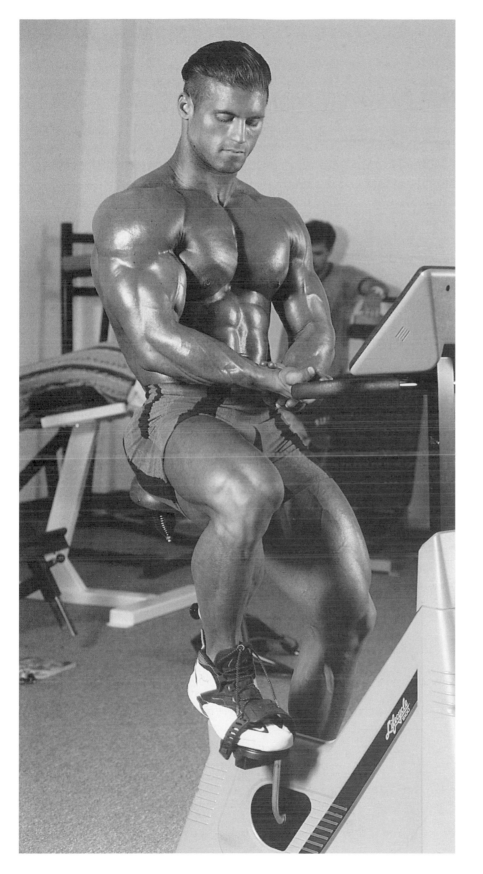

Mike Morris

without specific health-functioning claims allows for the countless number of items available on the market today.

JUST STARTED TRAINING?

If bodybuilding and all its outside-the-gym details are still new to you, consider the following: proper use of bodybuilding supplements is a discipline issue, more than an issue of finances.

Many of us cut our supplement teeth on multiple vitamins for quite a period of time and then followed with a protein powder. Listen to your body and take the supplements that best meet your individual characteristics. Start out with a multivitamin-mineral product and go from there as you learn more about what your body needs. You've then gone some distance in ensuring the ultimate success of your bodybuilding journey.

ROLES FOR BODYBUILDING SUPPLEMENTS

The needs of bodybuilders range from increasing muscle size to developing razor-sharp cuts displayed through plastic-wrap skin. In many ways this example illustrates the extreme opposites encountered in the sport. Not only is it unnatural to deliberately enlarge your muscle size, but doing so while attempting to minimize any increase in body fat makes the effort unnaturally difficult.

Further complicating a neat fix for the majority of bodybuilders are the tremendous variations that occur between individuals. Different structures with different metabolisms at different ages prevent development of an across-the-board product. The one-size-fits-all approach to bodybuilding supplements hasn't come along yet. The following is a casual list of some specific reasons for using supplements:

- to gain weight
- to offset negative effects of dieting and dangerous drugs
- to increase thermogenesis
- to aid in recovery from training or injury
- to boost immune response during periods of edge bodybuilding
- to decrease body fat
- to prepare for training or competition

No matter what your bodybuilding goals are, you will need extra protein in your daily food intake. You never want to become complacent and begin to overlook the amount of protein required to recuperate from workouts. Without exception, if you go by the name

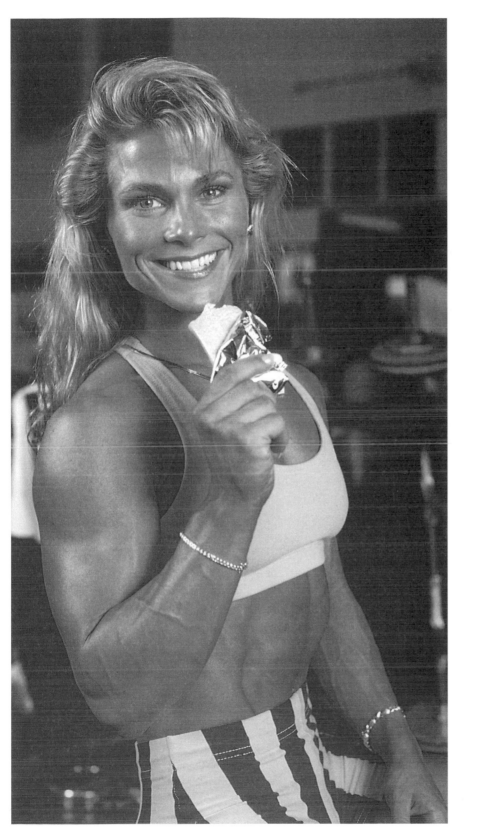

Carol Ann Hensley

"bodybuilder," you are mandated to utilize the best protein supplement you can afford. Your goal is increased muscle size; you must go into the building process with enough raw material to achieve that goal. Bodybuilding's raw material consists largely of proteins, and you will need to take in relatively large quantities on a daily basis—quantities of such volume that it will be difficult to meet your protein needs from food alone.

PRIMARY ROLE OF SUPPLEMENTAL PROTEIN

The largest single financial investment in your bodybuilding career will be protein supplements. Given that this amount of money could pay for a year of college, it's an area well worth paying attention to. There are some accepted aspects of protein supplements for you to be aware of. First is the type of original protein source from which the powder is manufactured. In best-to-least order, they are:

- whey protein
- caseinates
- eggs
- soya flour

This order is based on a protein's bioavailability. The most complete proteins are whey isolates and the least are soybeans. All of them get the job done—eventually. The trick is to gain as much muscle as you can in the shortest period of time. Who wants to peak at age 70?

Whey isolates are the top dog of protein supplements. Whey proteins are widely recognized for their superior nutritional properties. Whey proteins have an excellent amino acid profile, a high protein efficiency ratio, and contain some very interesting biologically active fractions. Undenatured whey isolates, such as those produced by cross-flow microfiltration, contain components that have antiviral and antibacterial properties. Studies have shown whey isolates to have a positive effect on some types of cancer.

A next generation of genetically engineered supplements might contain immunity-enhancing human milk proteins such as lactoferrin and lactoperoxidase. These are called immunoglobulins and are believed to be responsible for the prevention of some infections in babies nursed by their mothers. The immunoglobulins work wonders by binding to foreign bacteria and viruses, eventually eliminating them from the body. Of the whey isolates applicable to bodybuilding, the best is cross-flow microfiltrate, or CFM. This is a new process that uses high-tech ceramic filters to extract the highest quality protein available for muscle growth. In a natural process, CFM gently isolates undenatured whey proteins while excluding fat along with damaged or denatured proteins. This produces what is essentially a fat-free protein.

Marry Morti

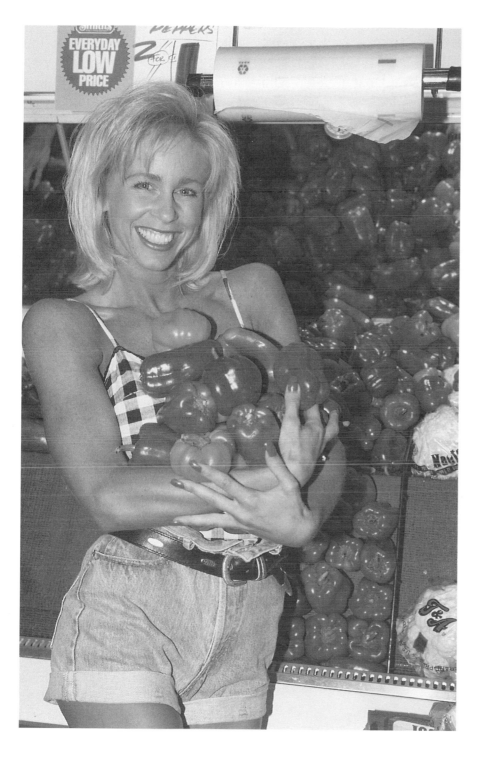

Denatured proteins are the equivalent of overcooked food. They have been physically altered by the process of protein extraction. CFM gives the highest percentage of the extremely desirable, pure, undenatured proteins. Protein should be purchased, in the largest size container available to minimize the price per serving.

SOME SUPPLEMENT TIPS

Here a few general suggestions for getting the best effect for every supplement dollar you spend in your quest for excellence: When you see the words Roid-Steroid Replacer, turn and run, clutching your wallet. Stay away from everything-under-the-sun–everything-but-the-kitchen-sink products. If the claims sound too good to be true, maybe they are. Cheapest is not often the best course of action in buying bodybuilding supplements—good ingredients cost more. It's a buyer-beware world, so do your thinking before you go to the store.

After you buy, spread your supplements throughout the day. Divide your protein shake into smaller amounts rather than drinking it all in one or two shakes.

There are hundreds of supplement companies in the world, if not thousands. The supplement marketplace is not like the Big Three in Detroit. There is, however, strong dominance by a few top players. Of all the supplement brands available today, some of the most utilized and trusted lines are offered by Gold's Gym, Weider Foods, and Now Foods.

CHAPTER 5 REFERENCES

Bucci, L., ed. 1993. *Nutrients as Ergogenic Aids for Sports and Exercise*. Boca Raton: CRC Press.

Friedman, M., ed. 1989. *Absorption and Utilization of Amino Acids*, Vol. 1. Boca Raton: CRC Press.

Latifi, L., ed. 1994. *Amino Acids in Critical Care and Cancer*. Austin: R. G. Landes.

Marles, R. J., and N. R. Farnsworth. 1995. "Antidiabetic Plants and Their Active Constituents." *Phytomedicine*: 2(2):137–189.

Wolinsky, I., and J. F. Hickson, eds. 1994. *Nutrition in Exercise and Sport*, 2nd ed. Boca Raton: CRC Press.

Types of Training

Training, nutrition, and supplements are the three big trouble spots for most bodybuilders. So far we've covered nutrition and supplements, so now let's knock off the last of bodybuilding's mine fields. This chapter will cover when, how long, and how hard to train.

Although bodybuilding is an individual sport, there is a striking similarity between many bodybuilders. Many bodybuilders start training with weights due to a strong desire to alter their physical structure. Maybe you started training because you were too skinny or too fat? The exact reason really doesn't matter. What matters is that deep down in our hearts, many of us just wanted to look different than we did. We wanted to restructure our external appearance.

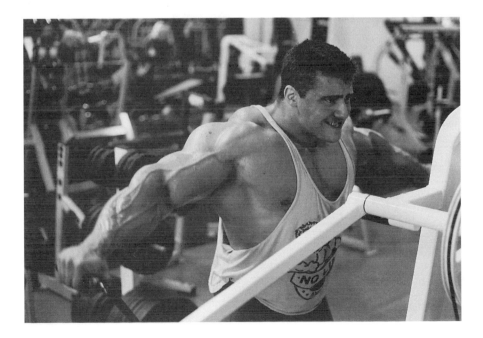

Jean-Pierre Fux

Jean-Pierre Fux

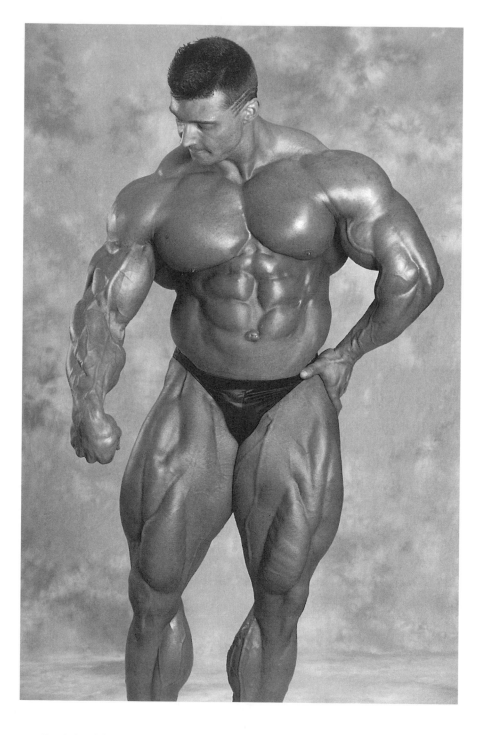

Bodybuilding is just the tool for the job. There is no better way to improve your self-image than by taking control over your life and becoming a bodybuilder. This is what it's all about, taking control and changing your circumstances for the better.

Successful bodybuilding is a real challenge. The enthusiastic novice bodybuilder probably has as sources of advice a thick stack of muscle magazines and his or her best guess. Bodybuilding suffers a lack of

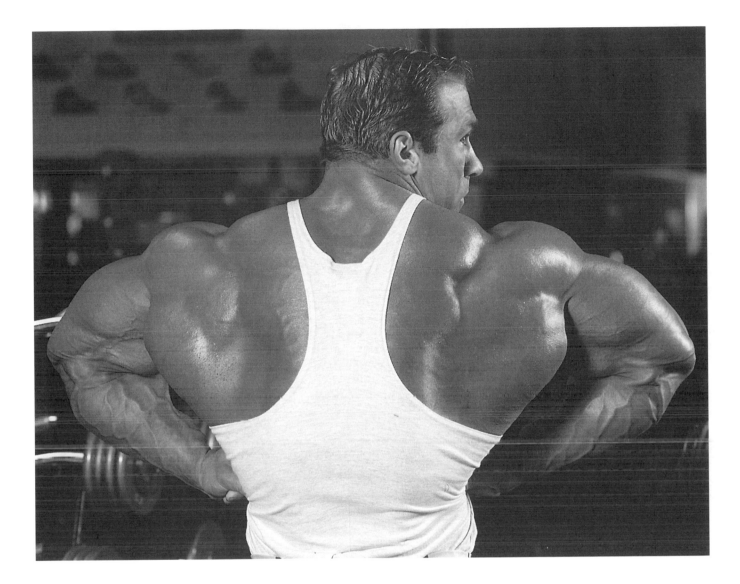

Mike Francois

coaches. Effective bodybuilding strategies need to be based on the practical application of technical information to individual metabolism. The role of the coach in sports cannot be overvalued. The athlete who is highly motivated to achieve only needs to follow sound instructions to become a better competitor, no matter what the sport. Where do bodybuilders get these instructions?

An incredible amount of bodybuilding information must be thoroughly understood before strategies can be planned. Information overload in bodybuilding has arrived. Without the ability to take in all the required material that would allow us to make the best bodybuilding decisions possible, we look to other areas of our lives for guidance. For example, work or school may be thought of as parallel to bodybuilding. Work and school are cause-and-effect relationships in that you work harder and longer to receive more compensation or positive feedback. It doesn't work that simply with bodybuilding.

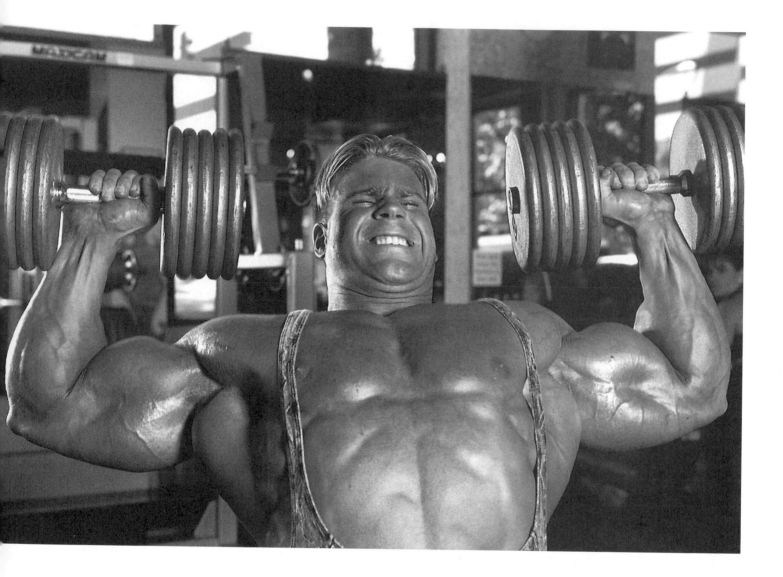

Jay Cutler

Bodybuilding is such hard work that too much of it will put you in reverse. A coach would be invaluable by monitoring the body-builder's work load and stress response. The coach would be aware of the signs indicating overtraining and could shift the workouts to allow for better recuperation. By avoiding this state of overtraining, the coach could help coax the gains along.

In the battle between enthusiasm and patient self-awareness, the bodybuilder often trains too often rather than too hard. There is a definite point where the amount of recuperation required increases until a lag time begins to spill over into the next training session with its new set of stressors. The role of training is to initiate a body response that produces new muscle structures as compensation to the impact of training. You cannot blindly continue to increase training time.

When you train with the correct intensity, your efforts become self-regulating. The effort is so intense that the body stops responding with reps and the sets are self-limiting. It takes an incredible degree of self-discipline to train this hard. The muscles being trained tingle deeply—it feels like a searing of a branding iron. It's rather hard to describe but you'll know when it occurs.

Bodybuilders want to get the biggest set of muscles as quickly as possible but are not sure how best to obtain them. At the moment bodybuilding coaches are rare. Without coaching, bodybuilders are left more or less to their own devices. However, this book can closely approximate a coach, so you're years ahead of those without it. The best thing to do is study the material in this book and use it to coach yourself.

This chapter will answer such training questions as:

How many days per week should I train?
How many sets should I do per exercise?
How many sets per body part?
How many repetitions per set?
With how much weight?
How do I decide which body parts to train together?
How long should a workout last?
How long should I rest between sets?
Is less more?

We live in a world where more is often perceived to be better than less. For many things this may be true, but for bodybuilding this approach is a virtual guarantee to stay small. The idea of more training being more productive is one of the hardest obstacles to get over. If your idea of bodybuilding means lots of muscle, then this "more training is better" attitude must go right now. Ditch it!

TRAIN LESS AND GROW MORE

Perhaps part of the difficulty stems from the early period of bodybuilding where much of the information was incorrect. In the early years of bodybuilding, some routines had trainers performing whole-body workouts a couple of times a week. This was training with a low degree of intensity but a lot of work volume—it rarely succeeded. The 1960s and 1970s saw the published training routines of the champions calling for large amounts of training. Some body parts were worked three days per week, with up to 25 sets per part!

When Arthur Jones came along in the late 1960s, he was called a revolutionary. He preached the sermon of one set. His Nautilus principle involved training each exercise in a single set with extreme intensity or 100-percent effort. The single-set-per-exercise approach resulted in low training volume that was performed in an all-out-until-total-failure

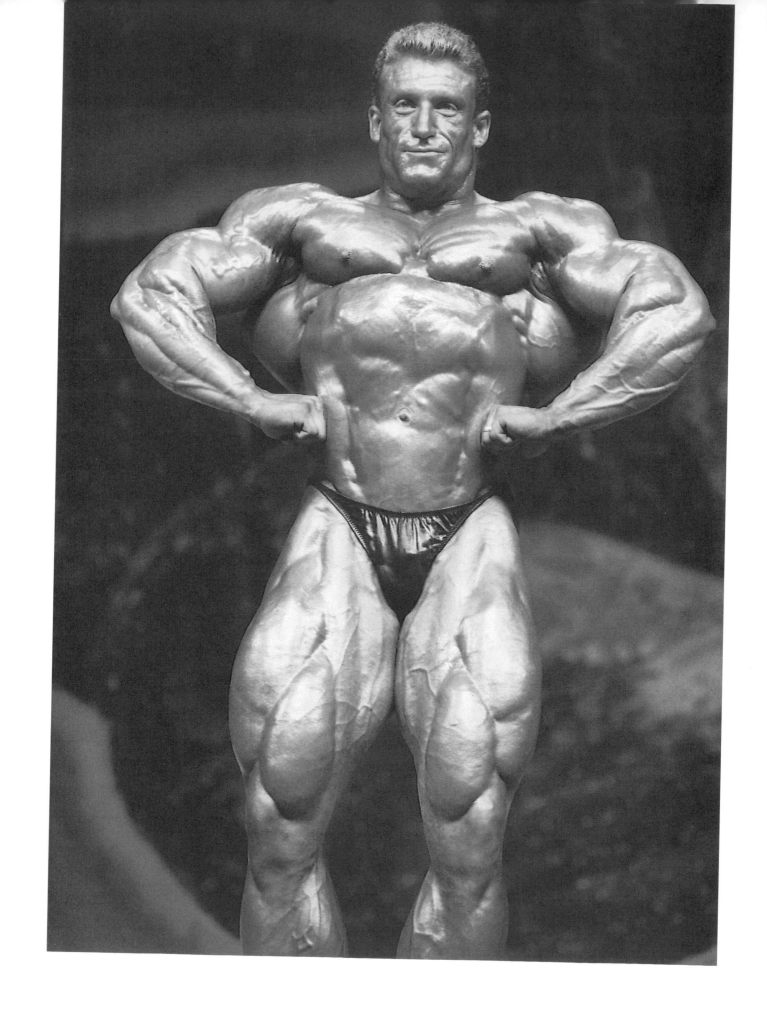

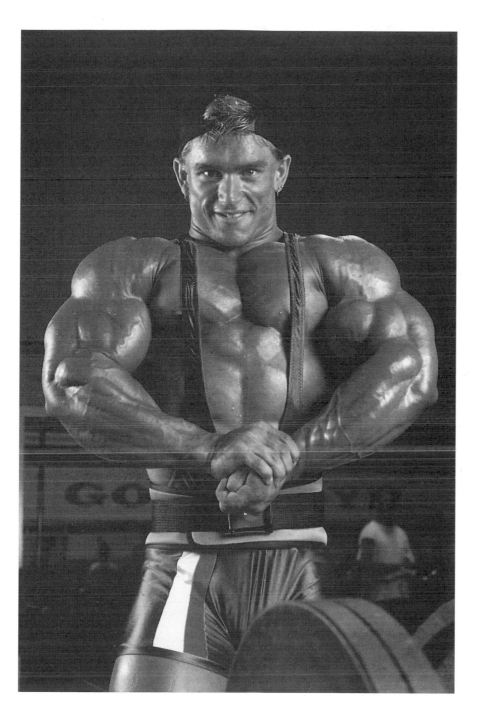

Mr. Olympia—Dorian Yates (opposite page)
Lee Priest

manner. Actual training sessions were less than 30 minutes each and took place three days per week—not much volume but tremendously hard work.

A slightly modified tactic was created by Gold's co-owner Pete Grymkowski in the early 1970s. (It is described in detail later in this chapter.) Only a few other perceptive bodybuilders picked up on the less-is-more concept. It fell out of favor until the early 1990s when it was revived by Dorian Yates.

Mr. Olympia—Dorian Yates

CHRONIC OVERTRAINING

Seen over an extended period of time, growth is a process of increasing body weight, increasing training weight, decreasing reps and sets, and increasing rest time between workouts. The bigger the bodybuilder becomes, the more food and rest he or she must have in order to retain the increased lean body tissue. The bigger you get, the easier it becomes to overtrain.

Overtraining is the state in which the stress of training, along with other stresses, accumulates beyond the body's ability to disassemble the damaged tissue, remove waste, and then rebuild the area of damage. In the face of this overload, the body shuts down and attempts to survive with a minimum of tissue turnover.

Many bodybuilders make the mistake of going to the gym far too often and exist in a sluggish fog of chronic overtraining. It is tricky to accept that you will get steadier gains by making yourself *not* go to the gym five or six days each week. Without the use of highly specialized lab tests, the status of your recovery process is pretty much left up to guesswork on your part. The question is when and how to train for maximum results. This is where experience and instinct become so important.

Training volume is the one area of bodybuilding that should deliberately be underestimated. If you train too little, you'll probably still grow. But just a little too much training will quickly stop all gains. Overtraining is stealthy and quiet. You may not feel a thing until your muscles are burned to a crisp. It's too late when you step on the scale only to realize in stark terror that you actually *lost* three pounds. You can keep an eye on your recovery status by using the following observations associated with overtraining as a checklist:

- You are more irritable than normal.
- You have trouble falling asleep, staying asleep, or waking up.
- You suffer from loss of appetite.
- You show signs of colds or mild flu-like symptoms.
- You are losing body weight.
- You are losing strength.
- You notice a reduction in training energy.
- You begin to waver on going to the gym.
- You are suffering injuries.

Cure for Overtraining

To begin to cure overtraining, skip two or three workouts. Don't worry—relax and be happy! A brief but complete layoff from the gym will resolve the trouble in about four to six days. Keep your food and supplement intakes at normal levels (or better yet, slightly above normal) during the time off.

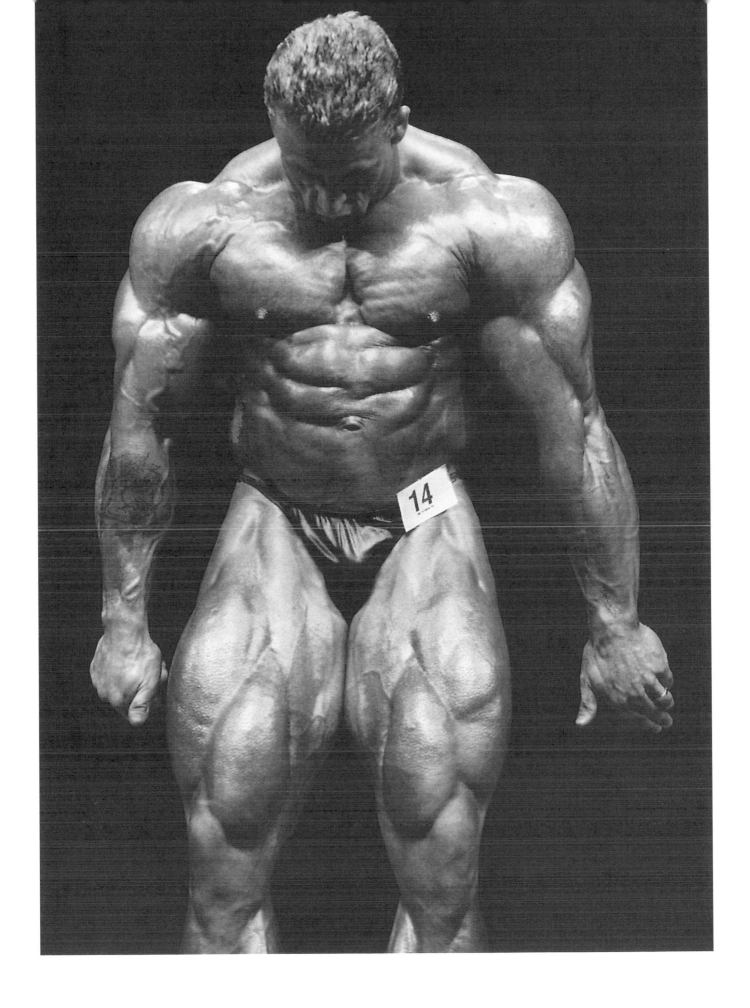

Debbie Muggli

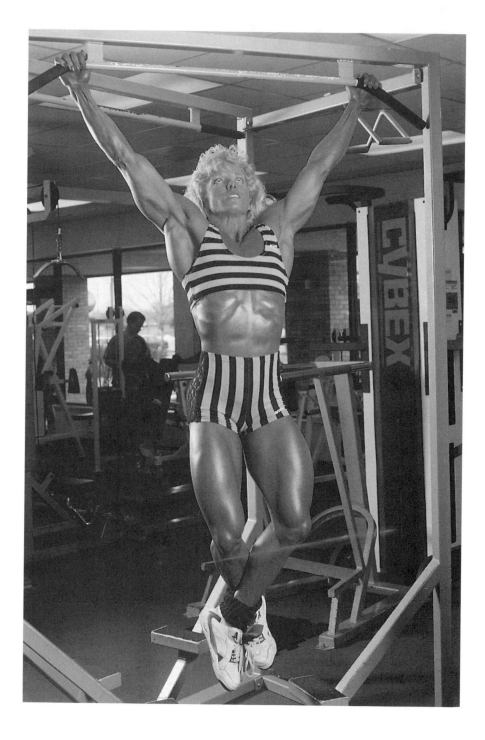

INTENSITY LEVELS

A workout for two people assisting each other should last about 75 to 90 minutes tops, assuming there are no additional rest periods than the two minutes or so it takes to load the weights. This is a tough pace to maintain but not at all impossible. Once you have developed discipline to keep out idle chatter, there will be sufficient time to rest between sets and still maintain this rate of training. If your workouts

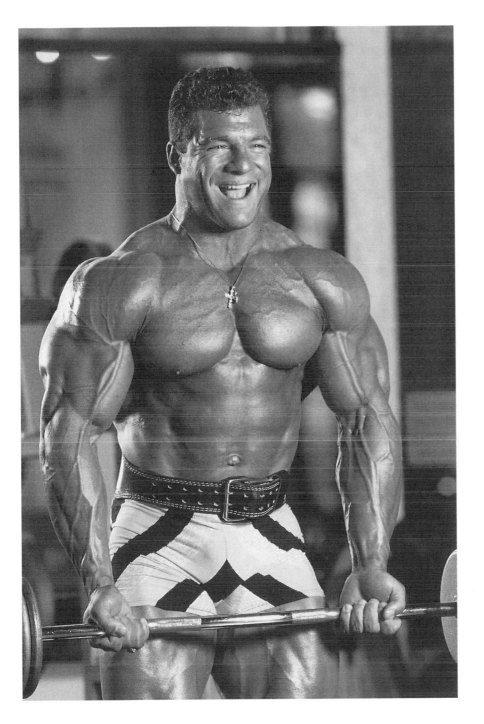

regularly take longer than 90 minutes, you should go back and take a look at how those minutes are actually spent.

TRAINING METHODS

There are many different ways to get the job of training done. However, some are more effective than others. When reduced to an essential characteristic, bodybuilding is the athletic endeavor to increase your existing degree of muscle size—bigger muscles for all. For the majority, significant muscle-size increase is attainable with consistent effort exerted in effective training and recovery. Of course, a few very gifted individuals have no difficulty increasing their muscular parameters, but they are rare. Often the genetically elite bodybuilders seem to only look at a barbell and eat some protein to gain weight.

THE PUMP

The pump is a favored approach to training that dominated the gym scene during the 1970s and 1980s. With this type of training, the ability to continue performing repetitions within a set is limited by the accumulation of blood and fatigue products. Failure is reached but not due to the same set of factors as eccentric-based methods of performance. Submaximum weights must be utilized to allow for sufficient repetitions to be performed to produce the degree of muscular fullness dictated by pumping reps, ranging from 10 to 20 per set.

Don Long

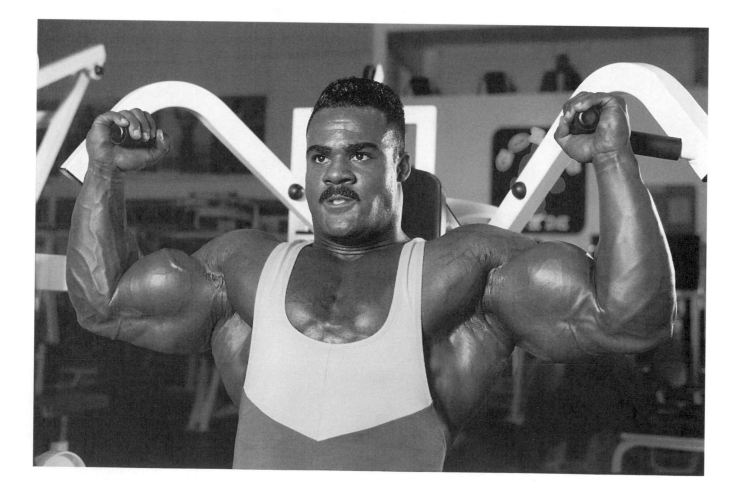

Pumping produces a tremendous feeling of outrageous engorgement for a period of time after the workout. It is, however, only a temporary state of muscular engorgement. This form of training produces little long-term gain for the vast majority of bodybuilders. A consistent observation is that, after time away from the gym, pumpers who have gained size over the years appear to rapidly lose much of their size increase. But when they begin pumping up again, their size rebounds quickly. Some of the best physiques ever developed were pumped into existence. In addition, pumping with higher than normal reps is the only way to rehab or train around an injury.

HIGH-VOLUME TRAINING

High-volume training is associated with the pumping method of training. You appear to be able to handle far more work when performing many reps with less weight. It is a method of training whereby the feedback mechanism for the perception of exhaustion centers on the engorgement of blood within the confines of a particular muscle group. The blood flow causes a pooling of fluids in the area being trained. Muscle becomes engorged and incredibly hard to the touch. (If you try and train this way, don't start with calves or you'll be hobbling around on crutches for the better part of a week.)

Individuals associated with the high-volume concept have been known to use industrial grade duct tape to prevent trainees from letting go of the bar when a set becomes too intense. Our suggestion: forget you ever heard of 100-rep sets.

LOW-VOLUME TRAINING

Heavy Duty or High Intensity

Before Dorian Yates there was Mike Metzner, before Mike Metzner was Pete Grymkowski, and before Pete Grymkowski were Arthur Jones and Casey Viator. It is not so much a point as who came first but rather that they all played a major role in developing the revolutionary method of obtaining maximum muscle size through low-volume, high-intensity training.

When multi–Mr. Olympia Dorian Yates appeared on bodybuilding's scene, the standard was permanently raised. He forced everyone to take a look at how he trained. What had Dorian done that was so different than all the other top pros? Some will seemingly never accept the fact that Dorian did the same thing Metzner, Grymkowski, and Viator did before him. They all trained as hard as they humanly could, harder

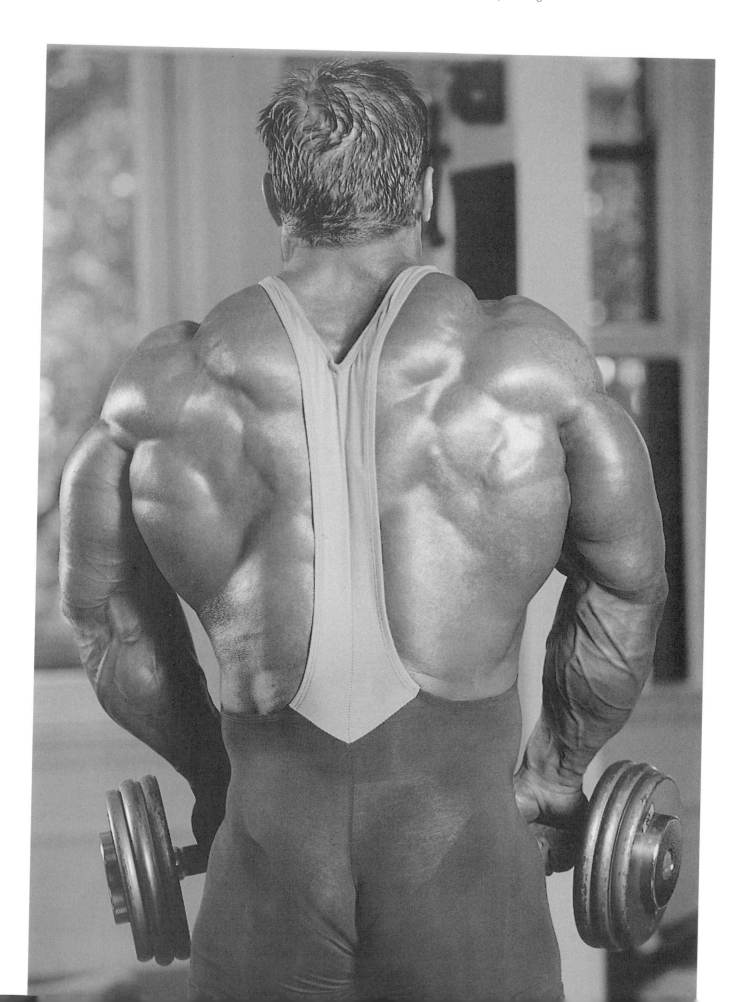

than any of their contemporaries, then they stopped and allowed time for repair and growth. They all trained harder but less. On average all four of these size monsters trained only three days per week.

There are many reasons why this type of training was so long in rising to the forefront. Probably it had to do with the message of sheer terror it sent to the subconscious after the first session had been endured. In addition to stressing short, brief, and intensely hard workouts, high intensity emphasizes the negative or eccentric portion of every movement. There is a noticeable difference to training with a focus on the eccentric aspect as compared to a looser technique seen in

Mike Francois (opposite page)

Jay Cutler

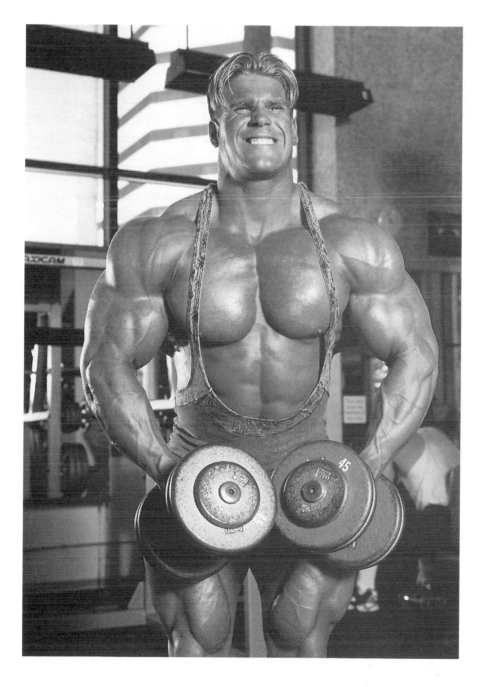

pumping or other less strict methods of performance. Training eccentrically is a study in motion control. The reps, though heavy, are controlled and resistance is applied at every angle and position of the movement. The following are some unique and effective low-volume–high-intensity training techniques.

Drop Sets

In drop sets, at the point of momentary muscular failure (or other pre-arranged signal) the lifter stops the movement long enough to allow spotters to decrease the weight by a certain amount. Grip and position are maintained while plates are removed or the stack changed. The extended set is then continued. Drop sets are very intense and it is relatively easy to overtrain. Use with caution.

Rest-Pause

Similar to drop sets, rest-pause may be done without the active assistance of partners. At the point of muscular failure, the lifter maintains grip or position with the resistance load as in drop sets. However, the weight remains constant without any adjustment from spotters. Hands remaining in the training position, the lifter rests or pauses for 15 to 35 seconds, then resumes the extended set. Tremendously intense and easy to overtrain with, rest-pause also should be used with extreme caution.

Partials and Half-Reps

Since this technique involves less than full repetitions, partials and half-reps use a shortened range of motion that allows for heavier than normal weights to be employed. Often partials and half-reps are performed in a weight rack or Smith-type machine. Half reps are reps without the top half of the movement, as in curls, or without the bottom half, as in squats. Partial reps are the same as half-reps but are performed with more or less percentage of completion according to the specified degree of performance.

Forced or Assisted Reps

Two extremely brutal training techniques for greatly increasing your level of intensity, forced or assisted reps are grossly overused by inexperienced bodybuilders. Both methods require a partner or two. Moreover, the training partners or spotters must have a clear understanding of what you need them to do.

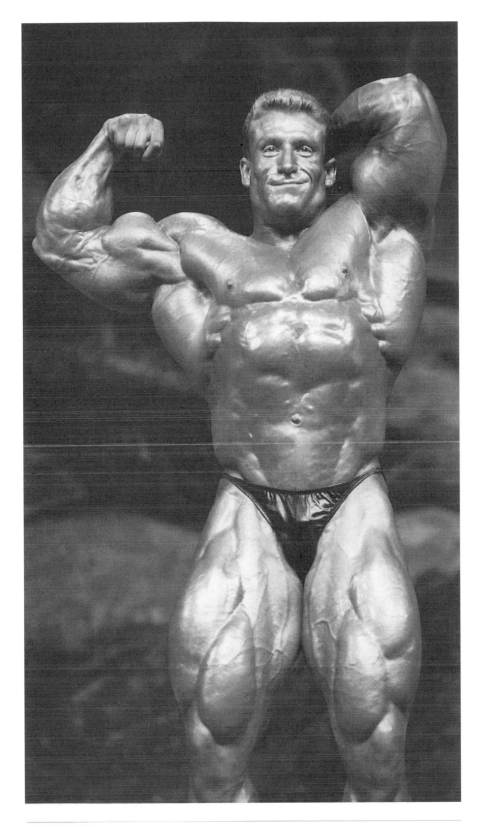

Mr. Olympia—Dorian Yates

Jean-Pierre Fux

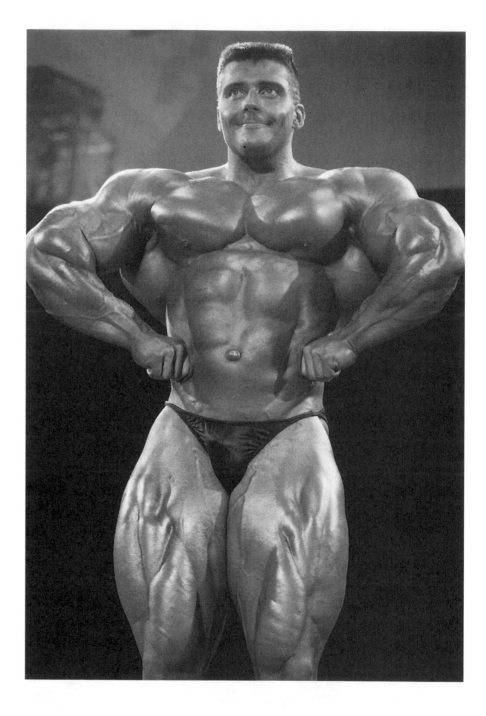

An assisted repetition is a technique where, as the lifter fails during the positive or concentric portion of the exercise, lifting partner(s) help complete the full rep. Correct application of this technique requires experience on the part of training partners. They must be able to apply just enough help finishing the rep. If they assist too much, they are doing the work. If they help very little and the lifter is still able to complete the rep, the weight is too light.

Having a partner assist in finishing a rep is greatly overused by underexperienced bodybuilders. Remember, if you are just starting out, there is no rule that says you must perform bench presses with nothing less than a 45-pound plate on each end. This is too heavy for many novices. Unfortunately for these bodybuilders, most of the other lifters in the gym are lifting considerably more weight, and with only the best of intentions, the new bodybuilder attacks the bar with a vengeance. The problem for new bodybuilders is they often attempt to use weights that are too heavy. Once the set is started and the struggle begins, their enthusiastic spotters grab the bar to help finish the reps. What is seen at the end of the set is a rep count of 3 for the bodybuilder and 7 for bodybuilder and partner.

Of course, this experience is borderline macho and quite pleasing to the sense of a powerful self. And without a doubt the eager lifter does get quite sore. But this is not a beneficial way to train. The very few, if any, gains that occur don't occur beyond maybe the first four weeks or so. This does not mean the practice of overspotting ceases at that time. All too often this self-deceiving mistake continues for the entire career of many anonymous bodybuilders.

If you are new to bodybuilding you must be certain you can get at least 6 to 8 reps on your own—without any help from spotters. If you're more experienced, it still pays off to make sure you're doing your own lifting.

A forced repetition is a similar intensity-increasing technique. The basics are the same as for assisted reps. In forced reps a training partner deliberately applies extra resistance to the reps. The difference between assisted and forced reps is very subtle and not always clear. In assisted reps the partner applies just enough help to finish the repetition. With forced reps the partner applies extra resistance by holding back against the bar or handles. The amount of extra tension placed on the muscle is generally sufficient to see the movement slow just short of actually stopping.

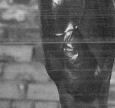

Don Long

ECCENTRIC ONLY

Eccentric is the aspect of contraction involving the lengthening of the muscle, also called the negative half of a full repetition. (The other half is called concentric or positive, wherein the muscle shortens.) Eccentric reps cause small microscopic tears in the muscle fibers themselves. These small tears are thought to be involved in the process of hyperplasia.

Obviously, eccentric-only reps have intense impact on your muscle structure and must not be overdone. Be very careful. In the case of eccentric-only training, lowering heavier weights can result in over-training as well as injury to the muscle, joint, or both.

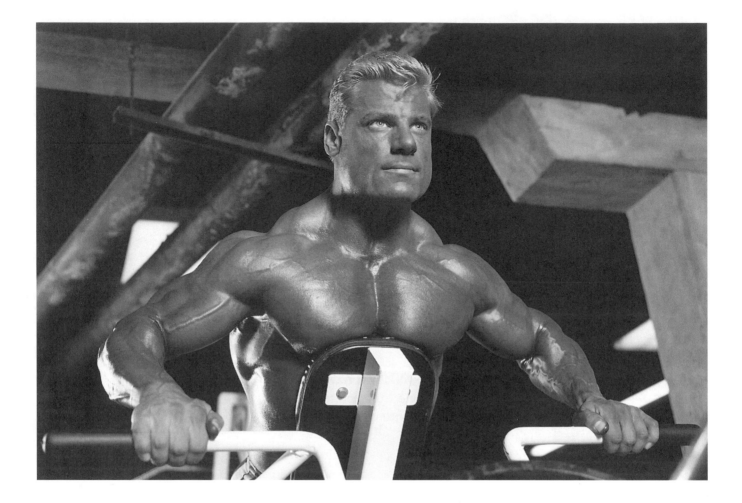

Joe Lazzaro

PRIMA-PRO PROTOCOL

In the early 1970s, Gold's Gym co-owner Pete Grymkowski took an extended layoff from training, which allowed his peak body weight of 230 pounds to drop to around 205. At this time Pete worked in the engineering department of General Dynamics, a creative environment that encouraged him to work to understand how he could become even larger than he had previously been. He eventually arrived at the concept that adequate recovery after training was the ultimate answer. He realized the body response that took place after training was the ticket to ultimate size. The solution was not to be found in drugs or special supplements. It was not the training so much as the recuperation period.

Shortly after Pete arrived at this concept of growth, he was fortunate enough to have many lengthy discussions with Dr. Michael Weintraub and Dr. Gilbert Forbes from the University of Rochester. In

PETE GRYMKOWSKI'S MASS-TRAINING ROUTINE
(Circa 1972)

Monday: Torso (chest, back, delts, traps)

Prima-pro pullovers: 3 warm-up sets and 1 heavy set of 6 reps

Bench press: 3 warm-up sets and 1 heavy set of 6 reps

Seated DB press: 3 warm-up sets and 1 heavy set of 6 reps

Wide-grip front chins: 1 heavy set 9 reps with extra weight

45° incline barbell press: 1 heavy set 9 reps with extra weight

Radical delt rack chins: 1 heavy set 9 reps with extra weight

Wide-grip front pulldowns: 1 heavy set 9 reps

55° incline dumbbell press: 1 heavy set 9 reps

Alternate DB laterals: 1 medium set 12 reps

Bent-over barbell rows: 1 heavy set 9 reps

45° incline dumbbell press: 1 heavy set 9 reps

Rear deltoid dumbbell raises: 1 medium set 12 reps

Seated low cable rows: 1 heavy set 9 reps

Flat-bench dumbbell flyes: 1 heavy set 9 reps

Upright barbell rows: 1 heavy set 9 reps

One-arm dumbbell rows: 1 heavy set 9 reps

Cable crossovers: 1 heavy set 9 reps

Dumbbell laterals: 1 medium set 12 reps

Wednesday: Arms (biceps, triceps, forearms)

Prima-pro compound biceps curl: 2 warm-up sets and 1 heavy set 9 reps

Prima-pro compound triceps extensions: 2 warm-up sets and 1 heavy set 9 reps

> Note: first two arm exercises were performed in a back-to-back, super-set protocol; both exercises were considered as 1 cycle, repeat cycles 2—3 times.

Barbell wrist curls: 1 warm-up set & 2 heavy set 9 reps

Friday: Legs (thighs, calves)

Leg extensions: 3 warm-up sets and 1 heavy set of 9 reps

Leg curls: 3 warm-up sets and 1 heavy set of 9 reps

Prima-pro seated leg press: 3 warm-up sets and 1 heavy set of 6 reps

> Note: first three movements were performed in a nonstop, pre-exhaust manner, with a 10-minute rest between a second cycle of these three exercises, if desired.

Standing calf raise: 2 warm-up sets and 1 heavy set of 12 reps

Donkey calf raise: 1 warm-up set and 1 heavy set of 12 reps

collaboration they decided an ideal post-exercise recuperation period is seven days. This period was based on brief but intense eccentric training sessions. A few brief sets taken to the point of total muscular exhaustion stimulated the recovery process. Less than seven days between working the same body parts prevented a full recovery. Repetitions were taken to complete muscle failure in order to ensure the exhaustion of each body part.

Pete started training again and quickly regained the 25 pounds he had lost *and* packed on an incredible 25 pounds of *new* muscle. For the Mr. America contest, he grew from a low of 205 pounds at 5 feet 10 inches to an all-time high of 255 pounds. Keep in mind that Pete, along with his contemporaries, had at one time trained six days per week for three to four hours a day. As Pete's instincts grew sharper, he began to decrease the amount of reps and sets and increase the weights. This shift yielded a consistent trend toward a heavier body weight.

In his first workout of the week Pete worked his torso. The week's second workout focused on arms, being far less intense and very short in duration, so as not to interrupt the recuperative process from the extreme stress of the torso workout. On Friday Pete worked on legs, and though short on numbers of sets, the intensity of Pete's leg training bordered on the limit of human endurance to pain.

This pattern of cycling the degree of training stress allowed Pete's metabolism to recuperate at the highest degree of functioning when the need was greatest. Likewise, this cycling of training intensity allowed his stress response to continue from the first workout while coping with the next two workouts each week.

Of course, just as important as the training was the amount and type of food consumed to fuel his recovery process 24 hours a day. For this mission of muscle repair and growth, Pete used tremendous quantities of milk and egg protein powders throughout the day.

TRAINING GUIDELINES

The following training suggestions are just that—suggestions for you to personalize according to your bodybuilding goals. The information is intended to apply to 95 percent of healthy bodybuilders. Exceptions to the rule are few.

How many days per week should I train?
The least number of workouts would be two days a week. You could set up your training schedule something like this:

- day one: chest, deltoids, triceps, thighs, and calves
- day two: back, hamstrings, biceps, abs, and forearms

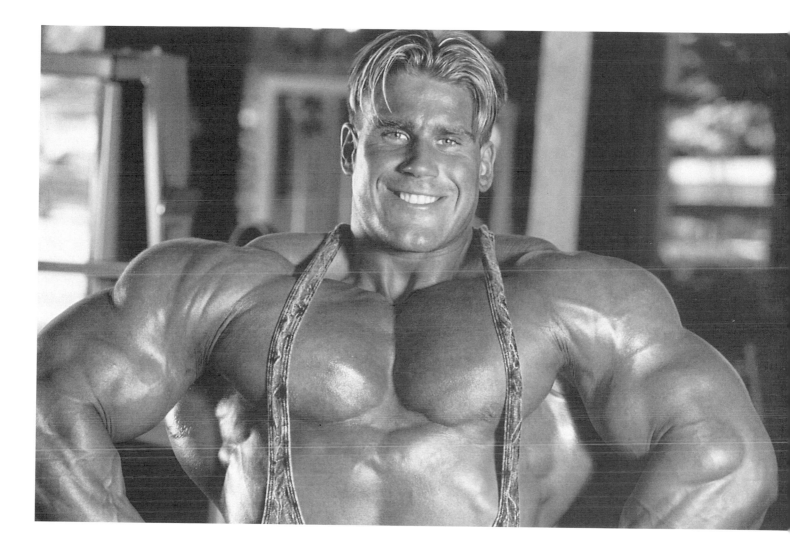

Jay Cutler

At the high end of weekly training sessions, you could still grow five days per week. Another approach might be to set the week up along the lines of:

- day one: back, traps
- day two: chest, abs
- day three: delts, triceps
- day four: biceps, forearms
- day five: thighs, calves

Either way you decide to train, it's the recovery after training that produces growth, not the workouts in isolation. Workouts, food, and recuperation are integral aspects to successful bodybuilding.

How many total sets should I do per body part?
A set range of 6 to 14 sets per workout for thighs, back, chest, and delts is appropriate for most bodybuilders. Of course, you should develop your own numbers according to the number of different

TRAINING SUGGESTIONS

Less Than 1 Year Training

- 3 workouts per week
- 2–3 body parts per workout
- 4 sets (after warm-ups) for biceps, triceps, calves, and abs
- 6–8 sets (after warm-ups) for thighs, back, chest, and deltoids
- 8–10 repetitions on average per set with enough weight to perform 10 fully controlled, unassisted repetitions
- don't go for partner-assisted repetition and other ways to increase intensity; be patient

1–2 Years' Training

- 4 workouts per week
- 1–2 body parts per workout
- 6 sets (after warm-ups) for biceps, triceps, calves, and abs
- 8 sets (after warm-ups) for thighs, back, chest, and deltoids
- 8–10 repetitions on average per set with sufficient weight to perform 8 controlled, unassisted repetitions

2–4 Years' Training

- 3–4 workouts per week
- 1–2 body parts per workout
- 2–4 sets (after warm-ups) for biceps, triceps, calves, and abs
- 4–8 sets (after warm-ups) for thighs, back, chest, and deltoids
- 6–12 repetitions on average per set with enough weight to become momentarily unable to perform a full repetition

muscle groups being trained on a particular day. The thighs, chest, back, and delts are considered large-muscle groups. The biceps, triceps, calves, forearms, and abs are the small-muscle groups. For the biceps, triceps, calves, forearms, and abs, a total set range of 3 to 8 per training session works tremendously well.

How many sets should I do per exercise?

Simply take the number of total sets per body part and divide by the number of exercises. For example: Your training routine calls for 6 total sets of biceps. You decide that the two exercises you will use are barbell curls and seated dumbbell curls. You would perform 3 working sets (3 sets BB curls and 3 sets seated DB curls) for both exercises after first completing your warm-up sets.

How many repetitions should I do per set?

When setting up your workouts, it is very important to pay attention to the range of repetitions per set of an exercise. As important as the reps is your training form. The repetitions must be smooth and controlled. There is a wide range of possible rep schemes in bodybuilding. A low rep count is 5 to 6 repetitions per set, a high count is 12 to 15. These are the suggested range of numbers for bodybuilding workouts, not training for a sport or other specific lifting protocol.

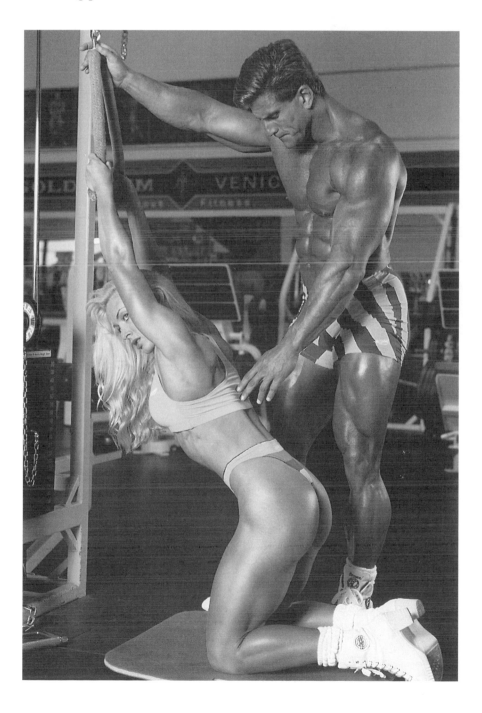

Debbie Kruck and Lee Apperson

Cathy LaFrancois

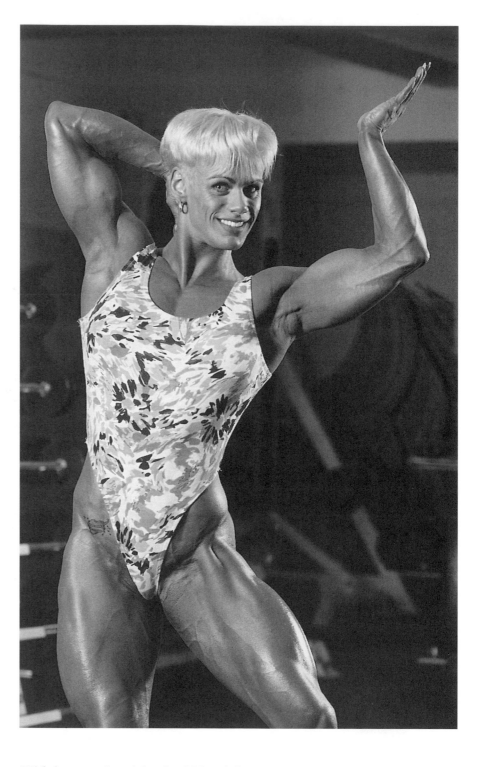

With how much weight should I train?

As the number of repetitions decreases, you will use more weight to perform the exercise. Likewise, as the number of repetitions increases, you'll have to use less weight. In general, the biggest bodybuilders used the heaviest weights in their training careers.

Which body parts should I train together?

You can group your body parts together according to their relative aspects of movement. This approach, known as push-pull training, works as follows:

- day one: back, biceps—pull
- day two: chest, delts, triceps—push
- day three: thighs, calves

Train the largest body parts first in your workout and work your way down to the smallest muscle for that day. Remember, this is not a hard-and-fast rule cut into a mountain in Tibet; this is only a suggestion. Please knock yourself out and tweak this push-pull routine to fit your needs. But never lose sight of the potential to overtrain.

Another manner of arranging your sets is in pre-exhaust training, an intense way to train in a condensed amount of time. This type workout is to be utilized for increasing your training intensity or if there is a need to train with a minimum of time available. Using deltoid training as the example, instead of training with a heavy pressing move first, such as BB presses, this type of compound, multi-joint exercise is performed last in the sequence of exercises. The first exercises are known as isolation exercises because they use a minimum of assisting muscles. Side DB laterals, front BB raises, and bent-over rear-delt DB raises are all isolation movements for the delts.

The idea is to pre-exhaust the delts with the isolation-only movements performed in a back-to-back sequence. These first isolation pre-exhaust movements are to be done with no rest whatsoever between sets. You quickly put down one set of weights and immediately pick up the next and begin. Train like this until all the pre-exhaust exercises are completed. The deltoids are then considered pre-exhausted by the three previous isolation movements. BB presses are next—the last in a series of four consecutive exercises. You are training the deltoids with the BB presses to total muscular failure beyond the degree associated with conventional training. Be aware that the amount of weight used in any exercise trained in a pre-exhaust manner will of necessity be less than normally handled in regular straight sets.

One way to ascertain if you are training hard enough in pre-exhaust fashion is to make certain you are unable to handle your normal amount of weight in the last, or compound, exercise. If you are able to train with the same weight you regularly use, you did not sufficiently pre-exhaust that body part with the isolation movements.

Tom Jimenez

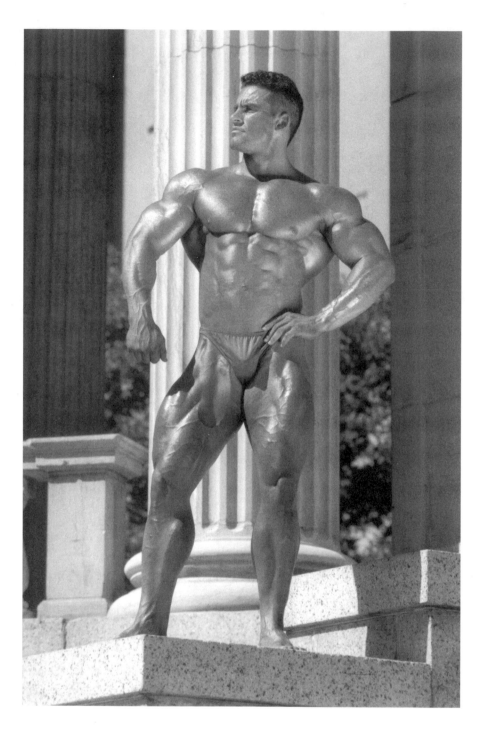

How long should a workout last?

In general, it may take about 50 minutes for an individual to train at a speedy pace. On average, training with one other partner, a two or three body-part workout lasts 60 to 90 minutes. The exceptions are leg workouts. Due to the tremendous amount of energy and oxygen consumed during leg workouts, in most cases, they

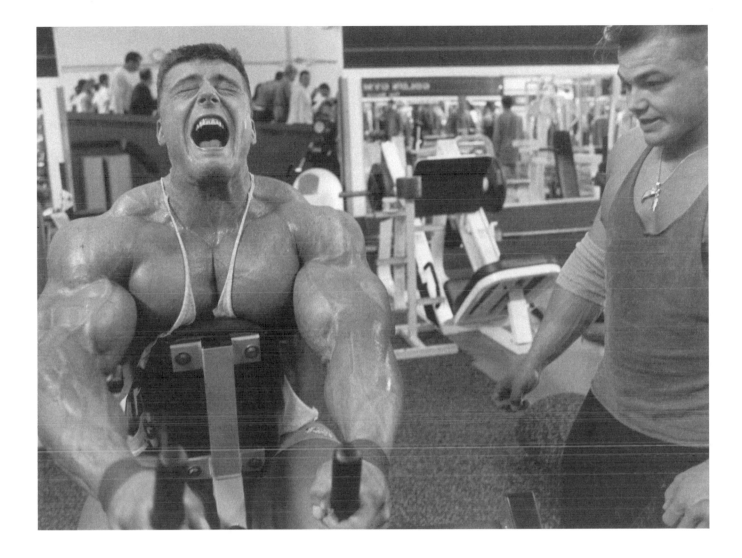

Jean-Pierre Fux (left) and
Daniel Sherrer

take the longest time to train correctly. An extreme of 100 to 150 minutes is not unheard of. More commonly the session will take less than 95 minutes. Training with a partner is recommended if at all possible. However, you must allow for a longer workout based on the partner's background and experience.

What about super sets?

Super sets are specific exercises trained back to back with as little time as possible between sets. You can perform super sets a number of unique ways. Put two exercises together for a super set, three together for a tri-set, and four separate exercises trained one after another for a giant set. There is also the option of training complimentary or opposing muscle groups. For example, train chins super-setted with bench presses as opposing exercises. The complimentary arrangement would be chins super-setted with BB bent-over rows. Unlike pre-exhaustion, the use of super sets is limited only by the exercises you decide to train. It is, however, similar to pre-exhaustion in its level of intensity. Take it easy with this training approach, as well as with all other radical training methods.

How long should I rest between sets?

This answer needs to be based on a number of factors. First, what type of physical condition are you currently in? If your health is good, then train as hard and as fast as you want. However, often there is some extra body fat that really needs to come off before you train at a fast pace. Get comfortable with yourself in the gym, and as your general conditioning improves—and it quickly will— pick up your training pace.

When getting ready for a contest, bodybuilders often pick up the pace of their workouts to a mere 30 seconds between sets. Now that is really hustling! Thirty seconds is very little time in the world of weights. On the other hand, when the training strategy calls for increased size and strength, rest periods last as long as five minutes between sets. This is designed to allow for the most complete recharging of the energy-producing systems of the body. The more power, the more weight lifted, and the more weight lifted, the bigger the muscles will become.

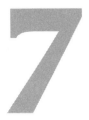

Thighs and Hips

The thighs, hips, and lower back are not just some of the largest muscles on your body but also among the strongest. Due to their ability to perform under heavy work loads, the thighs, hips, and lower back stress your total metabolic machinery toward the desired goal of increased muscle size like nothing else! Without the correct performance of the following exercises or appropriately heavy weights, you will not begin to see your true potential. Likewise, once you are a Squatting Master, the increased size will arrive sooner than ever imagined.

The sheer amount of muscle tissue stimulated, for example, with deep, heavy squats produces an incredible volume of metabolic by-products that cause the deep, throbbing burn associated with this exercise. This degree of bone-blistering pain is exactly what keeps all but the most determined and physically gifted from reaching their desired size. However, the rewards are there for those of you willing to withstand the self-imposed torment!

Truly amazing, almost cartoonlike thighs are becoming more common every year. Once the first thigh-mass monster broke through whatever size limit had been previously accepted as the upper limit for human legs, then others were sure to follow, and of course, many did. Until just a few years ago, a thigh measurement of more than 30 inches was unheard of, as compared to today when near 30-inch thighs are not at all uncommon in many large gyms.

ANATOMY AND KINESIOLOGY

The largest muscle group of the thigh is the quadriceps, which consists of four individual muscles. The quads contract to straighten the leg from a bent position, and to an extent, to pull the knees toward each other. The quadriceps femoris, called the great extensor muscle of the anterior thigh, is composed of the rectus femoris, the vastus lateralis, the vastus medialis, and the vastus intermedius.

On the back of the thigh is the biceps femoris muscle group, frequently referred to as the hamstrings or leg biceps. The leg biceps contract to bend the leg from a straight position. Actually this is a group of muscles consisting of three muscles at the back of the thigh—medially, the semimembranosus and the semitendinosus, and laterally, the biceps femoris.

Behind all this muscular power and torque are your gluteus maximi, which contract to move a straight leg to the rear. The glutes also contract to move your body to an erect position when you are flexed forward at the waist. No longer a holdover from the days of butcher shops when they were known as buttocks, glutes have joined the ranks of ultra-ripped body parts. So sought out is gluteal development that some manufacturers supply fake glute pads to be worn under your clothes. Skip those and get going on some squats!

THIGH AND HIP TRAINING

First, let's discuss an important difference between training the thigh and hip muscles and the rest of your body. What the best pictures and words can never capture is just exactly how hard correct leg training really is. For example: after a single 40-minute leg workout, a 275 pound top-five NPC national contender was so completely exhausted he was observed sitting on his gym bag and sliding down a long flight of stairs after his legs gave out underneath him!

The following are general comments and suggestions on how to best obtain your leg-training goals without injury and with a minimum of frustration:

▌ Unless there is a specific need or prescription for wrapping your knees, it is best not done until you have at least three full years of training under your belt and can squat one and a half times your body weight for 20 good reps. When you use today's high-tech knee wraps with their incredibly powerful elasticity, a mistake will surely send you face first to the floor. If you don't have a pre-existing injury, then skip the wraps. When performed correctly and consistently, squats will not hurt or damage your knees in any way.

▌ Using a block of wood or other means to raise your heel off the floor is no longer widely accepted. The only reason to use the heel-elevation setup would be lack of flexibility, so start stretching now. If one day you have become an above-average squatter and decide to

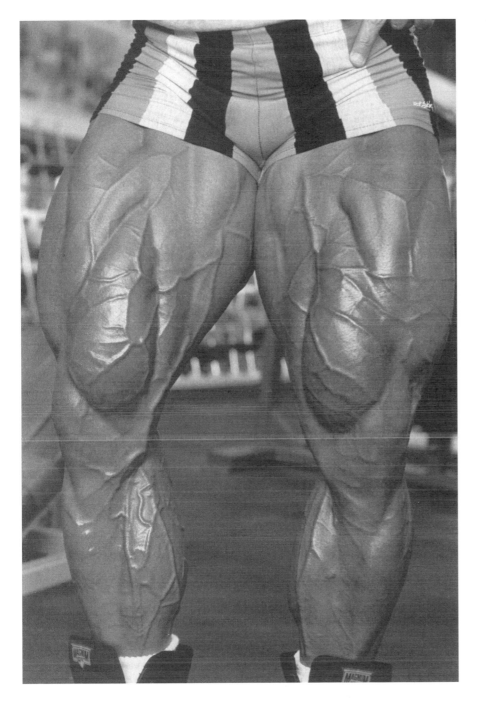

Roland Cziuriok

enter a powerlifting contest—no blocks here, baby! So why bother? With a little bit of time investment on your part, flexibility will soon be second nature and you'll be squatting like a runaway locomotive!

▌ Unless there is simply too much discomfort, skip wrapping pads and towels around the bar. Any discomfort will serve as a reminder how much more trap development you need! Skip it and get going on some squats!

Squats

Comments. You have now entered the PAIN ZONE, where real long-term growth resides. Once you have mastered the squat, you will be well on your way toward needing baggy pants instead of wearing them by choice. There is simply no better exercise for growing big and strong than squats!

Emphasis. Squats are widely considered the best lower-body exercise, as well as an incredible movement for stimulating a full-body, anabolic metabolism. Squats strongly stress the quadriceps, glutes, and lower-

John Caldarelli

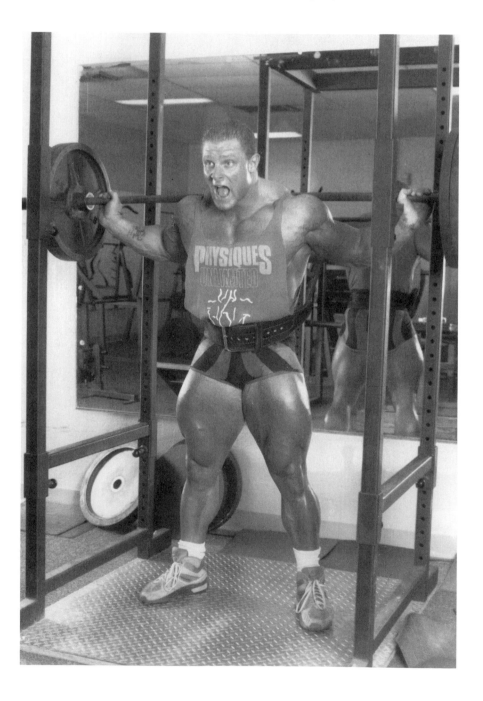

back muscles (erectors). Additionally, significant secondary stress is placed on the hamstrings, upper back, and abdominal muscles.

Starting Position. Squats in most commercial gyms today will be best performed from a power-rack apparatus. Facing the rack will allow you to visually assess your form. Set the pins or hooks at a point one inch or so below the top of your shoulders. With your eyes straight ahead and feet in a comfortable stance, place the bar across your upper back and trapezius. This may take a little bit of shoulder-area stretching at first to achieve a comfortable resting position without any undue shoulder strain.

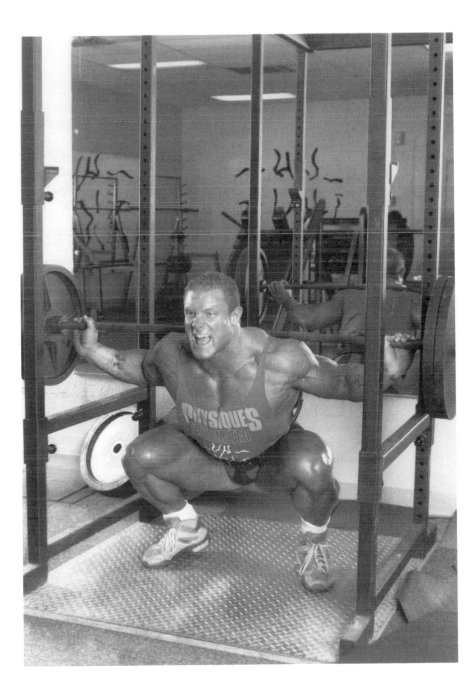

Movement Performance. Raise your head until your line of sight is straight ahead, arch your back, and stand up until you are under control. Slowly step backward only one or two steps to minimize any chance for injury. Place your feet almost shoulder-width apart for best stability and control. Point your toes toward their most natural position. Tense your back muscles throughout the movement to keep your torso upright during the exercise.

Now begin. Slowly and under complete control, lower yourself until the bottom of your glutes is lower than your knees, or to a full squatting position. As always, go *down* on a 6-second count and *up* on a 3 count. As best you can, keep your knees traveling out in the direction your toes are pointing. At the bottom point you should actually achieve a near pause without any bouncing. Now reverse your direction and travel upward. You have done 1 repetition. Repeat.

Tips. If you have difficulty maintaining an erect posture, try focusing your eyes on a spot on the mirror or wall in front of you and keep the

Amy Fadhl

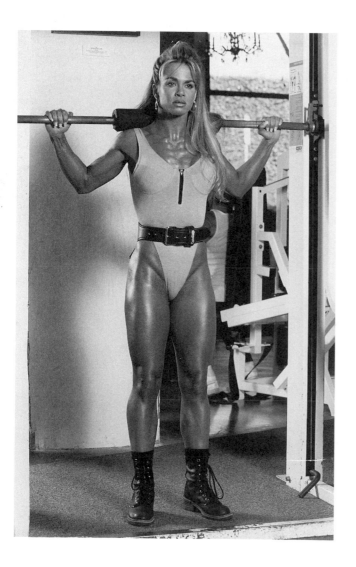
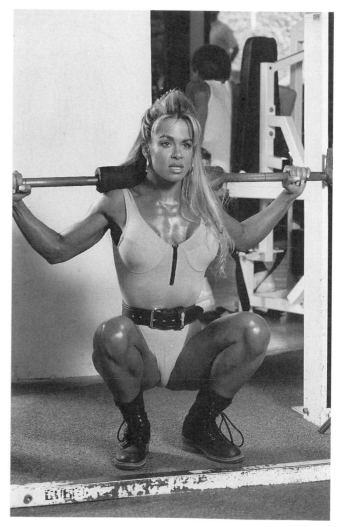

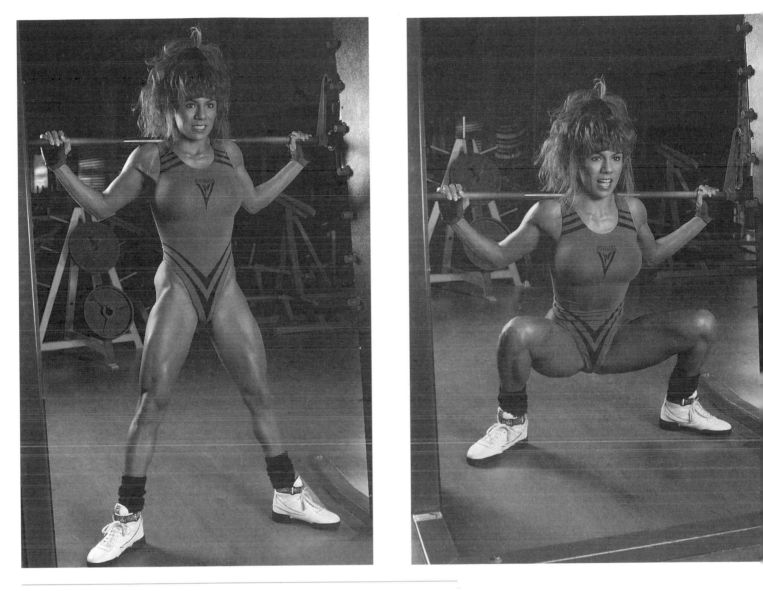

Lisa Ibarra

focus on this point as you perform your motion. Wearing a lifting belt is a good idea and strongly recommended.

As to how much weight you should begin with, the best answer is to proceed with patient enthusiasm. Form is the most important aspect of training effectiveness. All too frequently, poor form is due to the obsession with heavy weights before you are ready to use them. Poor form will lead to little progress at best, and at worst, a serious injury. It will never result in long-term size gains. Here is a general set of reasonable goals for deciding how much weight to use for squats:

- beginner: 50 percent body weight times 20 reps
- experienced: 100 percent body weight times 20 reps
- elite: 150 percent body weight times 8 to 20 reps

Roland Cziurlok

There is no need to hurry to squat with heavy weights right away. More than 15 individuals have already squatted more than 1,000 pounds in various competitions—good things come to those willing to wait. (By the way, 1,100 pounds includes the bar with collars and 11 sets of 45-pound plates on each side.)

Variations. For varying types of stress on your thigh muscles, you can squat with a narrower-than-usual stance in order to emphasize more thigh involvement. Alternatively, taking a wider foot placement serves to throw more work onto the hips. Partial squats are best performed in a power-rack setup due to the poundage overload often used with this technique. The performance is the same as for the full squats, except you go down either a quarter of the way to a full squatting position (quarter squat), or halfway down (half squat), three quarters of the way down (three-quarters squat), or only until your thigh bones reach a position parallel to the floor (parallel squat). Some additional variations are: bench or box squats, power-cage squats, jump squats, DB squats, and machine squats.

Leg Presses

Comments. Among some of the more incredible pieces of equipment are the new generation of leg-press machines. With literally dozens of different designs and aspects, they range from poor copies of one another to absolutely phenomenal designs that almost make the lift seem too easy at times. The most common types now found in gyms are the 45-degree-angle, sled-type units.

Emphasis. We will approach the performance of a leg press assuming a common sled design is available in your gym. There are many similarities between a full squat and a leg press, such as the shared stress placed primarily upon the quadriceps and glutes. A difference would be the lack of torso stabilization required in the leg press. The leg press almost totally isolates the lower body, which is not seen in squats.

Starting Position. For most, placing of the back of the leg-press backrest about halfway between top and bottom is best. Place your feet as in squats, with a narrower stance hitting more of the thigh directly while a bit wider-than-shoulder stance shifts more work to the hips. A major consideration is where you place your foot on the platform relative to the top or the bottom. By positioning your feet more to the top you cause work to shift from the thigh to the hips. A lower point will allow more direct thigh focus, although with less weight. As in squats, keep your toes pointed in the direction your knees follow. With your

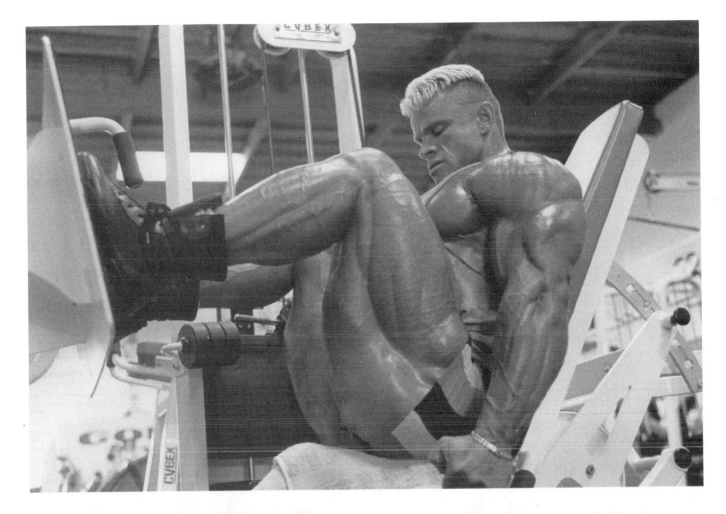

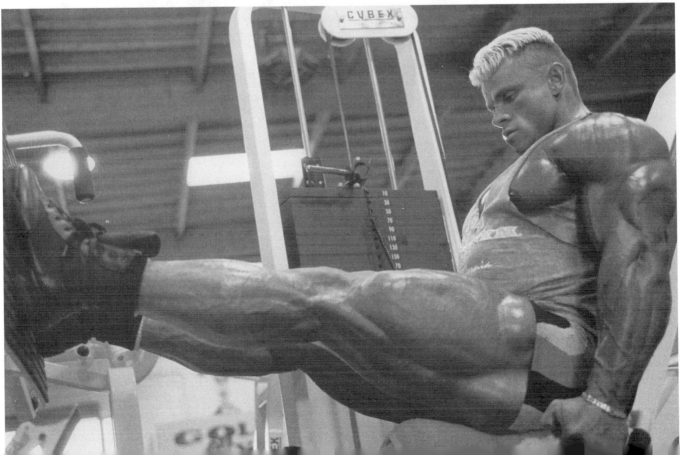

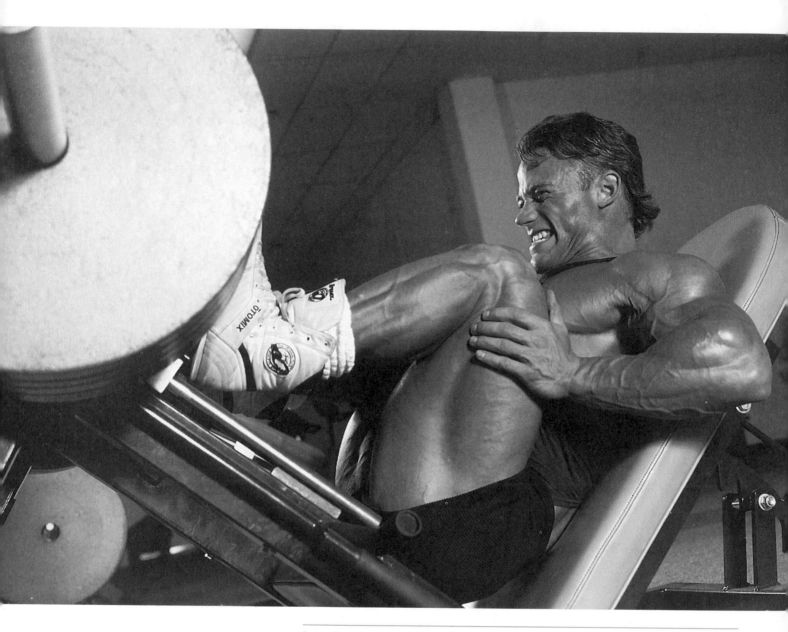

Jason Arntz

back arched and torso tight, take a deep breath and rotate the handles to unlock the weight sled or stack. The knees should be just slightly bent, not locked. There should be handles on the side of the machine to grasp in order to maintain position.

Movement Performance. Slowly, as in squats, lower on a 6 count and after a split-second pause, straighten your legs upward on a 3 count. Try to almost but not quite allow your hips to leave the back of the pad at the bottom position. This indicates a good and thorough range of motion. You have now done 1 repetition. Repeat.

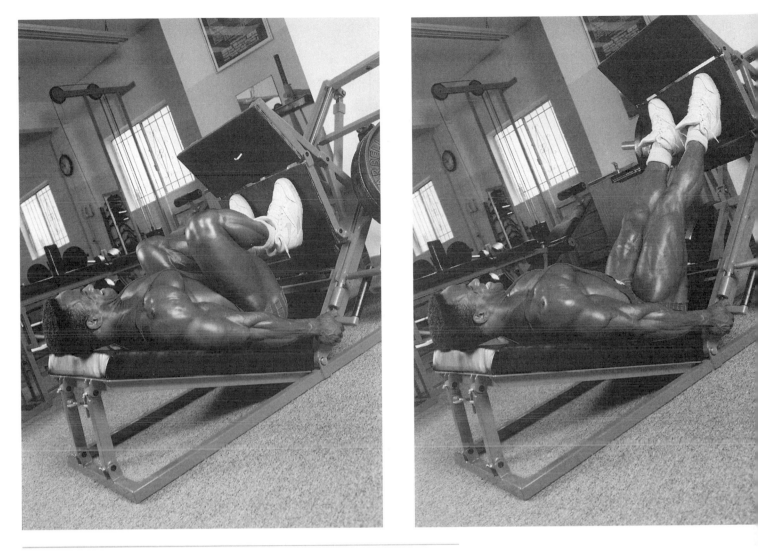

Al'q Gurley

Tips. It is essential that you never hold your breath while exerting against the weight, such as in the leg press. This would potentially build your blood pressure up to a harmful degree. With near maximum weights, it is a good practice to keep from fully straightening your legs each repetition, since this could eventually harm your knee joints.

Front Squats

Comments. Front squats position the bar across the top of a platform formed by crossing your arms from shoulder to shoulder.

Emphasis. As opposed to full squats, the primary emphasis here is on the quadriceps, particularly the lower part just above the knee. Secondary emphasis is on the glutes, abdomen, and back muscles.

Jamo Nezzar

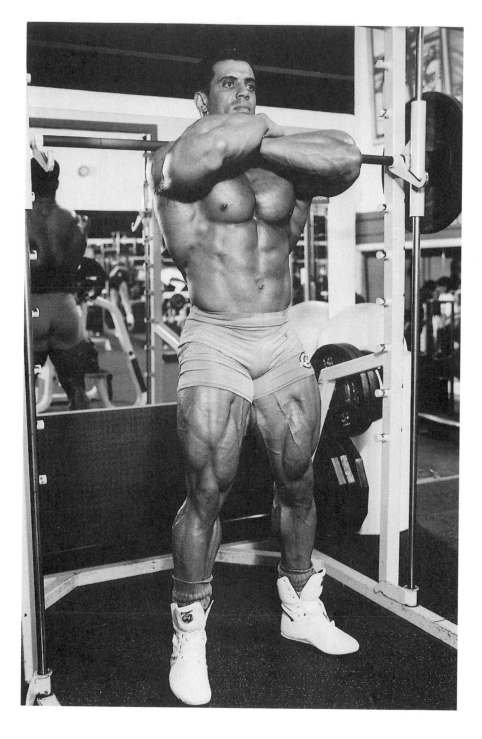

Starting Position. Approach the bar in the same fashion as when you squat. Your elbows are to be crossed to the opposite shoulder as shown in the photos. Keeping your elbows high will maintain the bar in a safe and balanced position.

Movement Performance. Keeping your torso as upright as possible, bend your legs, while pushing out and back with your hips. Slowly on

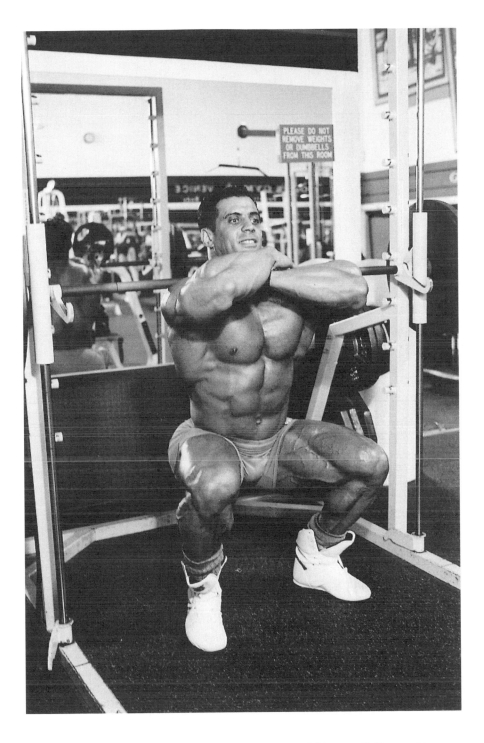

a moderate 6- to 8-second count, lower yourself into a full squatting position. Without bouncing at the bottom of the movement, return to the starting point and repeat.

Tips. Due to the stresses placed upon your lower back, it is essential that you wear a lifting belt tightly around your waist at all times when performing front squats.

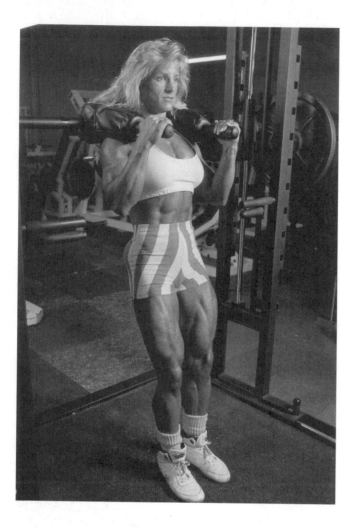

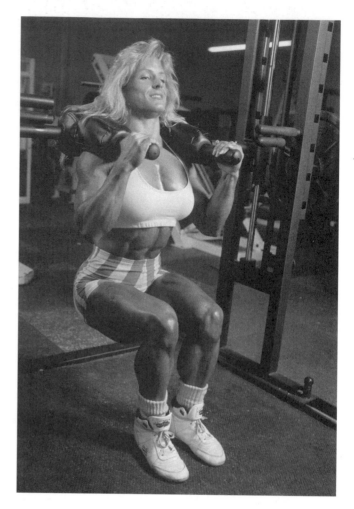

Sue Price (above)

Jay Cutler (opposite page, top)

Johnnie Morant (opposite page, bottom)

Hack Squats

Comments. The initial comments here are the same as for leg presses. To avoid any undue confusion, we will assume you will be using a high quality 45-degree-angle, sled-type hack machine.

Emphasis. Hack squats stress the quadriceps in relative isolation from the remainder of your body. Particular emphasis is placed on the quads just above the knee, and perhaps even more so, the outer-thigh sweep.

Starting Position. Place your feet on the angled footrest with your heels about eight inches apart and your toes angled outward. Place your back against the sliding platform of the machine and straighten your legs, standing up to release the safety catches.

Movement Performance. Slowly bend your legs and sink down into as low a squatting position as possible. Make sure your knees travel out over your feet as you do the movement. Straighten your legs to return to the starting position. Repeat.

Variations. For a superintense contraction of your quads, try to rise up with your hips thrust as far forward as possible. This type of hip position is analogous to sissy squats, described later in this chapter.

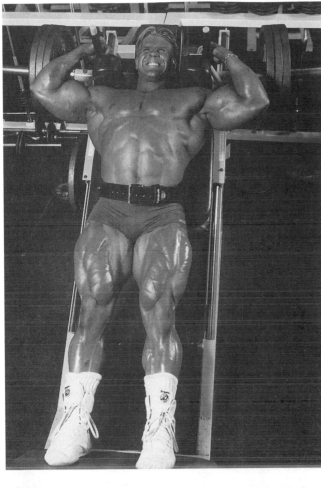

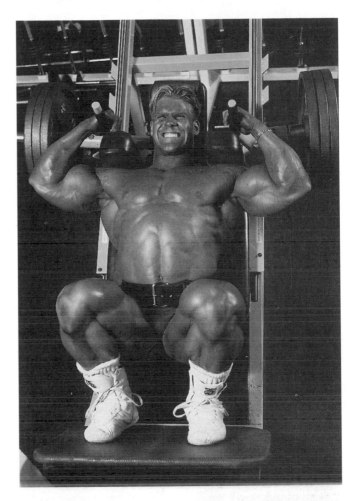

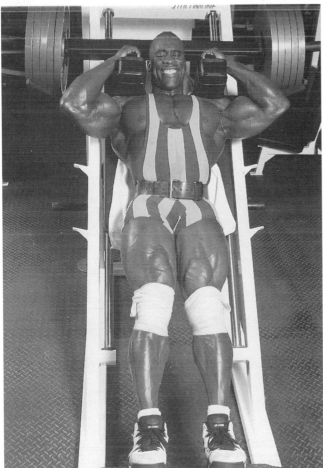

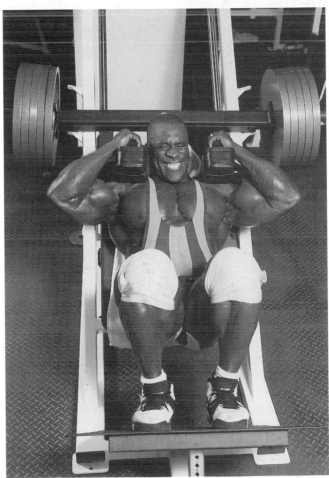

Leg Extensions

Emphasis. Leg extensions almost completely isolate the quadriceps muscles. The remainder of the body serves to merely stabilize and prevent throwing the weight.

Starting Position. Sit on the seat and comfortably rest the backs of your knees against the padding. Place your feet against the pads or otherwise as indicated by the manufacturer. Sit tall and straight with your back arched for support. Hold on to the side handles (if provided).

Movement Performance. Moving only your lower legs, straighten your legs to the top position. Hold at the top for a brief second to ensure peak contraction in your thighs. Then lower or perform the eccentric movement on a moderate to slow 6 to 8 count until you are once again at the starting position. Repeat.

Tips. If you're after the ultimate thigh burn, why not try a "21" leg extension. Choose a moderately heavy amount of resistance and begin with 7 half-reps from the bottom of the movement halfway up to the

Bob Cicherillo

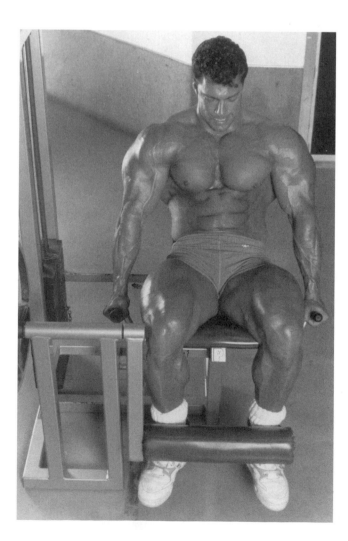
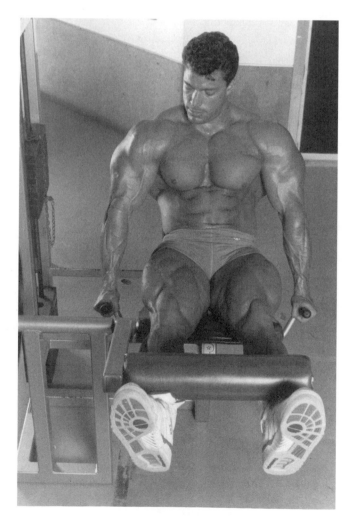

top position. Next, perform 7 half-reps from the midpoint to the finish of the exercise. Finally, do 7 complete reps to finish this brutally demanding and advanced technique. Your thighs will burn like never before, almost as if your training partner had just applied a blowtorch to them!

Variations. This exercise can be performed with one leg at a time or alternating back and forth between right and left. It's particularly valuable to do one-legged exercises when, for instance, you are rehabilitating an injured knee.

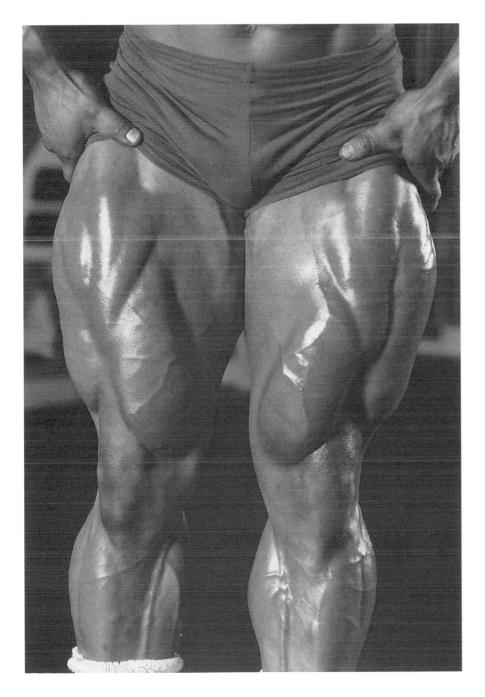

Jay Cutler

Leg Curls

Comments. Please refer to the section on leg presses concerning machine variety and differences.

Emphasis. This is a hamstring exercise. There will be minimal stimulation of the stabilizing muscle groups involved.

Starting Position. Lie facedown on the padded surface of the machine or assume the correct position as indicated by the manufacturer. Position your knees at the edge of the pad toward the lever arm of the machine. Hook your heels beneath the pads, or between the pads if on a Hammer Strength unit. Your legs should be in an almost straight position at this point. If a seat belt or strap is provided, make sure to

Guy Ducasse

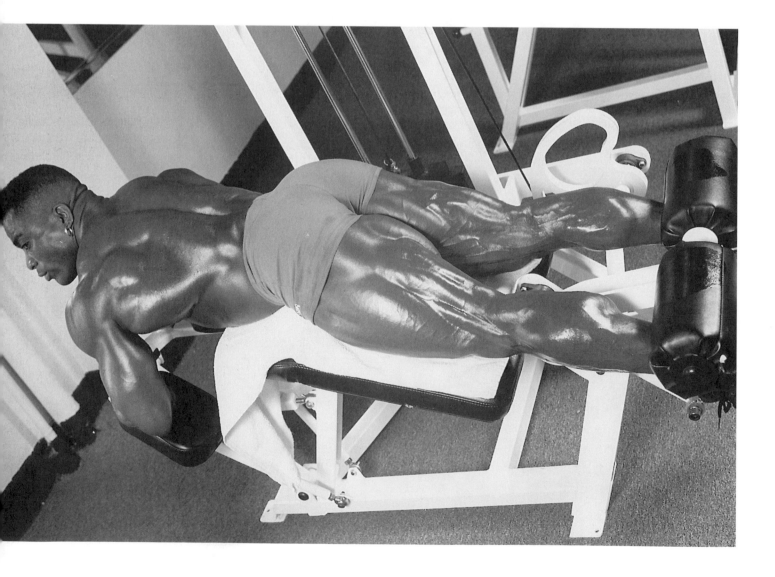

tighten it sufficiently to ensure you do not alter your alignment with the resistance. If two handles are provided as the means to maintain stability, then grasp them somewhat tightly.

Movement Performance. Slowly bend your legs as fully as possible, pausing at the top for a split second or two. This very brief pause allows for a total peak contraction effect in your hamstrings. Return to the starting position and repeat the movement.

Tips. It is advisable to alternate between doing leg curls with toes pointed slightly outward and from a pigeon-toed position.

Variations. The one-legged approach works as well here as it does under the same conditions in leg extensions.

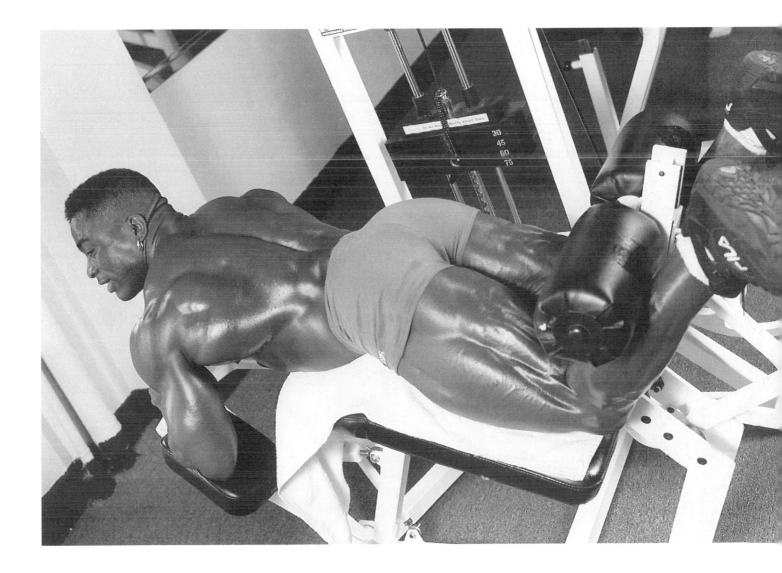

Standing Leg Curls

Comments. This type of leg curl is thought to allow for a tighter squeeze at the top.

Emphasis. This exercise provides relatively total hamstring isolation.

Starting Position. Stand either to the right or left and alternate sides as you work your way through this movement's sets. Your hands should be placed in a firm but comfortable position. Try to look straight ahead with an arched back and tightened abs.

Movement Performance. Without moving any other part of your body, slowly bend your leg as completely as possible. Try to attempt touching your heel to your glute. Lower slowly back to the starting position and repeat the movement.

Tips. Of course, you will need to pay attention to your reps here so there is a balance between your right and left legs.

Sue Price
Jeannine Cerny (opposite page)

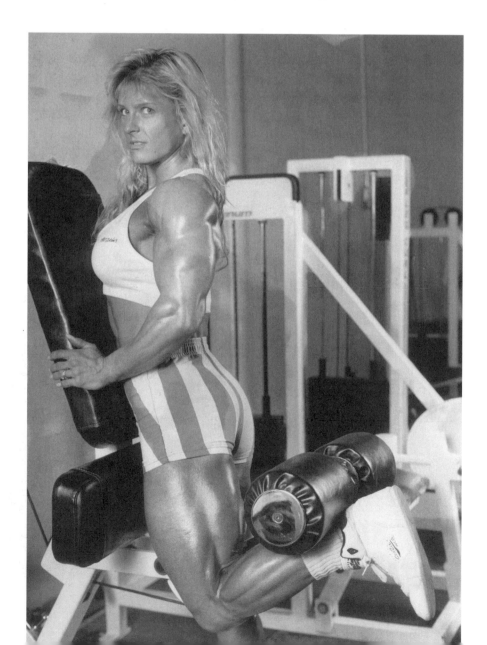

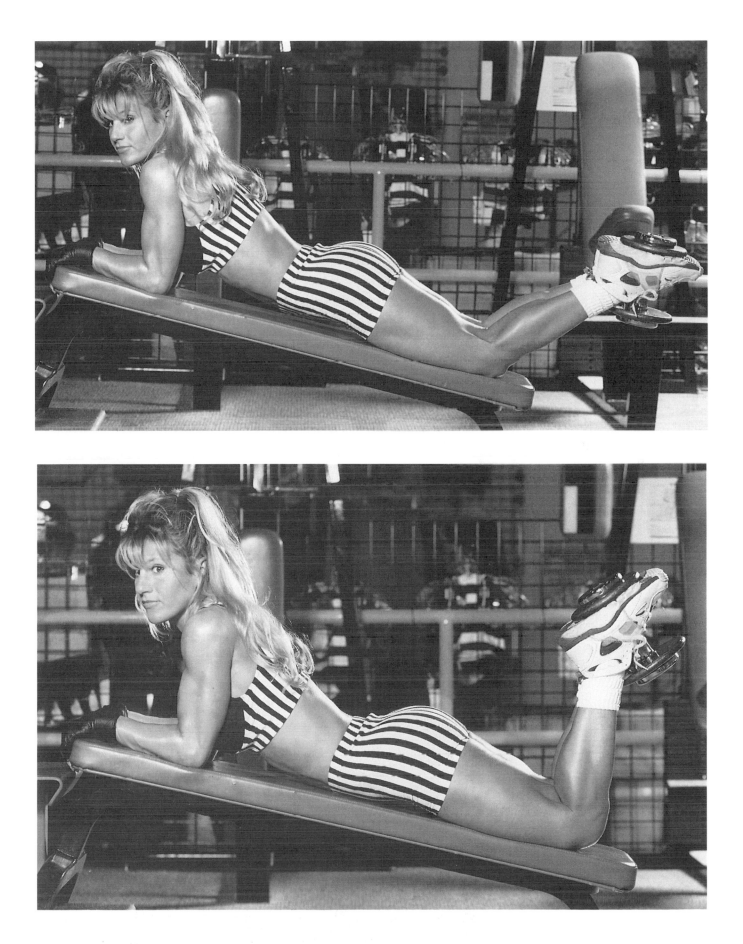

Lunges

Comments. This is a refining movement, and as such, is not intended to pack on significant mass.

Emphasis. This movement stresses the quadriceps, particularly the upper section near where the muscle originates near the pelvis. Nonetheless, significant stress is borne by the glutes and upper hamstrings near where they run into the glutes. Champion bodybuilders do plenty of lunges close to a major competition because the movement is excellent for separating the thighs.

Starting Position. Place a light barbell behind your neck as for a set of squats, holding it near the width of the plates. Place your feet about eight inches apart, your toes pointed straight ahead. Stand erect.

Movement Performance. Step forward two and a half to three feet with your left foot, being sure to position your foot firmly on the floor with your toes pointed directly forward. Keeping your right leg rela-

Lisa Allen

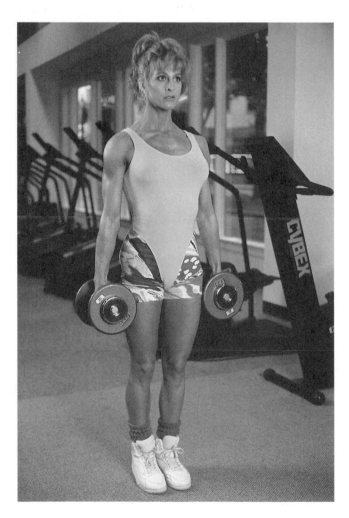
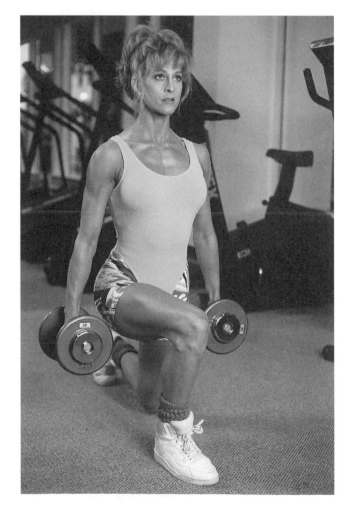

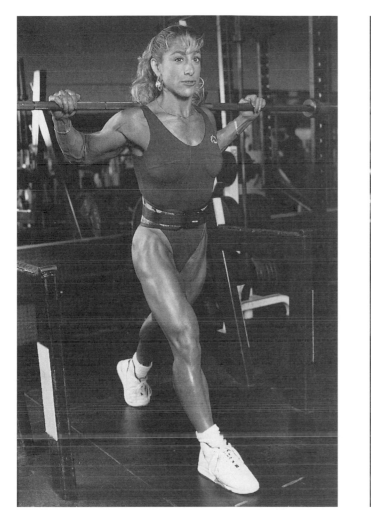 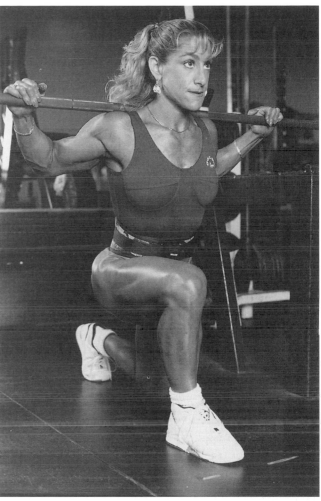

Jodi Friedman

tively straight, slowly bend your left leg as fully as possible. This will lower your body so your right knee will be three or four inches from the floor and your left knee will be three or four inches ahead of your left ankle. In this position, you should feel a powerful stretching sensation in your left glute and right quadriceps muscle. Push off with your left leg to return to the starting point of the movement and do the next repetition with your right foot forward. Alternate between legs until you have completed the desired number of repetitions.

Tips. Be sure to keep your torso as erect as possible as you do this movement. You may discover it's easier to keep your torso erect if you hold two dumbbells at your sides instead of a single barbell behind your neck.

Variations. Many bodybuilders prefer to do lunges placing their forward foot up on a four-inch-thick block of wood. You can also do a short lunge in which you step only about two feet forward with your front foot and bend both legs to lower your body toward the floor.

Side Lunges

Emphasis. This version of the lunge stresses virtually all the muscles of the thighs and hips, with a particular focus on the adductor muscles on the inner edge of the thighs.

Starting Position. Assume the same starting position as for regular lunges.

Movement Performance. Without twisting your torso to one side or the other, step directly to the right with your right foot about two and a half to three feet. In the correct position, both of your legs will be straight and at a 50- to 60-degree angle with each other. Keeping your left leg totally straight, slowly bend your right leg and return to the starting position. Do the next repetition to the left and alternate movements to each side until you have done the desired number of repetitions with each leg.

Machine or Cable Abductors

Comments. The use of cables in this move is somewhat more common than in thigh adduction movements. There are also specific items of training apparatus for hitting this area.

Emphasis. Leg-abduction work targets all your hip and side thigh-abductor muscles.

Starting Position. Follow the directions of the equipment manufacturer. If cables are the call, attach the padded cuff to your right ankle, rotating the cuff so its ring is toward the midline of your body. Attach the cable to the cuff and stand with your left side directly toward the cable so the cable runs across the front of your body. Brace yourself in a secure position and allow the weight attached to the cable to pull your foot well across the midline of your body. Be sure to keep your leg straight throughout the movement.

Movement Performance. Slowly move your right foot in a semicircular arc to the right and upward as high as you can. Hold the top position for a moment, then lower your foot back to the starting point. Be sure to do equal numbers of repetitions for each leg.

Tips. Some athletes prefer to stand on an elevated platform or thick block of wood when performing both these and thigh-adduction cable movements.

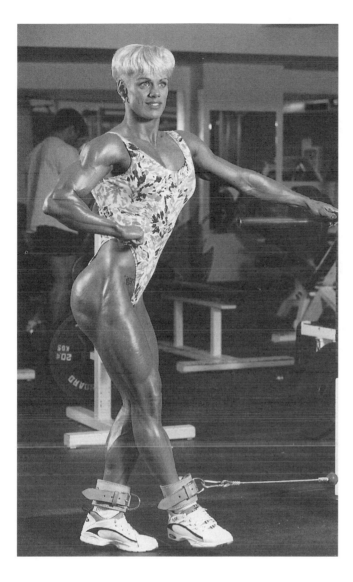 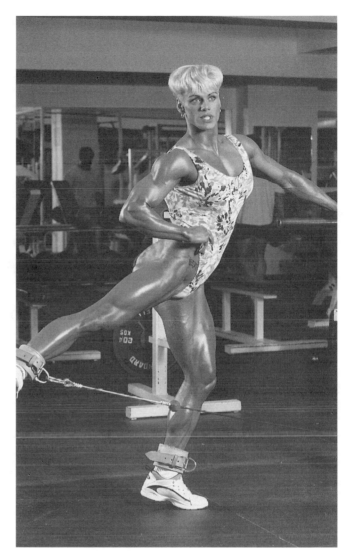

Machine or Cable Adductors

Cathy LaFrancois

Comments. The use of specialized equipment has become common in today's modern gym. Whether to use a cable-and-strap arrangement or a specific piece of equipment is a matter of personal choice.

Emphasis. Leg-adduction work targets all the thigh-adductor muscles.

Starting Position. The position adopted depends on what, if any, machine you are using. For cable adductions, make sure that in the upright position your working leg is pulled well away from your body by the cable.

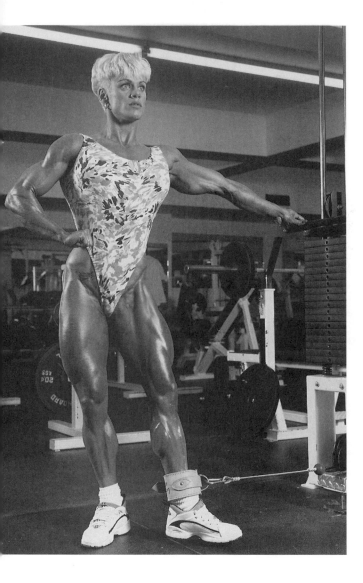

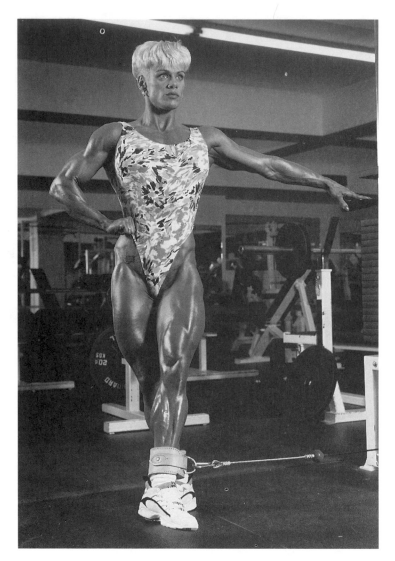

Cathy LaFrancois

Movement Performance. Keep your leg straight throughout the entire movement. Begin by slowly pulling your working leg toward the center line of your body (even across the midline if possible). Hold the contracted position for a moment, then slowly allow the leg to return to the starting point. If you are using a machine, then please follow the specific details indicated by the manufacturer. The essentials of the movement are consistent regardless.

Sissy Squats

Comments. Nothing in this book is for sissies!

Emphasis. This movement is often performed during a contest preparation cycle because it is great for carving deep cuts into the fronts of your quadriceps groups. You will also find sissy squats to be one of the best ways to intensely stretch your thighs.

Starting Position. You will find it easier to balance your body during sissy squats if you stand between a set of parallel bars or poles. Lightly grasp the uprights attached to the bars as you do the movement. Your feet should be about shoulder-width apart, your toes pointed directly forward. You will not likely need to add resistance to this movement for a while.

Movement Performance. You must simultaneously do four movements in order to reach the correct position at the bottom position of this exercise:

1. Rise up on your toes.

2. Bend your legs to at least a 90-degree angle.

3. Thrust your knees as far forward as possible.

4. Incline your torso backward until it is approximately parallel to the floor.

If you correctly perform these movements, you will feel a very strong stretching sensation in your quads. Reverse the procedure to return to the starting point, then repeat the movement.

Tips. If you eventually require extra resistance for sissy squats, you should securely belt a loose barbell plate against your waist.

Variations. While it is more difficult to balance your upper body, you can do sissy squats while holding on to a single upright with one hand. And to keep continuous tension on your quads, you can come only about 75 percent of the way up in the movement before you begin to descend again.

THE LOWER BACK—IT'LL HELP OR HURT YOU!

The weak link in your chain of growth may ultimately be your lower-back strength. A back injury either greatly slows down or even stops progress due to an inability to lift sufficiently heavy weights. The sacrospinalis, also called erector spinae, is a large, fleshy muscle of the back.

At this point, let's go over a fundamental aspect of becoming truly big. If you are able to learn to squat correctly, as indicated in the prior pages, then you will be 60 percent of the way toward your goal of huge

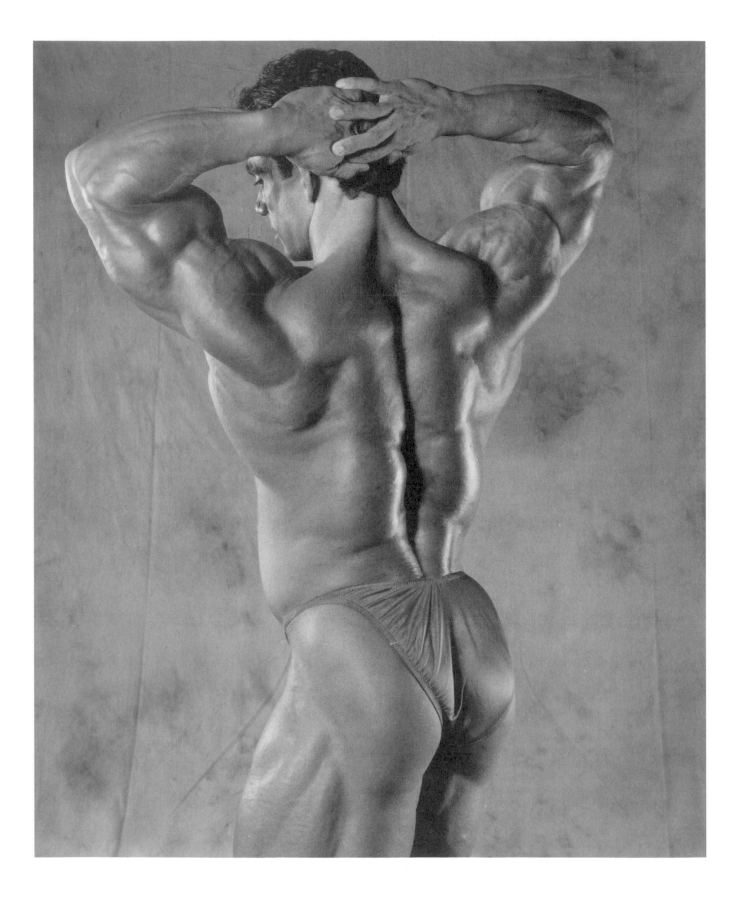

size. But often the trouble is that too many novices skip over the dead-lifts. The lower-back strength derived from doing deadlifts is essential for doing heavy squats. When your legs are ready but your lower back is not, under a heavy enough weight, you'll be good for three weak reps before the back gives out. Then you are finished training for a month minimum, probably more. You must be able to work through all the weak points in a movement if there is to be a steady progress.

This is the reasoning behind including deadlifts, stiff-legged dead-lifts, hyperextensions, and good mornings in the leg section. No back—no legs. So let's get on with deadlifts, where the men rise above the boys.

Deadlifts

Comments. Next to full squats, there is no other exercise that gives a physique big, thick chunks of fullness than deadlifts. One of the reasons deadlifts are not performed as often as squats is that in numerous ways deadlifts are harder to perform.

Emphasis. Many pros looking for the Dorian lower-lat look have obtained the training advice of top powerlifting coaches. The coaches told them to go home and do deadlifts. The primary stress is placed upon the erector spinae, with hips and glutes following a close second. Your thighs, and in essence, your entire body receives significant stimulation due to the stabilizing factor.

Starting Position. Squat down with a distance of six to nine inches between your feet. You must maintain a strong arch in your lower back through the entire movement to avoid injury. Grasp the bar on either side of your ankles and adjust your position by slightly rolling the bar toward the front of your ankles until it rests just against the front of your shins. You will, in all likelihood, need to spend some additional time stretching before you are able to become flexible enough to fully benefit from deadlifts. Your hips must be lower than your knees.

Movement Performance. Slowly begin to pull your shoulders back to begin the upward travel of the bar. The hips are to rise after the bar has left the floor. Always keep your back tightly arched and head upright with your shoulders pulled back, not rounded to the front. You do not want to stand angled beyond a point of 90 degrees to the floor. In other words, do not lean back whatsoever with the bar—it is dangerous and immediately brands you as someone very new to training. As you approach the upright position, stop just short of the 90-degree point. Slowly begin to to lower the bar back down to repeat the movement.

Joe Deangelis

Paula Suzuki

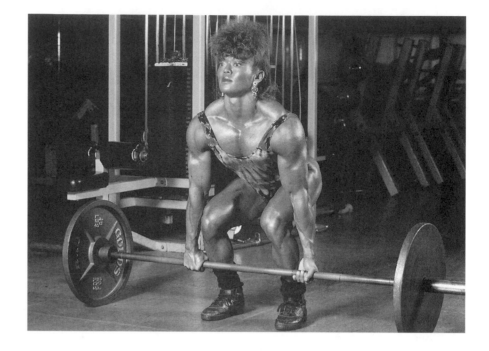

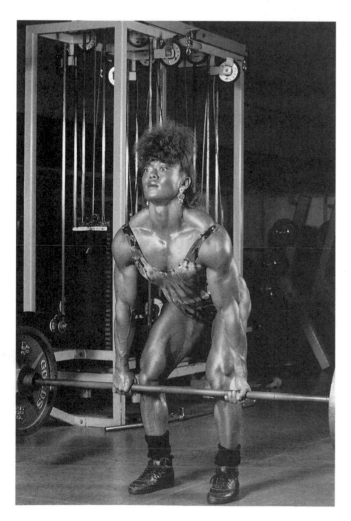

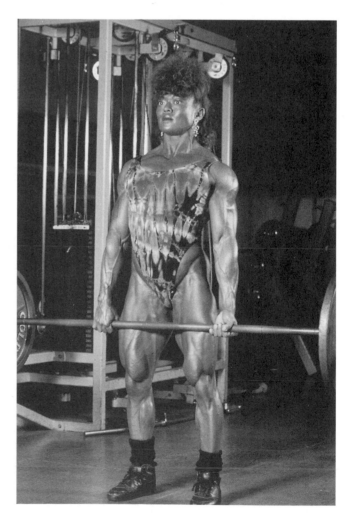

Tips. You may find it easier and more productive to begin with the barbell set upon a power-rack apparatus. This will allow you to lower yourself to initiate the movement, as lifting straight off the floor takes time before it can be done correctly. For heavier sets you may want to toss on a pair of straps to assist your grip. Always wear your belt and never wear knee wraps because they catch the bar on the way down.

Variations. Another variation is partial deadlifts in a power rack.

Stiff-Legged Deadlifts

Emphasis. This movement places very strong stress on both the lumbar muscles of your lower back and your hamstrings. Secondary emphasis is on your upper back muscles.

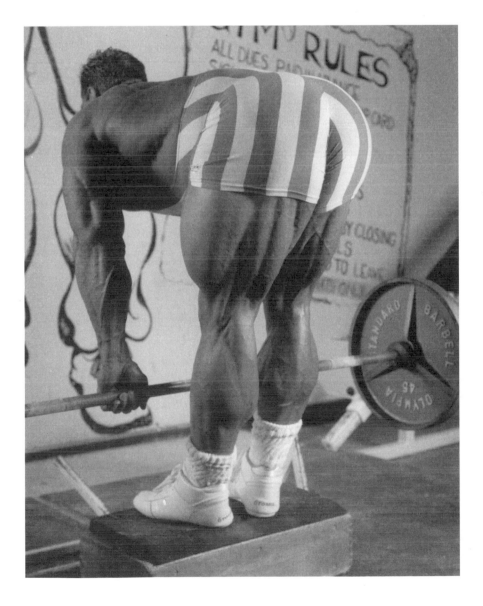

Mike Francois

Starting Position. The old practice of standing on a bench to perform this movement has grown out of favor the last few years. When performed correctly, there is no need for an exaggerated stretching of the hands past the top of your socks. A very strong arch in the lower back throughout the entire range of motion will give all the stress emphasis needed. Furthermore, any extreme stretching with a weight adding to the pull of gravity is simply not a good idea.

Movement Performance. Take a shoulder-width overgrip on the barbell and stand erect, your arms straight and the barbell resting across your upper thighs. Maintain a slight bend at the knee the entire time. With an arch in your lower back, bend forward at the waist and lower the bar downward until the plates just touch the floor. Do not rest but reverse the direction of the bar to once again stand erect. Repeat the move until the desired number of repetitions are done.

Tips. Unless you have very long arms, you will not need to elevate yourself. If you find the plates are touching the floor before you feel the correct stretch, you must simply arch your lower back even further. *Perform very carefully and slowly here, as your back is in a potentially dangerous mechanical position.*

Variations. Dumbbells may be used in place of a single barbell.

Hyperextensions

Emphasis. This excellent movement effectively isolates the stress on your spinal erectors, glutes, and hamstring muscles.

Starting Position. Usually this exercise is performed on a special bench constructed specifically for it. Stand facing the larger pad. Lean forward and grasp the handles in front of the pad to maneuver your body into a position with your hips across the larger pads and the backs of your ankles resting beneath the smaller pads at the back of the apparatus. Be sure to hold your legs straight throughout the movement. For novices or those who are injured, cross your arms over your chest. Others needing a more rigorous movement, place your hands behind your head and neck.

Movement Performance. Arch upward and backward until you rise just past the point where you are parallel with the floor. Undue or excessive arching of the back is not only ineffective but potentially injurious. Return to the original starting point (without rounding your back and losing any of the arch) and repeat the movement.

Remi Zuri

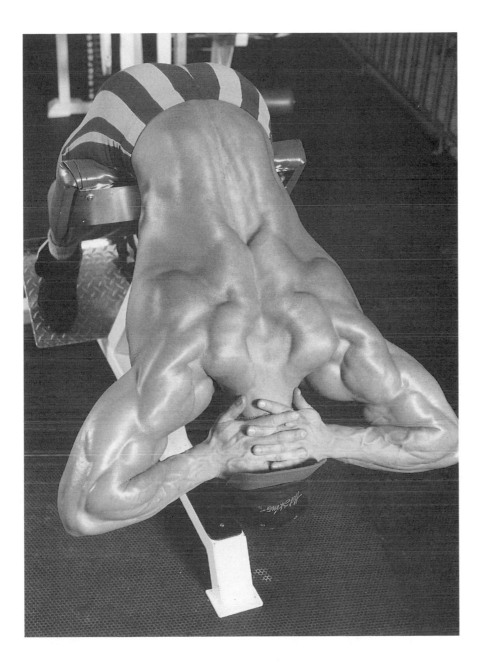

Tips. You can add resistance to this exercise by holding a light barbell or loose barbell plate against the back of your head and neck. The movement places a type of stress in the spine that fails to compress your vertebrae. In contrast, all deadlift movements compress your spinal vertebrae.

Variations. If you do not have access to a hyperextension bench for this exercise, you can still do the movement. Rest across a very sturdy high table or exercise bench. Have a training partner either sit or lie across your legs to hold you in place. Perform as on a bench.

Good Mornings

Comments. When performing this exercise, keep the weight light.

Emphasis. This oddly named exercise directly stresses the erector spinae muscles, and secondarily, the hamstrings.

Starting Position. Lift a very light barbell to a position across your shoulders and behind your head. Balance the bar in this position during the movement. Remember, the bar will try to slide down over your head so hold on firmly! Place your feet about shoulder-width apart and point your toes directly forward. Stand erect and hold your knees in a slightly bent position.

Remi Zuri

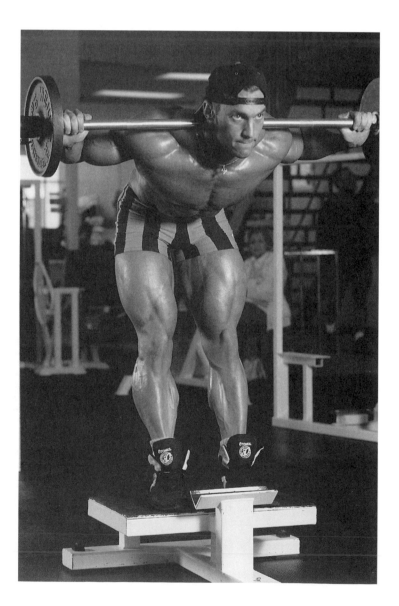

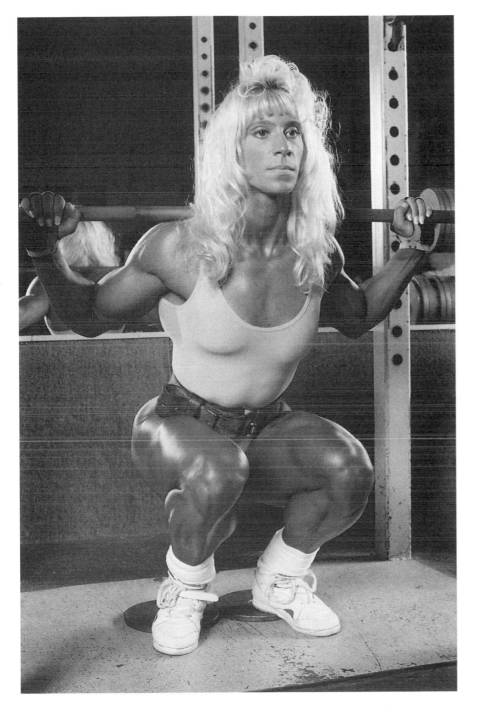

Movement Performance. Slowly bend forward at the waist, keeping your back firmly arched the entire time. As soon as your torso has descended past a position parallel to the floor, reverse the movement and travel back to a standing position. Repeat the exercise for the desired number of repetitions.

Tips. A workout belt should be worn during this exercise.

Cathy LaFrancois

Suggested Leg and Lower Back Routines

As we discussed in the opening chapters, your bases are covered with a repetition range of 6 to 10 reps for the upper body and 6 to 20 reps for your lower body. The only real exception is the deadlifts where, due to the tremendous work involved when correctly executed, the top end is 10 reps and a good range for heavy working sets would be 4 to 6 reps. For those who have been consistently training at this point less than six months, we will focus on the two primary moves, squats and deadlifts. The other exercises are to be considered later options, not for the less-than-one-year-training crowd. This workout is to be performed only once every five to seven days:

> *warm-ups and stretching*
> *squats: 3 to 4 sets of 8 to 20 reps*
> *deadlifts: 2 to 3 sets of 6 to 8 reps*
> *total sets: 5 to 7*

For those of you with six months to two years under your belt, the following might be helpful:

> *warm-ups and stretching*
> *squats: 3 to 4 sets of 8 to 20 reps*
> *leg extensions: 2 sets of 8 to 20 reps*
> *leg curls: 2 sets of 8 to 20 reps*
> *deadlifts: 2 to 3 sets of 6 to 8 reps*
> *total sets: 9 to 11*

After the two-and-a-half-year mark or so, you may have some competitive plans emerging and here's a killer routine to get you on your way to the top. This is a brutal and devastating way to punish your legs. When followed by sufficient rest and food, there will be so much growth you'll surprise yourself. This is a pre-exhaustion routine, so beware: the word *exhaustion* is a big one!

After the warm-ups, take 2 sets or so to arrive at your peak workout weight for leg extensions, then add about 20 or so extra pounds. Normally this extra amount of resistance is used at the end of the workout when you have less strength. By adding it at the beginning there will be more gas in the tank, so to speak, and accordingly, you'll need more weight to reach true failure.

Perform 1 set only—an all-out maximum, until-failure set. Stop and catch your breath for about one minute and no more. Repeat the same procedure for leg curls, then finish this leg section with the all-time-killer exercise—squats.

This is a four-movement cycle. If you want to go ballistic with intensity, try to repeat for a second cycle of four movements. You will

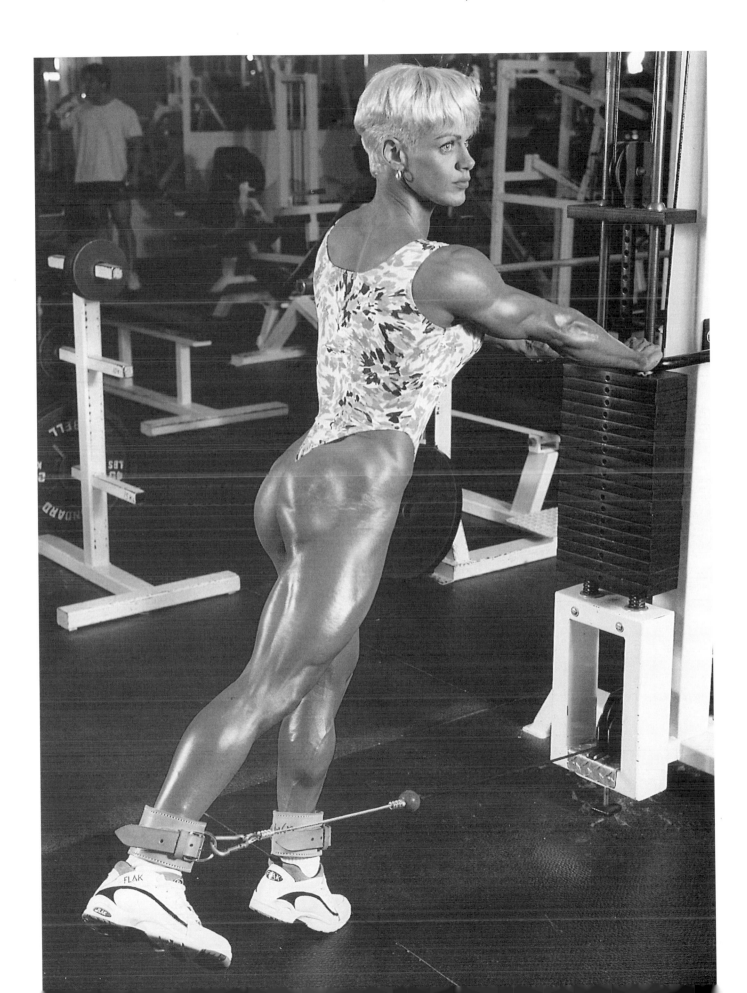

now need to rest for about 10 minutes before performing your regular deadlifts as before.

warm-ups and stretching
leg extensions: 1 set of 8 to 20 max-weight reps
leg curls: 1 set of 8 to 20 max-weight reps
squats: 1 set of 8 to 20 max-weight reps
deadlifts: 2 to 3 sets of 6 to 8 reps
total sets: 9 to 11

Tracy Smith

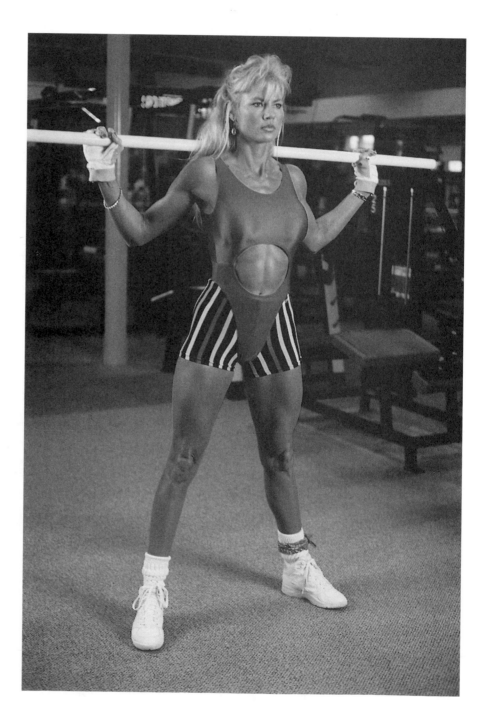

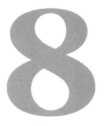 8

Back and Traps

The most widely recognized parts of the back are the wide, thick sheets that some attempt to mimic by assuming the *bodybuilder's walk*: "I'm too big for my own arms—that's why they always stick out so far when I walk around."

LAT AND MID-BACK EXERCISES

There are more than 20 back-expanding exercises detailed in the following section, with specific instructions for each. Those in the know here in Venice have seen countless times that the back is one muscle group that can be greatly improved past the initial genetic blueprint if there is narrowness here.

Machine Pullovers

Comments. This type of stress has been associated with incredible upper back and lat thickness. Machine pullovers were a favorite of Pete Grymkowski, who had one of the thickest torsos ever!

Emphasis. This exercise has been called the squat of upper body movements because of its phenomenal degree of total upper torso stress. As with the other types of pullovers, the major stress is on the latissimus dorsi.

Starting Position. The correct performance of this movement is similar among the various machines. The key element is to position yourself on the seat so that when your arms are in the overhead position your

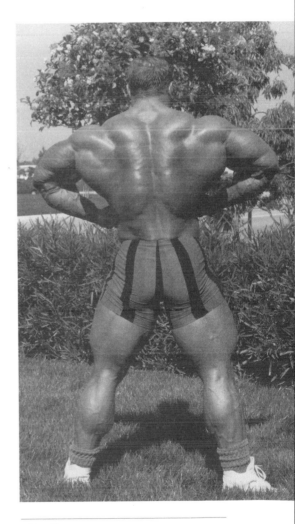

Mike Francois

Laura Creavelle

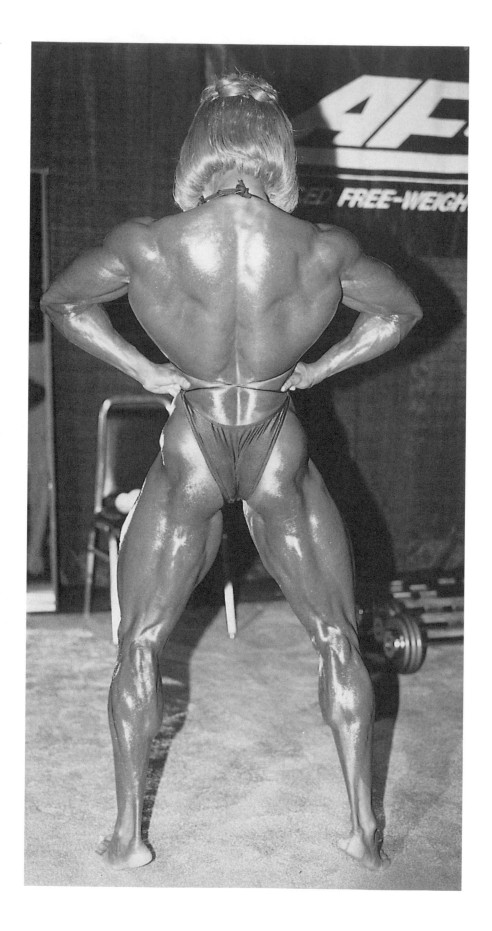

Derrick Whitsett

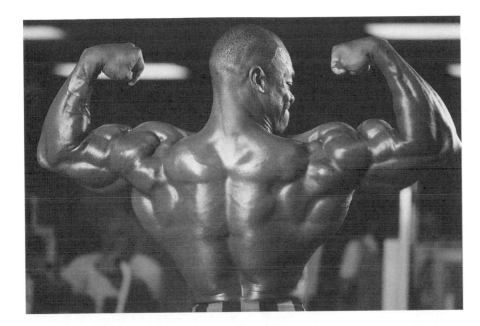

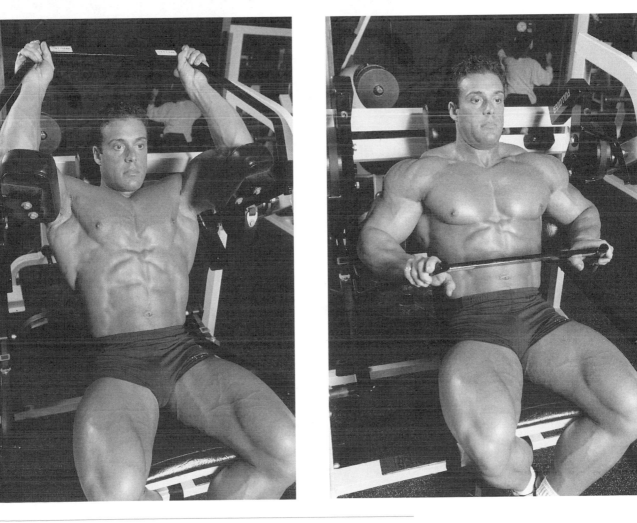

Lucio Paolini

shoulder joints are in line with the machine's center point or axis of rotation. The lower back should be arched throughout the movement. Be certain to utilize the equipment's seat belt or other means of restraint. Foot pads are generally provided to allow the arm-elbow pads to be brought to a starting position without assistance. Place the elbows against the pads and take a grip that is secure but not overly tight.

Slowly release the foot pedal or bar and allow the elbows to be drawn upward, above and slightly behind your head. A definite stretch is required to gain maximum benefit from the movement, but do not allow the machine's resistance to overwhelm your degree of flexibility.

Movement Performance. With your elbows pushing against the pads, bring the elbows down and in front of your torso as far as possible. Try

Sally Gomez

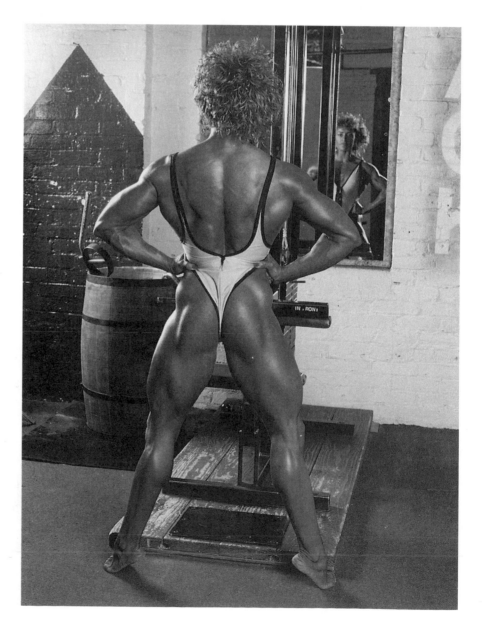

not to use your hands to pull on the bar, as in, for example, chins; bring the bar downward. The benefit to a machine pullover is that the lats are more completely isolated because pushing with the elbows removes the biceps involvement. The biceps are weak compared to the power of your lats. Hold the bottom position for a 1-to-2-second count to obtain a peak contraction. Slowly return to the top point and repeat for the desired number of reps.

Barbell (Bent-Arm) Pullovers

Emphasis. This free-weight movement essentially stresses the same muscles as the machine pullover. The upper arms displace some of the intensity from the lats, due to their lesser degree of strength.

Starting Position. Take a narrow thumb-over-bar grip on a barbell (six inches between your first fingers is appropriate). Be certain to use collars if the bar is not permanently set. Lie flat on a flat bench with your head off the end and feet securely positioned at the other end. Rest the bar across your chest with your elbows bent at your sides.

Lucio Paolini

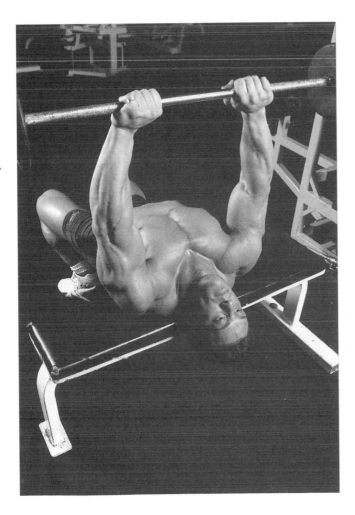
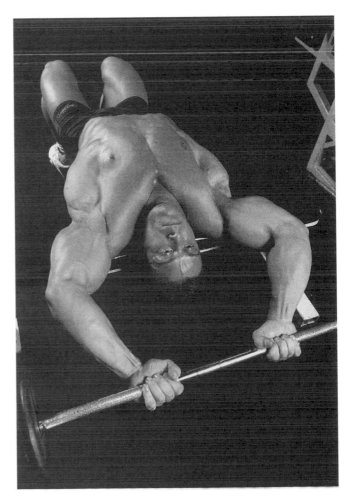

Movement Performance. Keeping your arms bent and your elbows as close together as possible, slowly bring the barbell in an arch across your face and down behind your head as far as a moderate yet comfortable stretch allows. Pull the bar up and reverse the arcing path until the bar once again rests across your chest. Repeat for the desired number of reps.

Tips. Keep your elbows as close together as possible throughout the movement.

Aaron Baker

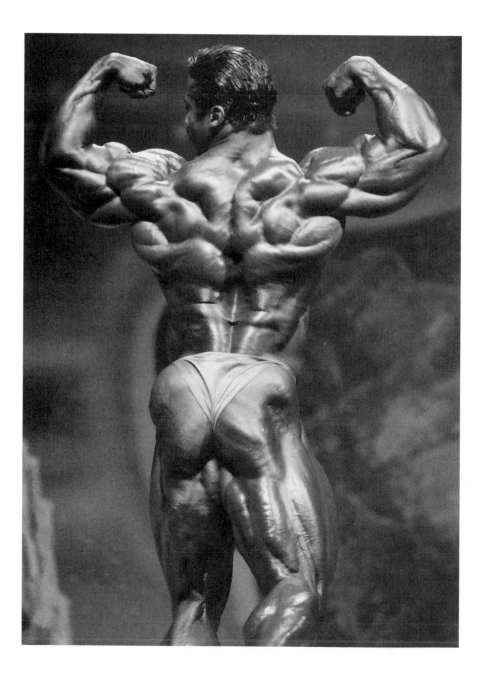

Dumbbell Pullovers

Emphasis. The areas of stress are essentially the same as for the other types of pullovers but with slightly more chest and triceps work.

Starting Position. Lie across the center of a flat bench in a perpendicular or T position. Your upper back and rear delts should be the point of contact with the bench, with your head well off the bench and your feet lower than your hips. Place your hands under the plates of the dumbbell so your thumbs are around the handle and your fingers are locked together and flat against the plates.

Movement Performance. Perform as for barbell pullovers but be certain to maintain the feet at a lower point than your hips without allowing the hips to rise more than one or two inches as you perform the exercise.

Barbell Bent-Over Rows

Emphasis. This is an excellent, if not the best, back thickness movement known to man. The major placement of stress is on the latissimus dorsi. Of course as in most back moves, there is significant secondary work forced on the arms, erectors, traps, and delts. As you perhaps know, all rowing-type back movements emphasize thickness, while in a general sense, the pulldowns and chinning-type moves are associated with increased width.

Starting Position. It is essential to wear a lifting belt and to keep your lower back tightly arched throughout the entire range of sets from the first warm-up to the heaviest stack of plates. Straps are useful if a strong grip is not available.

Stand about one-and-a-half feet back from a bar that, when loaded with a 45-pound plate on each side, rests near the midpoint of your shin. For years bodybuilders have stood on benches and blocks in the attempt to gain a greater range of motion for their lats. Unless your arms are so long that your knuckles drag the floor, your range of motion for the lats is more than adequate if you maintain a tight lower back and stand about two inches above parallel. Standing on a bench is a great example of monkey-see, monkey-do! The best backs belong to those who take a minute and question, "Am I really stretching my lats or is this more like playing a game of touch my toes with my rows?"

Bend over and grasp the bar with a shoulder-width, thumbs-over grip. Keeping the arch in your lower back, straighten your legs until your knees are slightly bent. Your upper body will be just above parallel

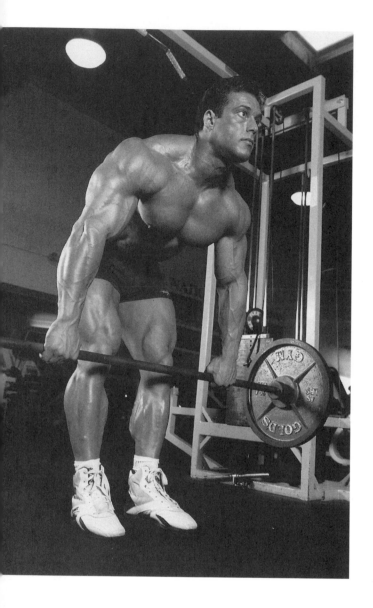
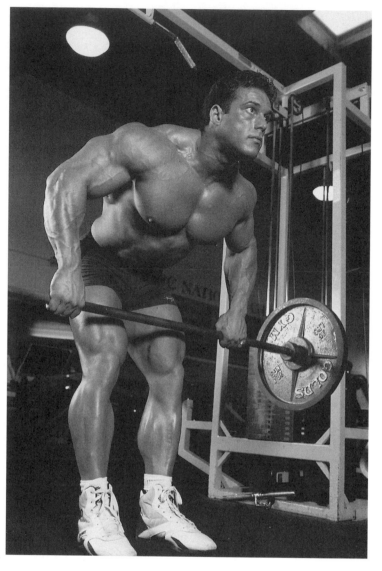

Lucio Paolini

to the floor. This will bring your bar to a point of the plates clearing the floor so there is no resting of the bar at the bottom position.

Movement Performance. Moving only your arms, slowly pull the bar back at a slight angle so that it touches the buckle on your belt. As you pull the bar toward the buckle, your upper arms should travel out away from your torso at 45-degree angles. As the bar touches the buckle, begin to lower it back to the starting position without exaggerating the stretch by allowing the lower back to move from its starting point. In other words, at no time during the movement should you bend at the waist. By maintaining your back in an arched position and not allowing the waist to bend, you will keep the stress on the lats and off the lower back! As you reach the starting position, attempt to feel your lats being stretched. Repeat the movement for the desired number of reps.

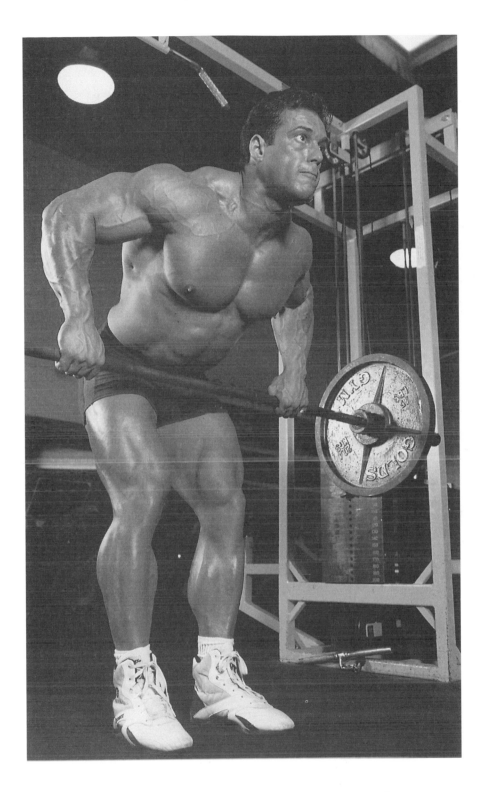

Variations. You can use a variety of grip widths as you perform your bent-over rows. Your grip can be as close as having your thumbs touching each other in the center of the bar, or a collar-to-collar width. For those with a lower-back injury, you may utilize a bench at the correct height to rest your head against for additional support.

Reverse-Grip Bent-Over Rows

Emphasis. Here the emphasis is increased in the lower lats, near the waist, as opposed to the midback area. Secondary stress is felt by the trapezius, posterior deltoid, erector spinae, and biceps muscles. The use of lifting straps de-emphasizes the forearms.

Starting Position. With either a straight bar or an EZ-curl bar, take the same starting position as for regular bent-over rows, with the major

Lucio Paolini

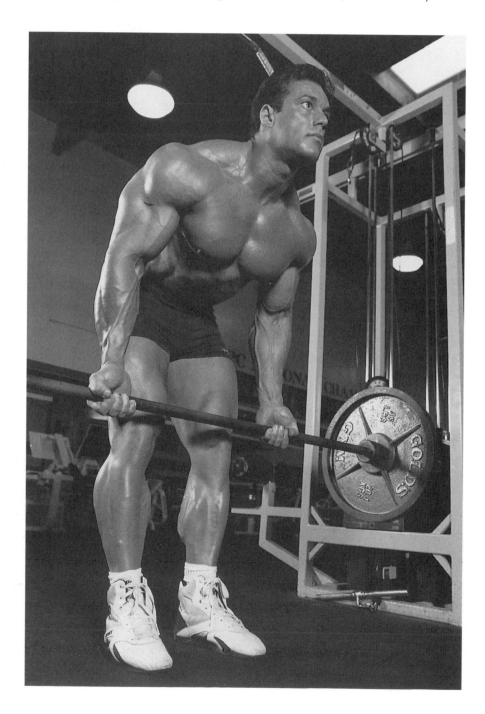

exception of reversing your grip so your palms are facing away from your shins. (The use of lifting straps is a good idea here.) Straighten the legs to a point where your torso is slightly above a 45-degree angle to the floor. Increase the bend of the knees over that which you use for a regular bent-over barbell row.

Movement Performance. You will repeat the same execution of the movement as in conventional bent-over rows with the following differences: (a) the elbows are actually drawn back toward the waist as opposed to straight up and down because of the increased bend in your knees; and (b) you will lower the bar back to the starting point with a slower negative or eccentric motion due to the increased elevation of your upper body beyond parallel.

Tips. *Safety* and *caution* are key words with this movement. The areas of concern are the biceps, in that the ability of the back to handle massive poundages can quickly overwhelm the lifting capacity of the biceps, resulting in either immediate muscle tearing or setting the stage for future muscle tearing.

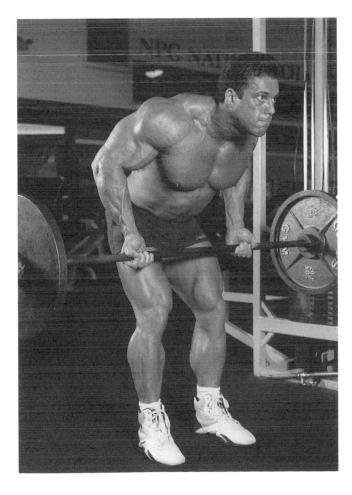
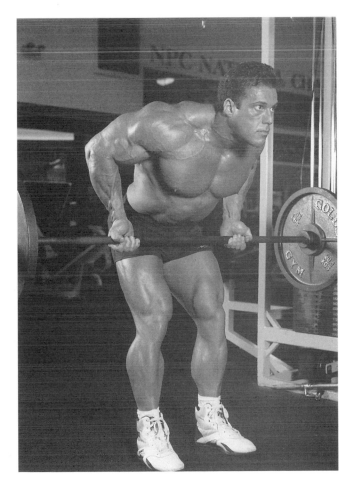

Dumbbell Bent-Over Rows

Emphasis. Performing bent-over rows with two dumbbells instead of a barbell allows you more freedom of movement with your hands as you stress your lats, biceps, brachialis, and forearm flexor muscles. Secondary stress is felt by the trapezius, posterior deltoid, and erector spinae.

Starting Position. Choose two dumbbells that when added together weigh approximately 80 to 90 percent of your training weight for barbell bent-over rows. Place them on the floor in front of you and stand with your feet about shoulder-width apart and your toes angled slightly outward. Unlock your legs throughout the entire movement, and as in all types of rowing movements, maintain the lower back in an arched position.

Movement Performance. Keeping your elbows close to your sides, slowly pull the dumbbells directly backward until they touch your lower-rib-cage–oblique-muscles area. Lower them back into the starting position and repeat for the desired rep count.

Variations. You can perform this movement with palms facing your legs or facing each other.

One-Arm Dumbbell Bent-Over Rows

Emphasis. As in the previous movement, one-arm dumbbell bent-over rows strongly stress the latissimus dorsi, biceps, brachialis, and forearm flexors. Secondary stress is felt by the trapezius and posterior deltoid. Due to the support provided by resting on a bench or other type of support there is somewhat less stress upon the erector spinae muscles.

Starting Position. Place a dumbbell of slightly more than 50 percent of your training weight for barbell bent-over rows at one side of a flat bench. Kneel with your right knee and lower leg on the bench and place your right hand about two feet ahead of your right knee. Reach down and grasp the dumbbell with your left hand. Completely straighten your left arm and slightly rotate your left shoulder downward to fully stretch your left lat muscle group. You may want to consider using lifting straps here due to the emphasis placed upon gripping strength.

Movement Performance. Keeping your elbow close to your side, slowly pull the dumbbell directly upward and roll your left delt area

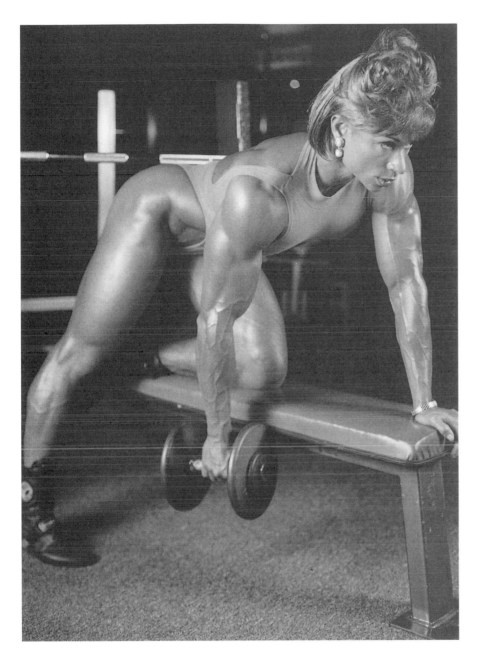

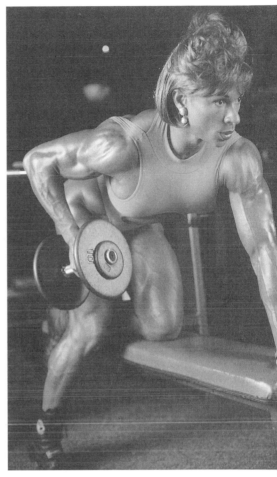

Laura Creavelle

as the dumbbell touches the edge of the lower ribs. Lower the weight
back to the bottom position and repeat for the desired rep count.

Machine Bent-Over Rows

Emphasis. Major emphasis is placed on the target muscle of the latissimus dorsi due to the isolation of the back and supportive posture
incorporated into each piece of well-designed equipment. Significant
work is performed by the biceps, brachialis, and forearm flexors.

Laura Creavelle

Secondary stress is placed upon the trapezius and posterior deltoids. The muscles of the erector spinae are isolated out of the movement to any significant degree.

Starting Position. Lie facedown with your chest resting on the pads as provided and firmly grasp the handles. Make sure your lower body is securely positioned.

Movement Performance. Release the weight by raising the handles or bar upward to begin the movement. Slowly lower the weight to a fully extended point and you'll feel the essential stretch. From this starting point, slowly pull the weight upward until you have reached the fullest possible degree of muscular contraction. Squeeze the muscles of your upper back, then reverse the movement with a controlled lowering. Repeat the sequence for the desired number of reps.

Tips. Most machines allow for a variety of hand widths for a total back attack, so find the best for your physique and begin the blasting process.

T-Bar Rows

Emphasis. T-bar rows place very strong emphasis on the latissimus dorsi, erector spinae, biceps, brachialis, and forearm flexors. Less intense work is performed by the posterior deltoids and the trapezius.

Starting Position. According to your degree of strength, load the apparatus and place your feet on the platform behind the handles. Bend over at the waist, always with a strong arch to the lower back, and remember to use your belt for this movement. Grasp the handles and straighten your legs just short of completely locking them, leaving a slight bend at the knees. This will elevate the bar off its resting point and raise your torso slightly above parallel.

Movement Performance. Slowly pull the weight upward, keeping your elbows tight against your sides, until it touches your chest. Squeeze the shoulders together at the top of the movement for an intense contraction. Slowly reverse the movement and lower into the bottom starting position. Repeat until the desired number of reps are completed.

Tips. If you're interested in looking like a goof, then you can always take an Olympic-size bar and jam it into the corner of the gym wall. This is a sure way to get tossed into the street once the owner sees you wrecking his corners.

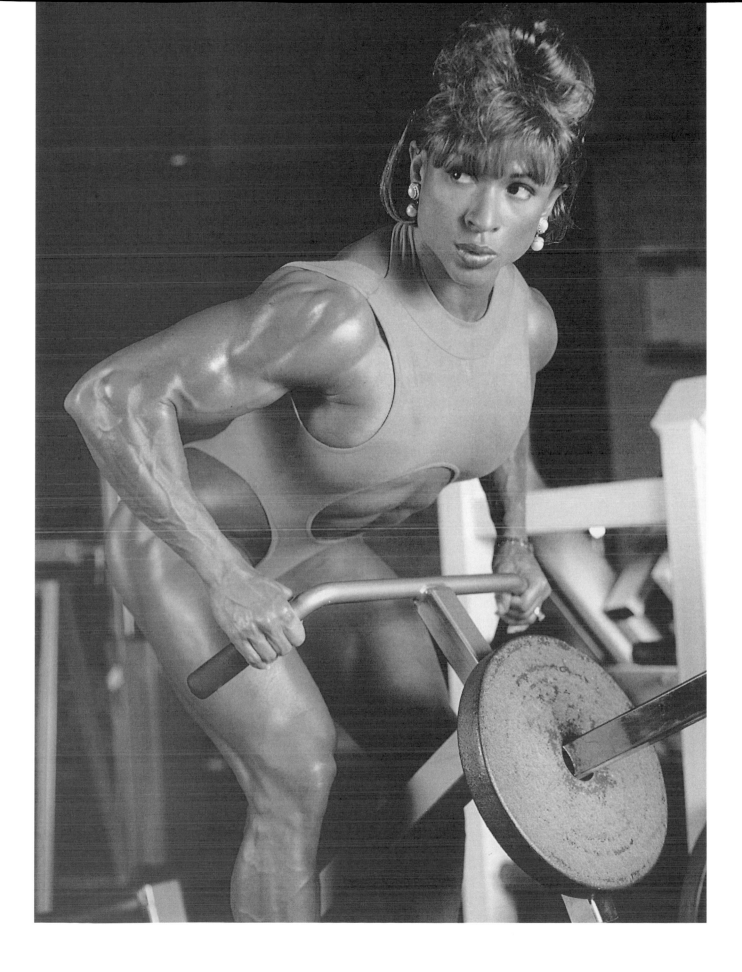

Seated Cable Rows

Emphasis. This is an excellent movement developing all the back muscles: trapezius, latissimus dorsi, and erector spinae. Strong stress is also placed upon the posterior deltoids, biceps, brachialis, and forearm flexors.

Starting Position. Most commonly this movement is performed with a handle that allows you to take a narrow grip with your palms facing

Ronnie Coleman

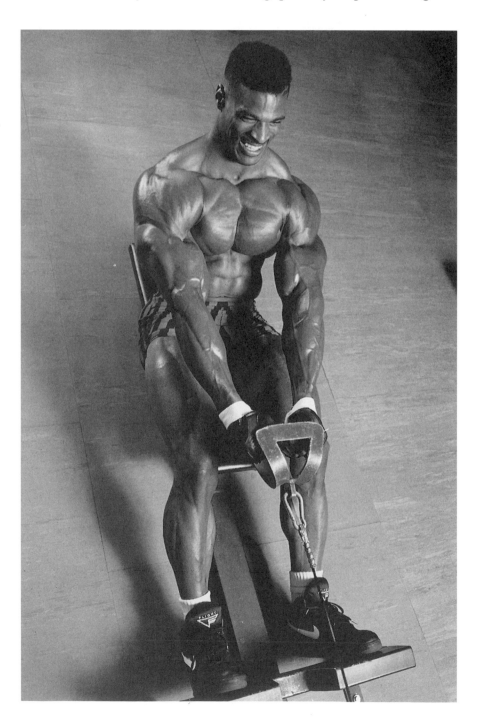

each other. Grasp the handle in this manner. Place your feet against the foot bars at the front end of the apparatus seat, straighten your arms, and sit down on the seat with your legs slightly bent throughout the entire movement. Sit upright at a 90-degree angle to the floor. Remember to always wear your lifting belt and maintain an arched back.

Movement Performance. Keeping your elbows tight against your sides, pull the handle back toward your lifting-belt buckle. Once the handle

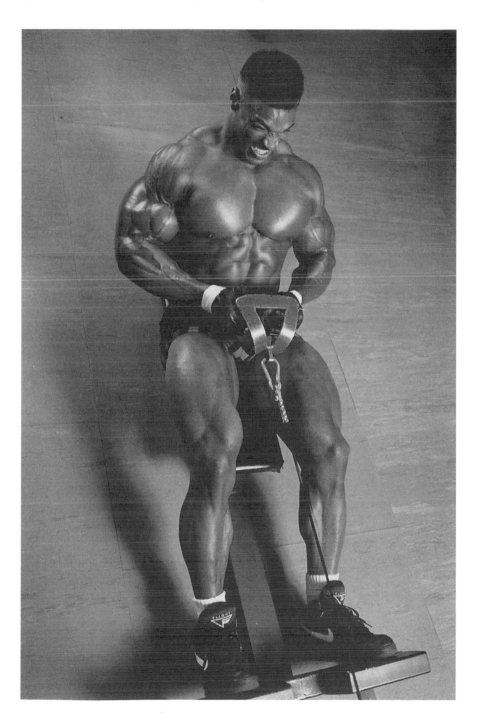

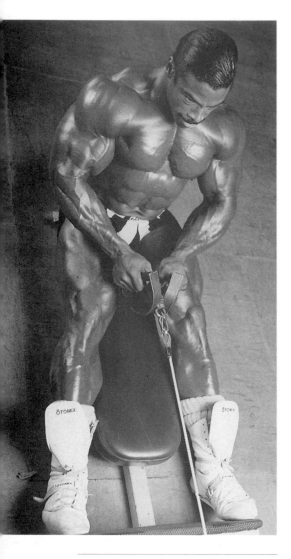

Aaron Baker

touches the buckle, squeeze the upper back together and slowly, under control, lower the weight back to the starting point.

Many opinions exist as to how far forward you should lean toward the actual weight stack. The best advice is that, since any excess bending of the waist in other moves such as bent-over rows is not good for the longevity of your training years, neither is bending forward at the waist to perform seated pulley rows. It stands to reason that you are attempting to build thickness in the latissimus dorsi area, not to perform a modified deadlift. In general, don't lean forward past a point slightly beyond 90 degrees. There is no mistaking the stretch placed on your upper and midback areas when this exercise is performed correctly as indicated.

Variations. This movement is most frequently performed from a low pulley machine, but it can also be performed from a high pulley set three to five feet above the floor. There are also several types of handles that can be used, the most common of which is a V-shaped handle where the grip has the palms facing together about six to eight inches apart. Using a straight bar two to three feet long allows you to use a thumbs-over or -under grip of many different widths. Finally, there are arrangements with two handles connected by a cable which is then attached to the pulley cable itself.

Seated Machine Rows

Emphasis. In this particular movement, the manufacturers have done an outstanding job of designing highly effective machines in a wide variety of styles. Common to all of these great designs is tremendous isolation of the latissimus dorsi, with secondary emphasis on the posterior deltoids, trapezius, biceps, brachialis, and forearm flexors. The erector spinae muscles have largely been isolated out of the movement.

Starting Position. Assume a position on the machine's seat facing the upright padded area. The seat is to be adjusted for your height so that when your arms are extended straight in front of you they are in line with the gripping area on the equipment. Position your feet firmly and lean forward so your chest is touching the upright pads. Grasp the handles firmly and sit erect by leaning slightly back in order to engage the machine's resistance.

Movement Performance. Keeping your elbows below shoulder level, slowly pull your elbows as far back as comfortable. Momentarily squeeze your shoulders together for peak contraction and reverse the movement to lower back into the starting position. Repeat the exercise for the desired number of reps.

Chins

Emphasis. The wide variety of chins you can perform all place very strong stress on the latissimus dorsi, biceps, and brachialis. A good rule of thumb to keep in mind is that rowing-type movements build thickness, while chins and pulldown exercises yield more width development.

Starting Position. Use a stool or other means of assistance to elevate sufficiently to grasp the bar. Unless your grip is very strong, lifting straps are normally called for. Take a thumbs-around-the-bar grip of anywhere from two inches to as wide as possible. The closer the grip, the lower the emphasis on the latissimus dorsi. Likewise the wider your grip, the more you will stress your upper lat area. The only concern is that you must be able to bring your torso up to a height at least where your chin is above the bar itself.

Jean-Pierre Fux

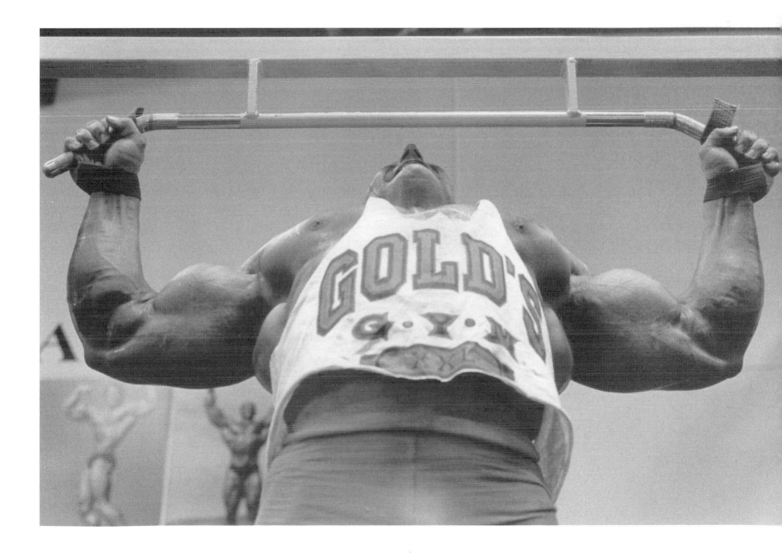

Lucio Paolini

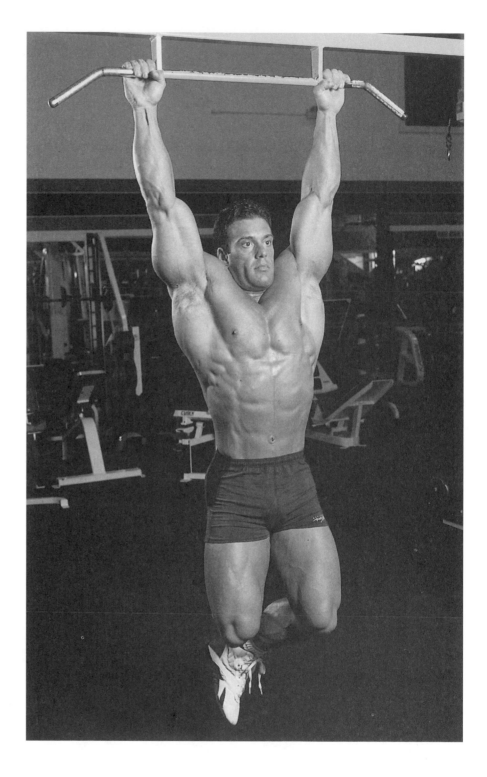

Movement Performance. Once your grip is firmly set, take your feet off the stool and allow your arms to reach a full extension. Now begin to pull yourself up to the correct level and arch your back at the top before beginning to descend. Reverse the motion and return to a full-

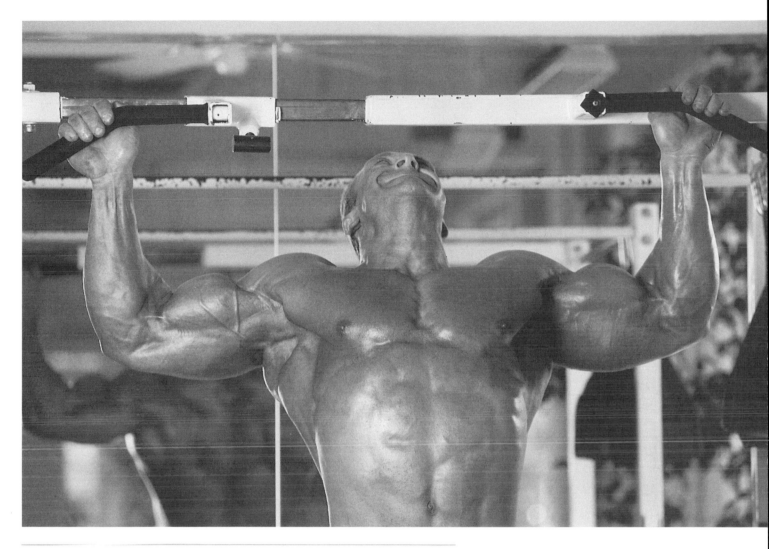

Ian Harrison

stretch starting point. Be careful not to overly relax yourself at the bottom or you could injure your shoulder joints.

Variations. Chins may be performed in a variety of ways according to your training goals. Hands positioned close together work lower lats and hands positioned wide work them higher. Decide how to approach this classic exercise according to how your physique is structured.

Chins may also be performed with a reduced range of motion in the more difficult behind-the-neck style. Reversing your grip so your palms face toward the torso, as in barbell curls, allows the biceps a more powerful pulling position.

Tips. A goal of 6 to 8 reps chinning your body weight is a reasonable gauge to ascertain whether you're in a position to get the full benefit

Jeremy Freeman

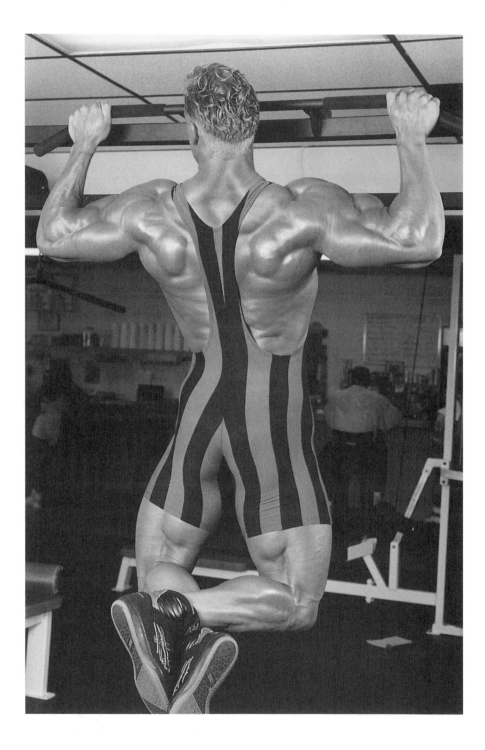

from this exercise. If you're not able to reach that repetition number, perform pulldowns until you build up the required strength for chins. If you are gifted or advanced in the number of reps and you're able to grind out more than 12 to 14 perfect reps, then it's time to start adding extra resistance after your warm-ups are completed. Some equipment manufacturers such as Nautilus have designed specific pieces of equipment that provide the needed extra resistance.

Lat Pulldowns

Emphasis. Lat pulldowns directly stress the latissimus dorsi, posterior delts, biceps, brachialis, and forearm flexors.

Starting Position. Adjust the seat height in front of the weight stack so your legs are firmly anchored under the pads provided. Now stand

Jean-Pierre Fux

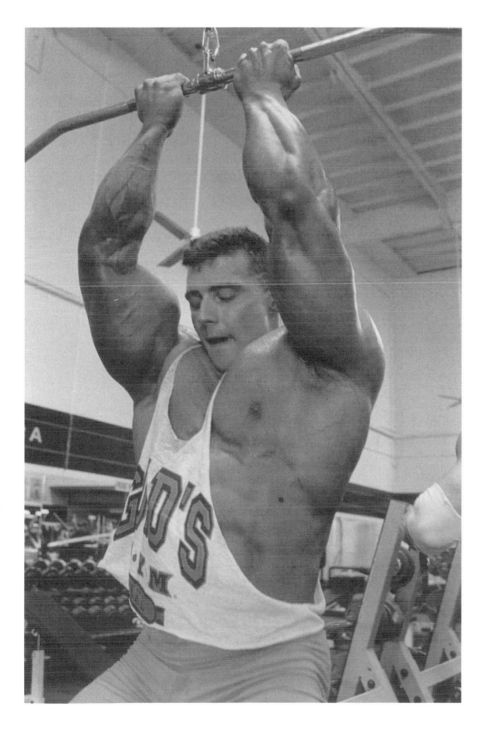

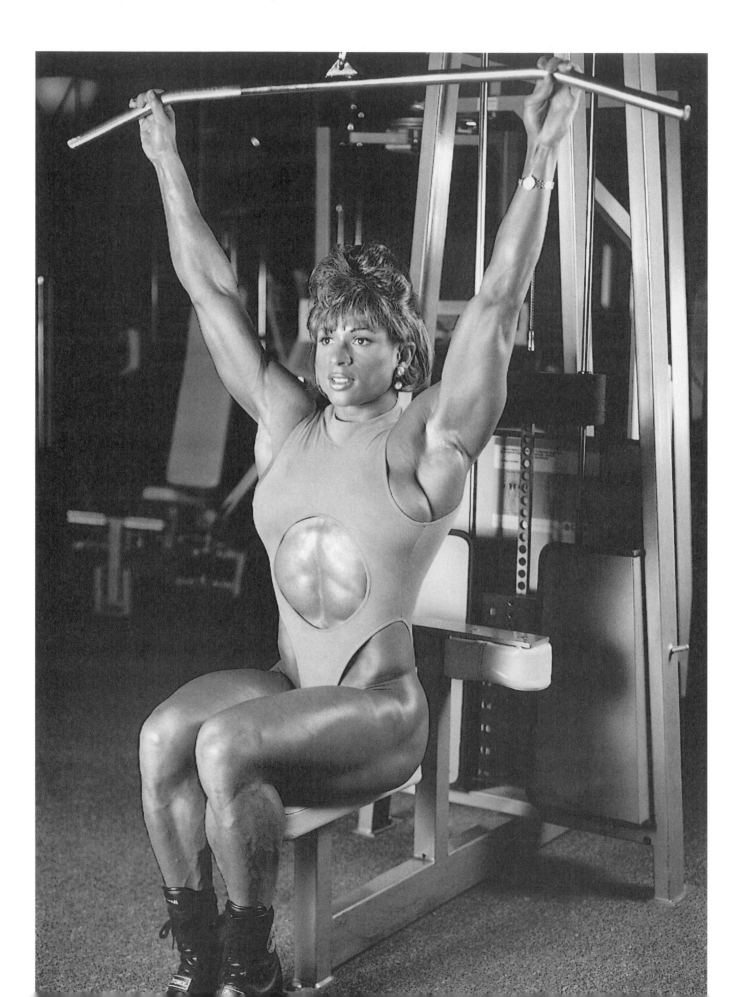

up and place your hands with palms facing away from you in a thumbs-under-the-bar grip. Your hands should be about shoulder width or slightly wider on the bar. Firmly grasp the bar, straighten your arms, and sit down, while simultaneously locking your legs under the restraining pads. Arch your back and keep it slightly arched during the entire movement.

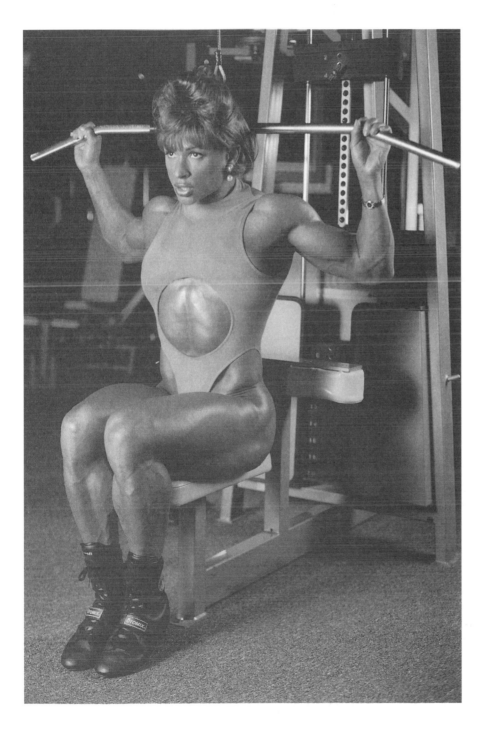

Laura Creavelle

Derrick Whitsett

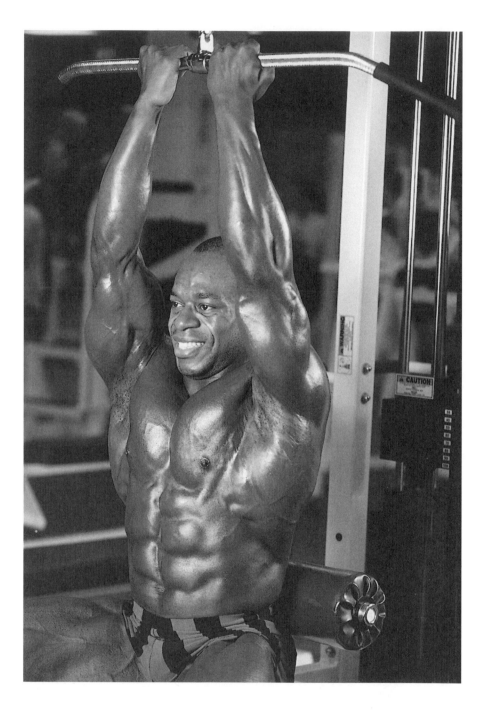

Movement Performance. Concentrate on pulling your elbows down-ward and backward as you pull the bar down in front of your neck to touch the upper portion of your chest. Slowly return to the starting position and repeat the movement for the desired rep count.

Tips. If you are strong enough to use heavier than body weight resis-tance in this movement, then have a spotter assist you into the start-ing position by pushing firmly down on your shoulders and traps.

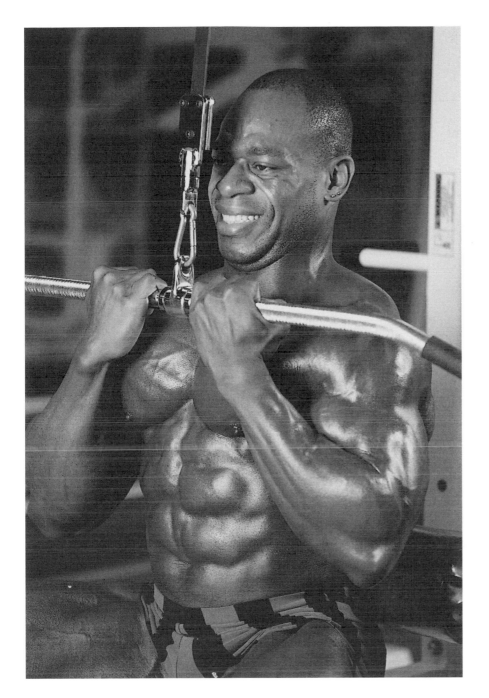

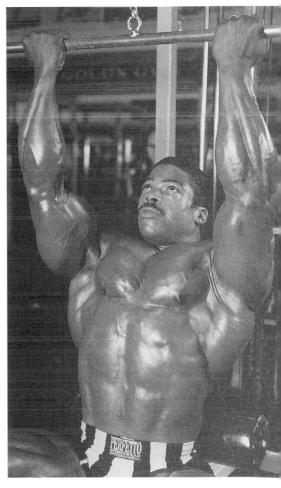

Variations. As with chins, merely changing your grip on the bar will shift the focus of muscular stress when doing pulldowns as follows: wide grip hits more of the upper lat, while a relatively close grip (four to six inches) stimulates the lower lat area. Again, as in chins, pull-downs may also be performed in a more challenging behind-the-neck movement. Placing the hands at various widths in a parallel fashion is also a way to change the variety of exercise for the lats.

Aaron Baker

TRAPS AND UPPER BACK

Barbell Shrugs

Emphasis. Barbell shrugs are a very direct movement for stressing the trapezius and other upper-back muscles. Secondary stress is on the gripping muscles of your forearms.

Starting Position. Wear your lifting belt. Assume a standing position in front of a power rack with the pins set so the level of the bar is at the tip of your fingers. Set your feet firmly on the floor, slightly less than shoulder-width apart. Grasp the bar at a width so that your hands are touching the outside edge of your legs. Use a thumbs-around grip with your palms facing away. Use straps if your grip is insufficient. Raise your head upward while arching your back.

Roland Cziurlok

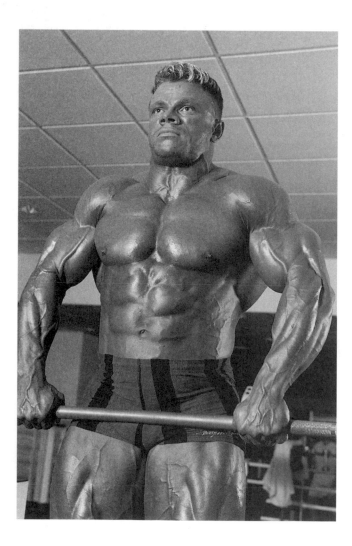
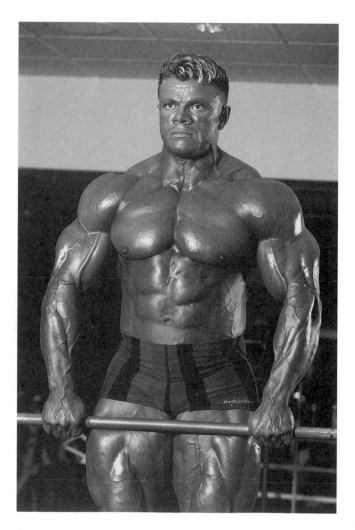

Movement Performance. Stand up by straightening your legs and maintaining the tight back-arched and head-up position. Once you are powerfully upright, allow your shoulders to relax. Then pull them upward and slightly atop the back, or in other words, just shrug your shoulders high. Do not bend forward or lean backward. Maintain the arched lower back. Squeeze at the top for peak contraction. Reverse the movement and repeat for the desired repetition count.

Variations. Widening or narrowing your grip lends different angles to challenge the area.

Dumbbell Shrugs

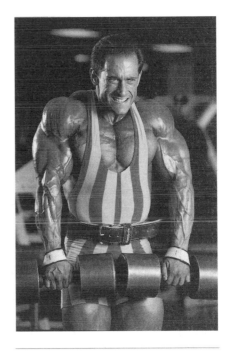

Emphasis. Dumbbell shrugs are also a very direct movement for stressing the trapezius and other upper-back muscles. Secondary stress is on the gripping muscles of the forearms. You will have more mobility in the shoulders when using a pair of dumbbells, so in some ways dumbbell shrugs are superior to barbell shrugs.

Starting Position. Wear your lifting belt. Grasp two heavy dumbbells, assume the basic pulling position, and lift the weights to the front of your thighs. Hold your arms straight and your torso securely erect. Allow your shoulders to relax and sag downward as far as comfortable.

Movement Performance. Slowly shrug your shoulders upward and backward as far as possible. Hold this peak contracted position for a moment, then lower the dumbbells back to the starting point. Repeat for the desired number of reps.

Variations. Rotating your shoulders in a semicircular shrug adds incredible variation to this effective movement.

Craig Licker

Machine Shrugs

Emphasis. As with all shrug-type movements, shrugs performed on specially designed benches or machines place tremendous primary stress on the trapezius and other upper-back muscles. Secondary stress is felt by the forearm flexors.

Starting Position. Elevate the seat height so that when your arms are resting at your sides your hands are slightly above the level of the gripping handles. Keep your back arched firmly and your head elevated throughout the entire movement. Wear a lifting belt. Lean forward and grasp the handles firmly, then sit up straight.

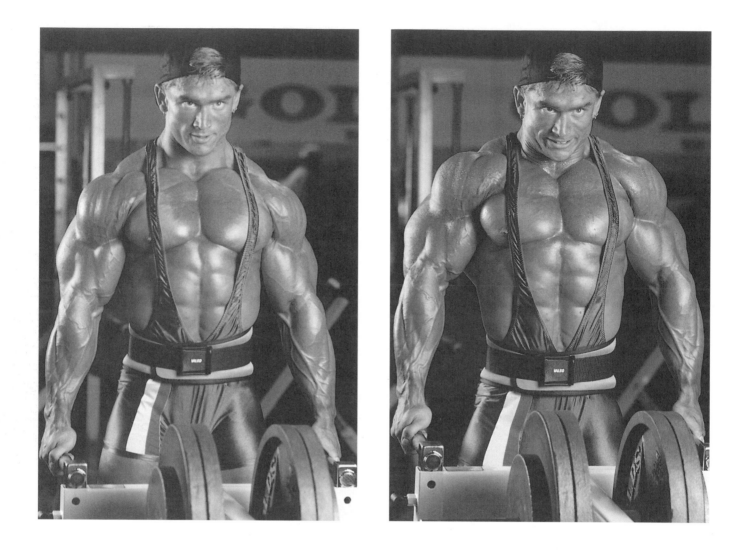

Lee Priest

Movement Performance. Slowly allow your shoulders to be pulled downward to a maximum comfortable stretch. At the bottom point of the stretch, begin to slowly shrug upward and backward as high as possible and hold for a peak contraction. Repeat for the desired number of reps.

Barbell Upright Rows

Emphasis. All variations of upright rows exercise the trapezius and deltoid muscles. Secondary work is performed by the biceps, brachialis, and forearm flexors.

Starting Position. Wear your lifting belt. Take a narrow overgrip in the middle of a barbell about six inches between index fingers. Stand erect with your arms straight down at your sides and your fists resting on your upper thighs.

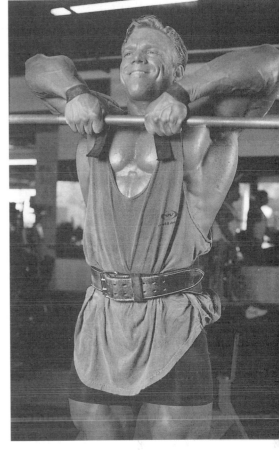

Dave Fisher

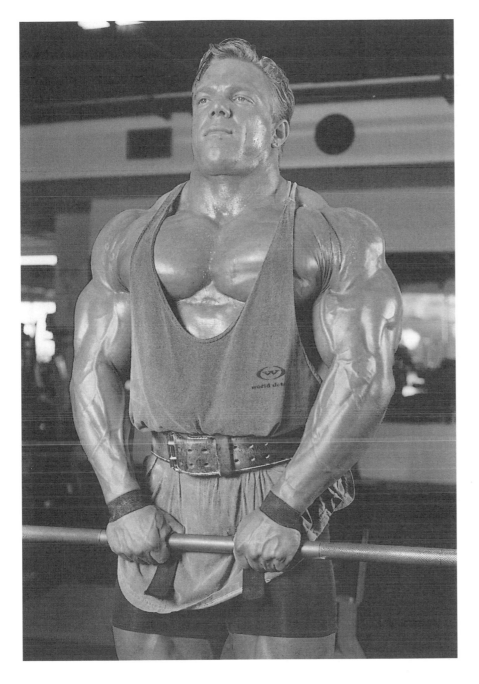

Movement Performance. Being sure to keep your elbows well above the level of your grip on the bar at all times, slowly pull the barbell directly upward close to your body until the backs of your hands contact the underside of your chin. In the top position, roll your shoulder blades backward and squeeze them together. Lower the weight slowly back to the starting point and repeat for the desired number of reps.

Variations. Moving your grip outward to various degrees allows the muscles to feel different stress.

Dumbbell Upright Rows

Emphasis. Dumbbells give you somewhat more freedom of movement than barbells when performing upright rows. Primary stress is felt by the trapezius and deltoid. Secondary work is performed by the biceps, brachialis, and forearm flexors.

Starting Position. Wear your belt. Grasp two moderately heavy dumbbells and stand erect with your arms hanging straight down, your palms facing the front of your body, and the dumbbells resting across your upper thighs.

Lisa Ibarra

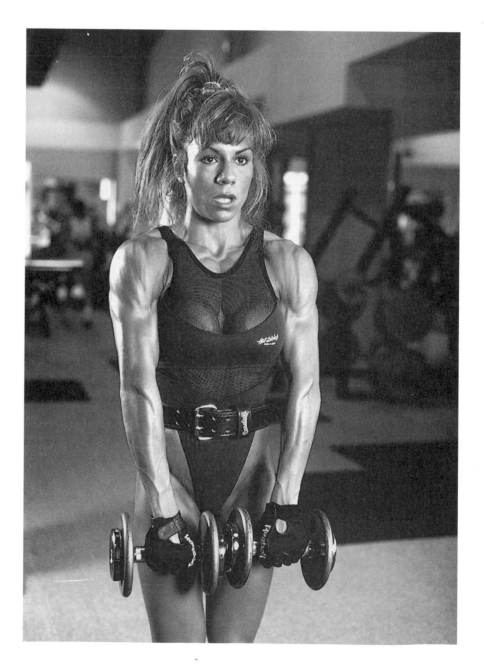

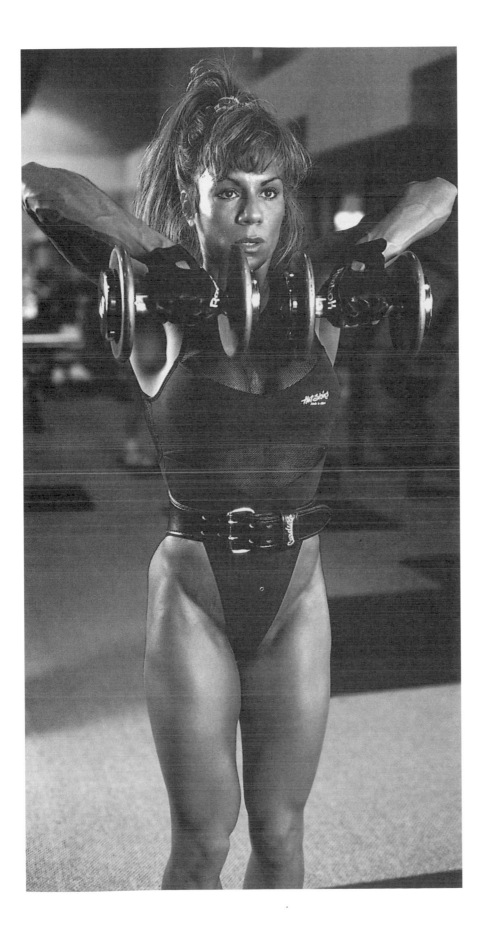

Movement Performance. Being sure to keep your elbows well above the level of your hands, slowly pull the dumbbells directly upward along the front of your body until they are just below your lower pectorals. Lower the dumbbells slowly and deliberately back to the starting position. Repeat the movement until desired reps are completed.

Variations. This type of rowing motion also can be performed with a low cable–pulley machine. A narrow, straight pulley handlebar about 12 inches long works well.

Shoulders

Side Dumbbell Raises

Emphasis. This movement is often incorrectly performed. Correctly executed, side dumbbell raises stress the medial heads of the deltoids in nearly total isolation from the rest of the body. Very minor secondary stress is placed on the anterior delts and trapezius.

Starting Position. Wear your lifting belt. Grasp two light dumbbells, place your feet about shoulder width apart, and stand erect. Bend

Yolanda Hughes

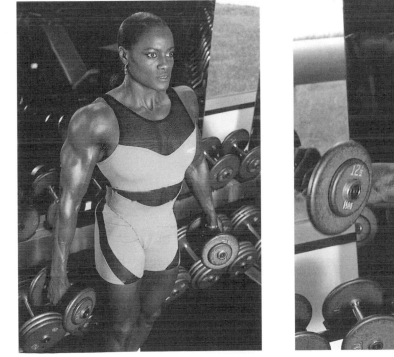

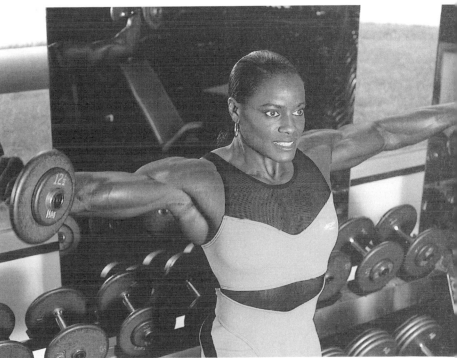

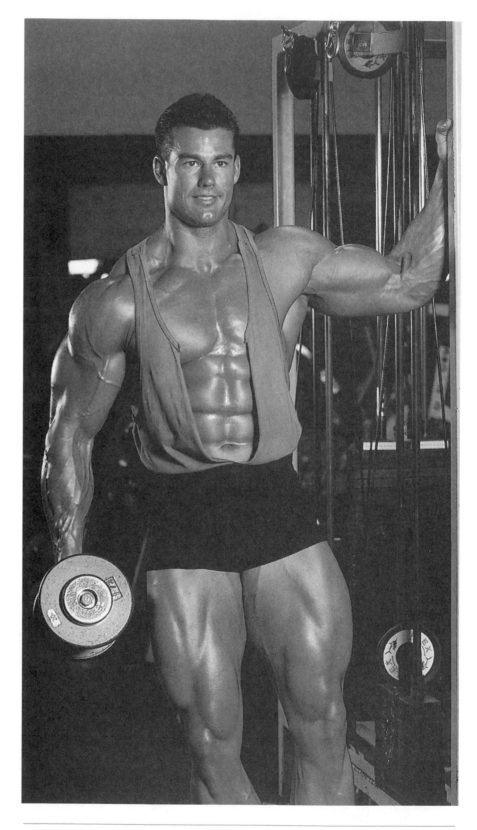

Bill Davey

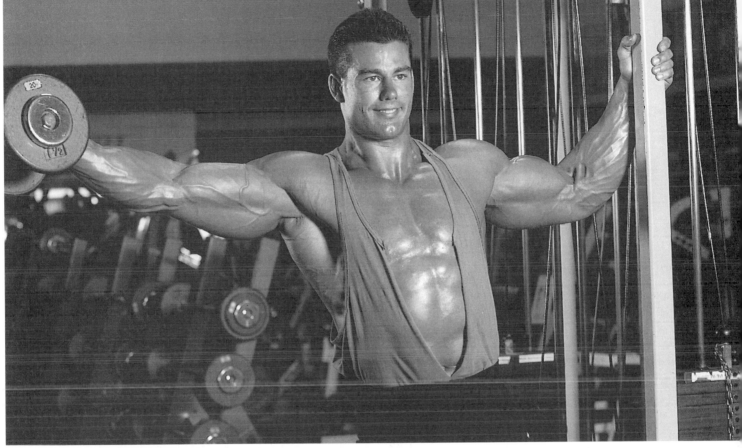

slightly forward at the waist and press the dumbbells together, palms facing each other, about six inches in front of your hips. Bend your arms slightly and keep them rounded like this throughout the movement.

Movement Performance. Using deltoid strength and keeping your palms toward the floor throughout the movement, raise the dumbbells in semicircular arcs out to the sides and slightly forward until they are just above the level of your shoulders. At the top of the movement, it's essential that you rotate the front ends of the dumbbells below the level of the back ends for a moment to isolate stress on the medial deltoid heads. Lower the dumbbells slowly back along the same arc to the starting point and repeat the movement for the desired number of reps.

Variations. To obtain even more deltoid isolation you can perform this movement while seated at the end of a sturdy bench. This exercise is

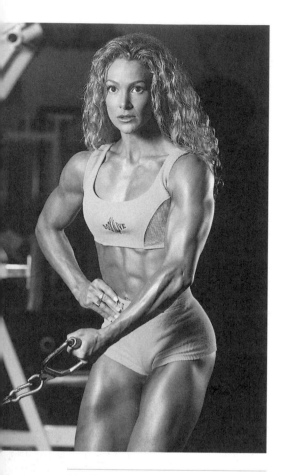

Mia Finnegan

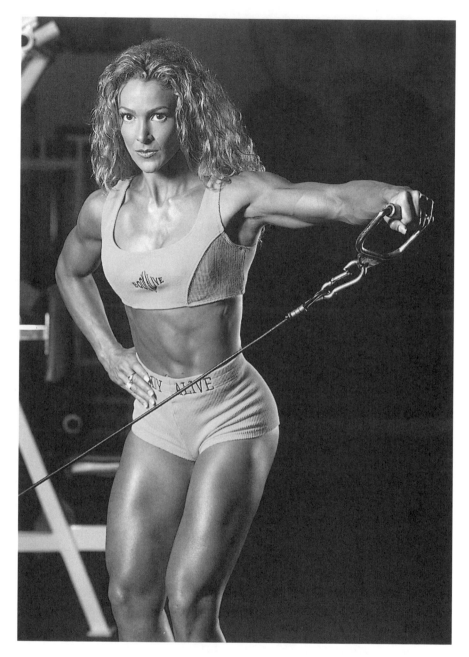

also known as seated side dumbbell raises. From the seated position, you start the movement with the dumbbells resting just below your hips, arms directly at your sides. Side cable raises are another alternative to side dumbbell raises. The cable handles should be in a crossed or X position in front of your upper thighs. Raises performed on a machine provide smooth movement and control.

Front Dumbbell Raises

Emphasis. Front raises isolate stress on the anterior deltoid heads, with minor secondary stress placed on the medial deltoids and trapezius.

Laura Bass

Starting Position. Wear your lifting belt. Grasp a pair of light dumbbells and stand erect with your hands facing the fronts of your thighs.
The two dumbbells should be touching with ends together. Set your
feet about shoulder-width apart and look straight ahead.

Movement Performance. Moving just your arms, slowly raise the dumbbells in a semicircular arc from your thighs to the height of your shoulders. From the position at shoulder level, slowly lower the dumbbells
back to the starting position and repeat for the desired number of reps.

Don Long

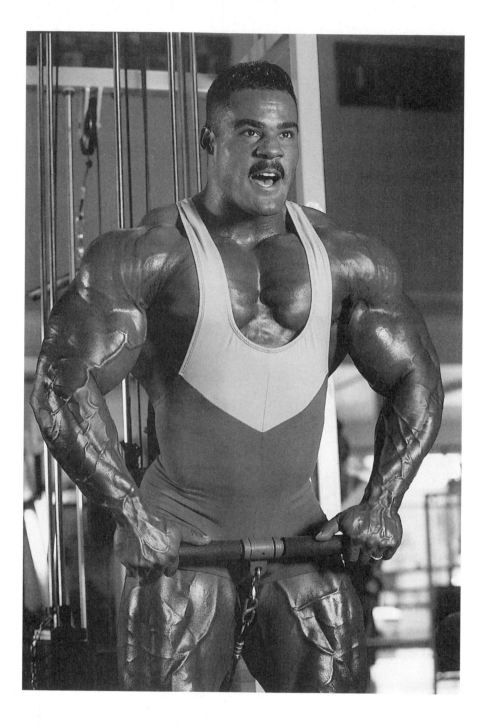

Tips. Many very successful bodybuilders like to flex their wrists slightly so their hands hang downward during the movement.

Variations. A barbell may be used in place of two dumbbells. Another variation is to alternate your right and left arms when using dumbbells. You may also add new areas of deltoid stress by performing front cable raises.

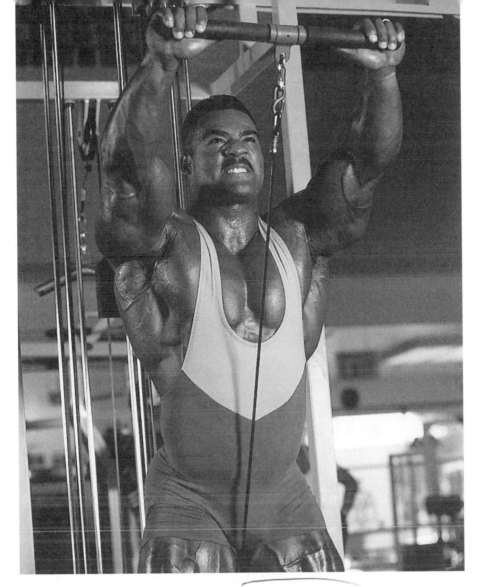

Monica Brandt (below)

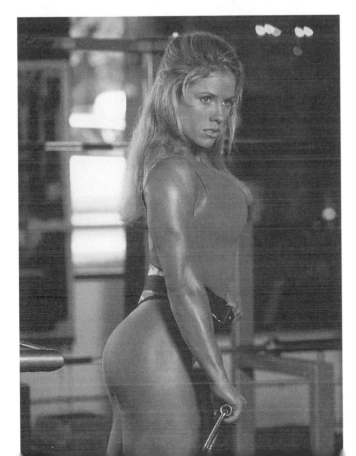

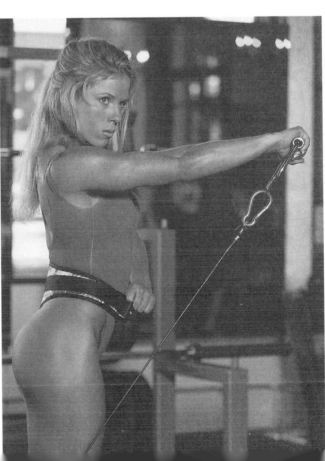

Dumbbell Raises—45 Degrees to the Front

Emphasis. Due to the 45-degree angle of the dumbbells relative to the front of your torso, the stress is shared by the anterior and medial deltoids.

Starting Position. Take the same position as in front dumbbell raises.

Movement Performance. Instead of raising your arms in front of you, move them approximately halfway between your side and front. At shoulder level, your arms are in a V shape.

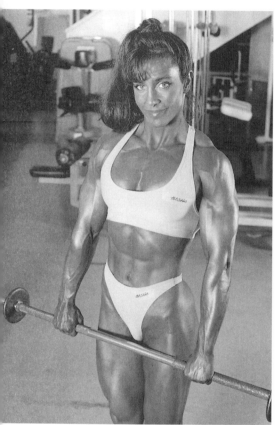

Laura Bass

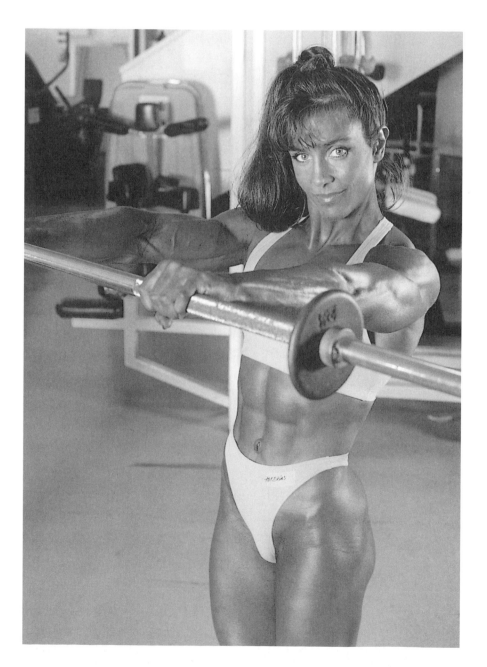

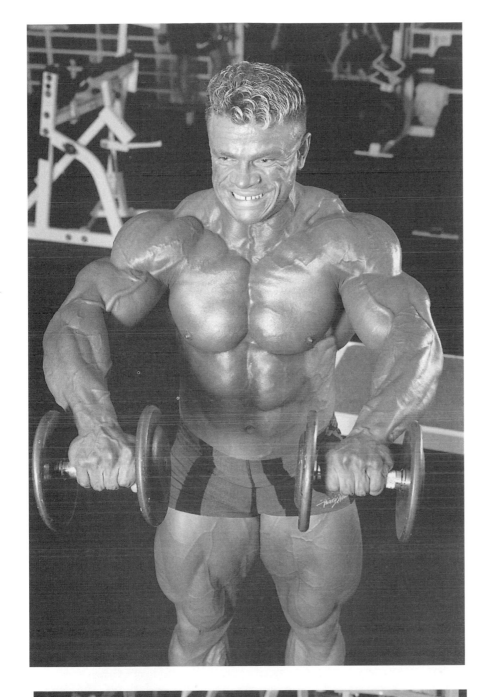

Roland Cziurlok

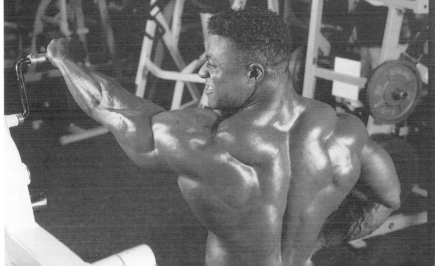

Garrett Downing

Grymko Dumbbell Raises

Emphasis. A dual level of stress is placed on the anterior and medial deltoid heads.

Starting Position. Take the same position as in standing dumbbell raises.

Movement Performance. First perform a conventional side dumbbell raise, and upon returning to the starting position, immediately perform a conventional front dumbbell raise. Alternate raises to the side with raises to the front. Repeat in this fashion for the desired number of reps.

Incline Dumbbell Raises

Emphasis. Incline dumbbell raises directly stress the medial deltoids, with significant secondary stress on the anterior deltoids and trapezius.

Starting Position. Grasp a light dumbbell in your left hand and lie on your right side on a 30- to 45-degree incline bench. Bend your arm slightly and keep it rounded throughout the movement. Allow the weight of the dumbbell to pull your left hand to the level of the bench, if not one or two inches below.

Movement Performance. Slowly raise the dumbbell directly out to the side and upward in a semicircular arc until it is directly above your left shoulder joint. Lower the weight back to the starting point and repeat the movement. Be sure to complete an equal number of reps for each arm.

Rear Dumbbell Raises

Emphasis. Primary stress is placed on the posterior deltoids, upper back, and trapezius muscles. Secondary stress is carried by the medial deltoid heads.

Starting Position. Grasp two light dumbbells and sit at the very end of a flat bench, facing away from the length of the bench. Place your feet close to each other about two feet from the end of the bench. Bend over at the waist and rest your torso along your thighs, with your arms pointed directly down toward the floor. Your palms are to face each other. Bend your elbows slightly and maintain this position throughout the movement.

Movement Performance. Without moving your torso, slowly raise the dumbbells in semicircular arcs directly out at your sides until they are at shoulder level. Lower the dumbbells slowly back to the starting point and repeat for the desired rep count. Do not allow your torso to move from its starting position.

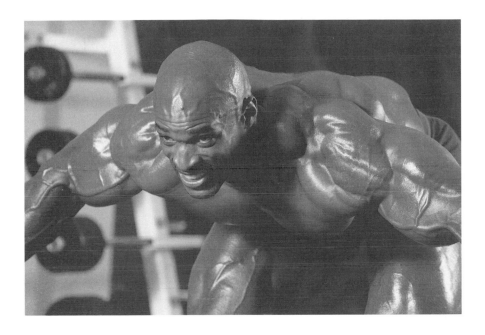

Ronnie Coleman (left)
Craig Licker (below)

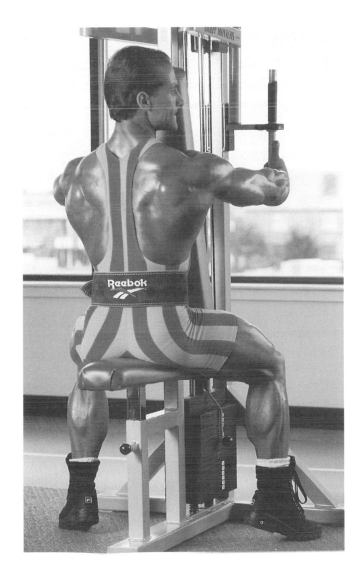

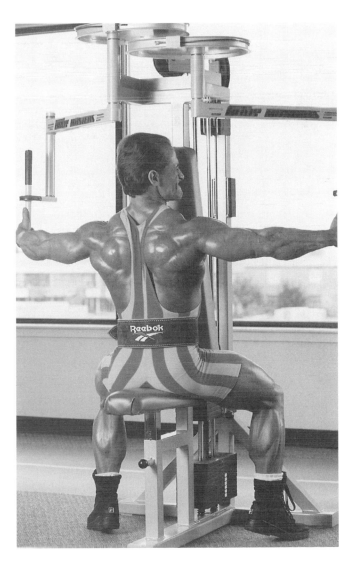

Variations. For a unique stress on your posterior deltoids, you can bring the dumbbells slightly forward as you raise them out to the sides. The cable crossover machine provides the ability to perform a tremendous alternative to dumbbells with rear cable raises. For even more of a change in your training, try pec-dec rear raises. Face the seat pad and proceed as in conventional rear raises.

Radical Grymko-Rack Delt Chins

Comments. Unless you have a rather large or unusually strong grip, this movement will be difficult due to the size of the uprights on power racks. Expect to find new calluses on your palms after about three weeks of performing this incredible exercise.

Emphasis. There is a radically intense degree of medial deltoid stress, with secondary work performed by the posterior and anterior delts, trapezius, latissimus dorsi, and biceps.

Starting Position. Stand facing a power rack with pins that are just below the top of your reach when your arms are overhead. Grab the uprights with your palms on top of the pins and facing each other. Your hands will be above your head in a wide V shape, with your feet curled up enough to keep from touching the floor.

Movement Performance. With your hands locked in place around the upright and resting on top of the pins, allow your feet to slowly come off the floor and at the same time hold your grip firmly around the posts. Slowly pull yourself up and somewhat back. Slowly lower yourself back to the starting point and repeat.

Barbell Press

Emphasis. Overhead pressing movements strongly stress the anterior deltoids and triceps. Secondary emphasis is placed on the medial deltoids, trapezius, and other upper-back muscles. If performed from a standing position, significant work is placed on the erector spinae muscles.

Starting Position. Wear your lifting belt. Use a power rack or other weight-support rack from which to take the bar. Place a moderately heavy barbell across the top of your chest with hands and wrists under the bar about shoulder-width apart. Step back with the bar across your shoulders and take a shoulder-width stance.

Movement Performance. Without allowing your torso to bend backward, slowly push the bar directly upward, close to your face, until it is

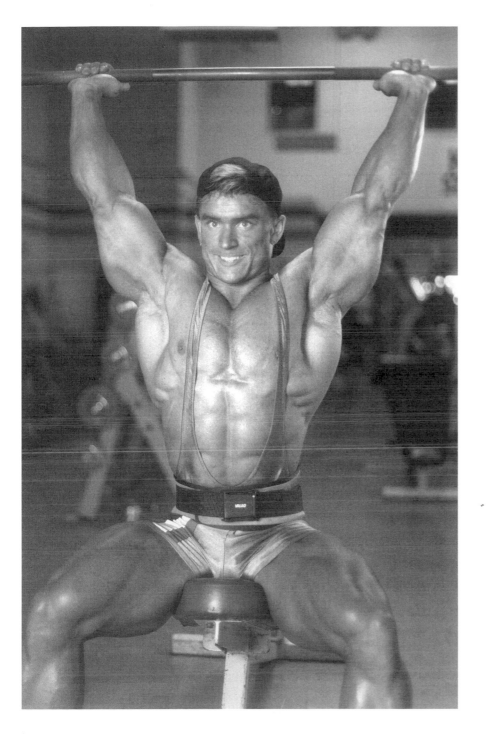

Lee Priest

at straight-arm's length directly overhead. Slowly lower back to the starting point without bouncing and repeat for the desired number of reps.

Variations. You may want to try doing barbell presses from a seated position. It is a good idea to use one of the many benches that have been specially designed for performing this movement, also known as the seated barbell press.

Garrett Downing

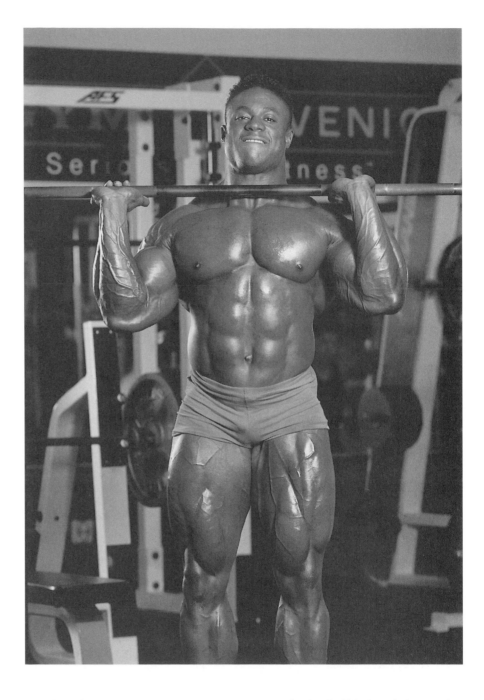

Another amazing pressing variation is the barbell-behind-the-neck press. However, as effective as they may be, behind-the-neck presses are associated with increased risk for shoulder injuries. You must be very flexible to get by for long without injury. The bench used for seated front barbell presses also is recommended for the behind-the-neck variation.

To perform the behind-the-neck press, load with a moderately light weight, and as always, wear your belt. Take a slightly wider-than-shoulder-width overgrip on the barbell. From a secure position on the

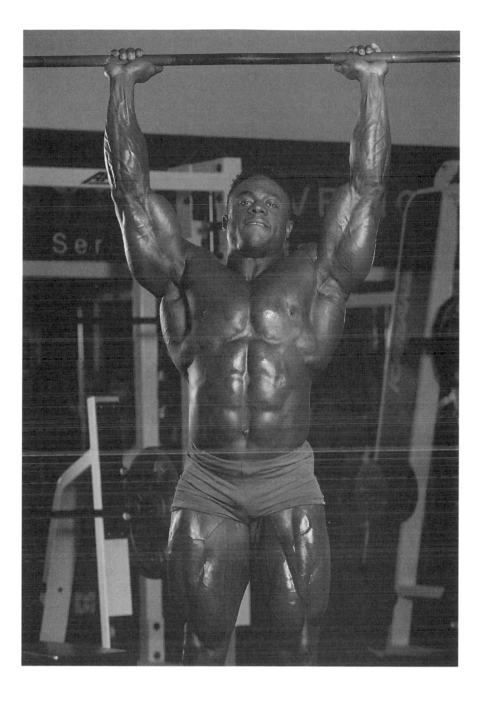

seat, carefully extend your arms to a point directly over your head, then very slowly lower the bar behind your head to a point even with the top of your ears. This is a reasonable degree of movement; lowering the bar past this point forces the shoulders into a position of poor leverage. From the bottom position, press the bar back to the starting point and repeat until the desired reps are completed.

All these variations and conventional presses can be more safely performed in a Smith machine as opposed to standing or using a free bench.

Machine Barbell Press

Emphasis. There is near total deltoid isolation designed into the latest generation of machine press equipment. The ability to cheat has been removed.

Starting Position. Set the resistance on the machine to the required load. Adjust the height of the machine's seat so your hands, when in the bottom pressing position, are just above the machine's handles.

Movement Performance. Sit in the machine and lock yourself in position with the restraint. Take a comfortable grip on the handles and slowly straighten your arms to a point straight over your head. Then slowly reverse the motion to the initial starting point and repeat for the desired rep count.

Dumbbell Press, Seated or Standing

Emphasis. This versatile deltoid movement stresses the anterior and medial deltoid heads along with the triceps. Secondary stress is placed upon the posterior deltoids and other upper-back muscles.

Starting Position. Wear your belt and grasp two moderately heavy dumbbells. Sit on a sturdy bench with a supportive back for balance during the movement. Bring the dumbbells to your shoulders with a powerful and controlled effort. Rotate your palms so they are facing forward, and begin the movement with your upper arms pressed against the sides of your torso.

Movement Performance. Slowly push the dumbbells directly upward until they touch each other at a straight-arm's length directly above your head. Slowly lower the weights to the starting point and repeat the movement.

Variations. The use of dumbbells allows for variety and creativity when planning your workouts. For a change from conventional dumbbell presses, you can press with your palms facing each other instead of away from your body. You can also bring the posterior delts into primary stress buffers by performing a reverse dumbbell press in which your palms face back toward your body as in the top position of a completed dumbbell curl. Twisting the reverse press about halfway to being fully extended, so that at the top the dumbbells are facing back away from your body, is called the Arnold dumbbell press.

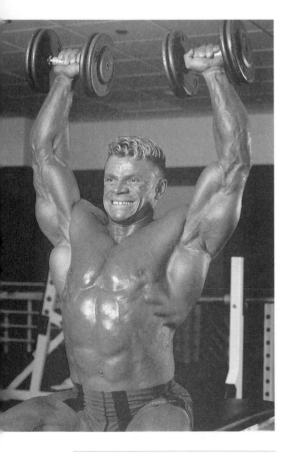

Roland Cziurlok (above)
Chris Cormier (opposite page, top)
Laura Bass (opposite page, bottom)

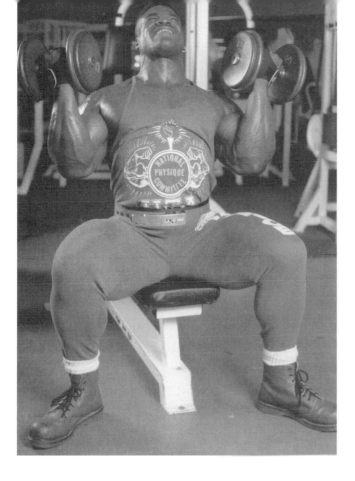 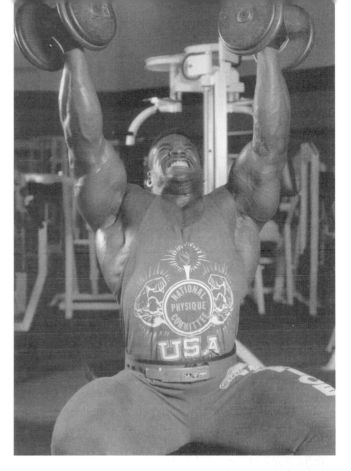

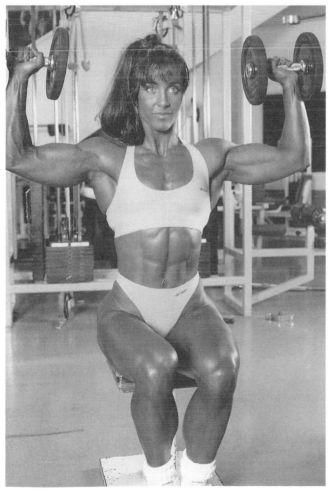 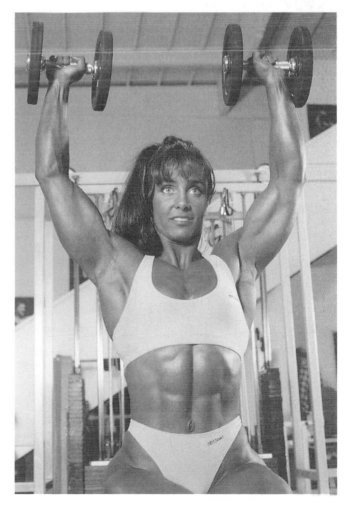

10

Chest

The large, fan-shaped pectoralis muscle group lies over the upper rib cage. Originating from attachments on the rib cage, it attaches via a large tendon to the humerus, or upper arm bone. The pectoral muscles contract to pull the humerus from a position with the elbow well behind the body to one in which the elbow is forward and well across the midline of the body.

By pulling your arm across the body at various points you can selectively stress different parts of your pec muscles. For example, pulling your arm across your torso below shoulder level stresses the lower portion of the pecs, while pulling it across your torso above shoulder level places greater stress on your upper pecs.

GENERAL CHEST-TRAINING POINTERS

Getting dumbbells off the floor and into the correct starting position to perform any type of dumbbell press or flye can be a chore and the ultimate joint wrecker.

For flat benches, assume a position at one end of a heavy-duty bench, dumbbells resting on end against the top of your thighs. Keeping your legs flexed toward your torso, roll backward onto the bench with your arms straight. This will bring the dumbbells to arm's length. To return to the starting point, simply draw or curl up your legs, placing your lower thighs against the ends of the dumbbells, and roll forward into an upright position.

The technique for incline dumbbell work is to assume the same position on an incline bench as in flat flyes or presses. The dumbbells are then lifted one at a time by lifting one knee at a time to a point where the dumbbell is resting at shoulder level. Repeat for the other arm.

Jean-Pierre Fux

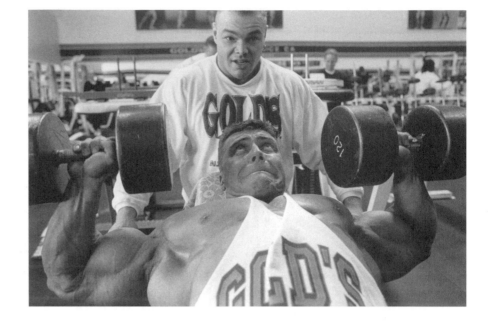

In the decline use of dumbbells, you should roll back from the initial starting point as in flat flyes or presses. Here you should have a training partner or spotter stand at either side. When you have completed your rep goal, the spotters can simply firmly grasp the appropriate weight at either end.

Bench Press

Comments. This exercise is responsible for the tremendous degree of chest development seen in today's champions. Bench presses are considered one of the best exercises for the upper body.

Emphasis. Benches strongly stress the pectorals (particularly the lower and outer portions of the muscle group), anterior deltoids, and triceps. Secondary emphasis is on the medial heads of the deltoids, the latissimus dorsi, and other upper back muscles that impart rotational force on the scapulae.

Starting Position. Load the bar on the bench's uprights to a moderately heavy weight. Lie back on the bench with your shoulder joints about three to four inches toward the foot end of the bench. Place your feet on the floor to balance your body on the bench as you do the movement. Take an overgrip on the bar with your hands set about two to four inches beyond shoulder width. Straighten your arms to remove the barbell from the rack and move it to a supported position directly above your shoulder joints.

Movement Performance. Making sure your elbows travel directly out to the sides, bend your arms and slowly lower the barbell from the sup-

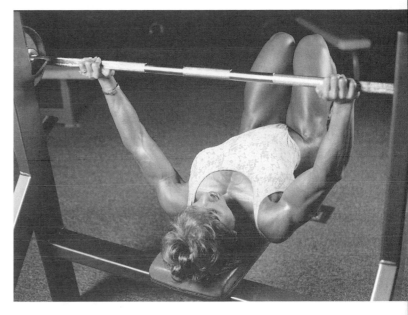

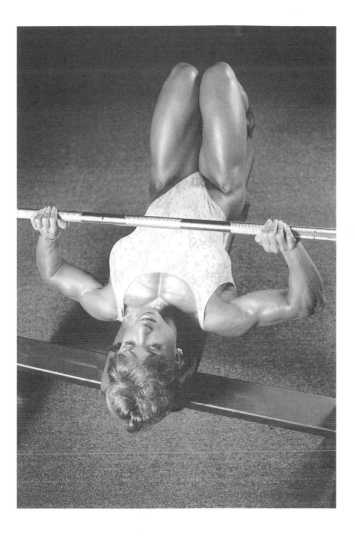

Laura Creavelle

ported position downward to lightly touch your chest two or three inches above the lower edge of your pectorals. Without bouncing the weight, slowly push it back to straight-arm's length. Repeat the movement until the desired number of reps.

Variations. The most common variation in this movement is moving your grip inward or outward. When you use a grip of less than shoulder width, you shift the stress more to the inner pectorals and triceps. A wider-than-normal grip places more stress on the outer pectorals and anterior deltoids. In addition to changing your grip, there are a number of other very effective twists on a conventional bench press. You might try using heavier than normal weights on a machine bench press because of the added leverage and decreased need for secondary muscle stabilization.

For those of you with sturdy joints, there are the always challenging dumbbell bench presses. With dumbbells, be extra careful regarding control and be well warmed up. The performance is basically the same as for barbells, once you have rocked the bells off the floor into the starting position.

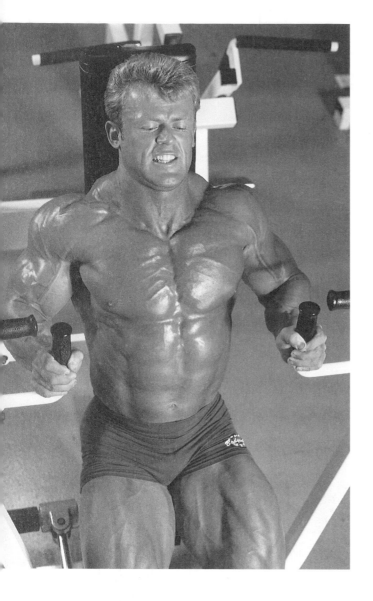
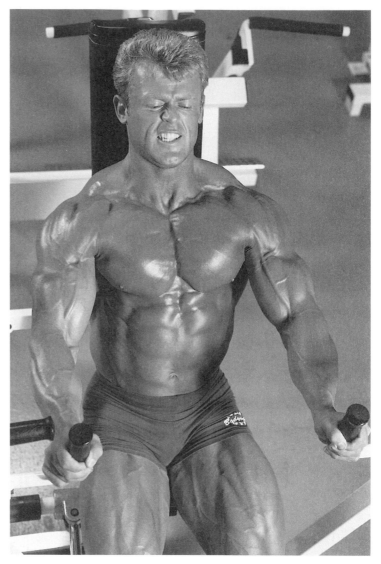

Art Dykes

An extra level of controlled smoothness and safety is provided by the Smith machine bench where the training technique is essentially the same as for conventional bench presses. Pay attention to the position of the safety catches on the Smith when training solo.

Incline Press

Emphasis. Incline presses performed with either a barbell, two dumbbells, or on a machine strongly stress the pectoralis major and minor, anterior deltoids, and triceps. Significant secondary stress is on the medial deltoids and the upper-back muscles that rotate the scapulae.

Starting Position. Place a barbell on the upright support racks at the tall end of the incline bench and adjust the weight on the bar to the

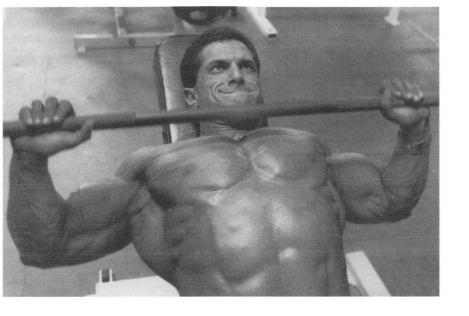

Joe Spinello

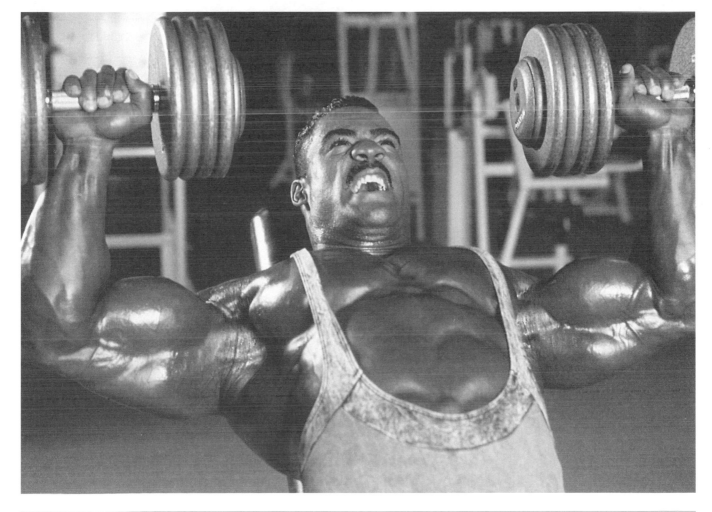

Don Long

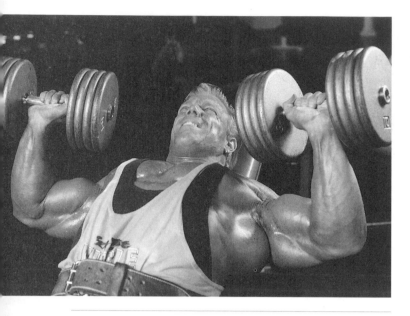

Dave Fisher

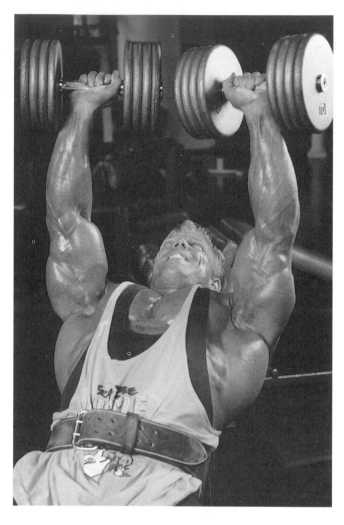

appropriate poundage. Sit on the bench's seat and lie back. Maintain a slight arch in your lower back and keep your feet firmly on the floor. Take an overgrip on the bar with your hands set three to five inches wider than shoulder width. Straighten your arms to remove the barbell from the rack and bring it to a supported position directly above your shoulder joints.

Movement Performance. Being sure to keep your elbows back as you do the exercise, slowly bend your arms and lower the barbell down to lightly touch your upper chest at the base of your neck. Without bouncing the bar off your chest, steadily push the barbell back to the starting point. Repeat the exercise for the desired number of reps.

Variations. As with bench presses, you can vary the width of your grip when performing incline barbell presses. If the gym you belong to is sufficiently large, there are likely to be a couple of differently angled incline benches. Using a different bench every so often will keep chest development massive and correctly proportioned. If you have trouble

Garrett Downing

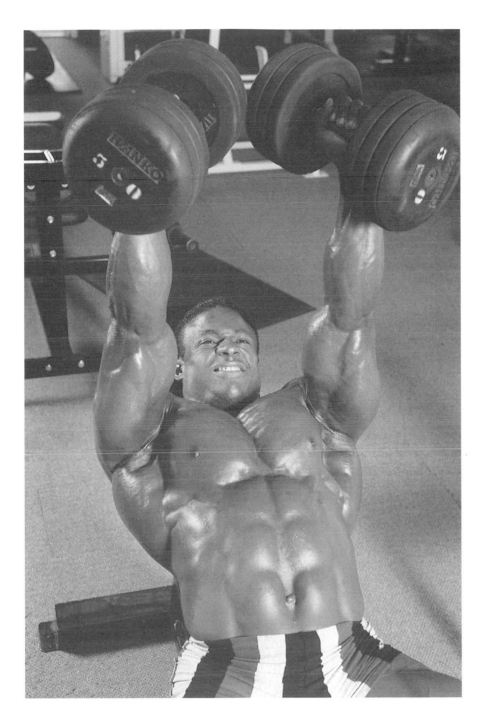

making the adjustment from flat benches to inclines, give some con
sideration to incline machine presses. The angle change can be tough
until you get the hang of it and the machine movement provides the
needed "groove."

Another similar variation of incline barbell presses, Smith Machine
inclines allow for even more incline angle adjustments. For an additional stretch, dumbbell incline presses are recommended but you
should use a spotter for extra safety.

Decline Press

Emphasis. Decline presses, whether performed with a barbell, dumbbell, or on a machine or Smith rack, strongly stress the lower and outer portion of the pectoralis major, anterior deltoids, latissimus dorsi, and triceps. Secondary stress is felt by the upper back muscles and medial deltoids.

Starting Position. Adjust the support racks on the decline bench so you will be able to rack the bar upon completion of the movement without any undue difficulty. Rest a barbell loaded to the appropriate

Edgar Fletcher

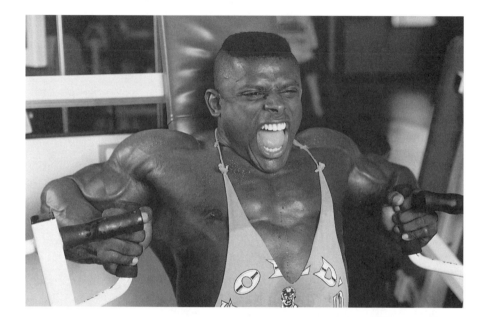

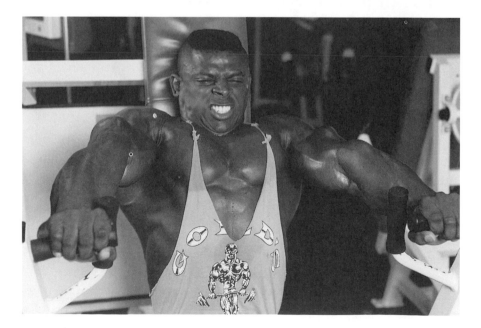

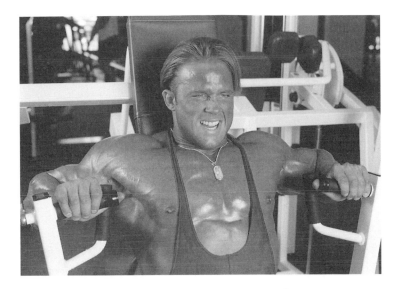 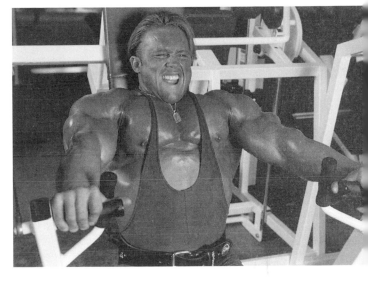

Craig Titus

weight on the supports and be certain to place collars on each end. Sit on the end opposite the support racks and hook your feet under the restraining bar. Carefully lie back, and without slicing your scalp open, slip your head under the bar and attain a slight arch to the lower back. Take an overgrip on the bar with your hands three to five inches wider than shoulder width. Straighten your arms to lift the bar off the racks and directly over the line of your shoulder joints.

Movement Performance. Keeping your elbows back, slowly bend your arms and lower the barbell down to touch the lower part of your chest at your pec line. Without bouncing, slowly push the weight back to straight-arm's length. Repeat the movement for the desired target.

Tips. Be sure to have a spotter at the rack end of the bench to protect against crude plastic surgery if you get stuck and can't lock out the weight. Remember, the only place the bar will roll is directly onto your neck and head.

Variations. As with both barbell bench presses and barbell incline presses, declines also lend themselves nicely to a number of variations, depending on your personal needs. There are decline machine bench presses, decline dumbbell bench presses, and declines on the Smith Machine. The instructions hold true for all three basic moves: benches, inclines, and declines. You may alternate your grip width as well.

Parallel-Bars or Machine Dips

Emphasis. This is an excellent upper body movement that stresses the pectoralis major and minor, anterior deltoids, and triceps with incredible

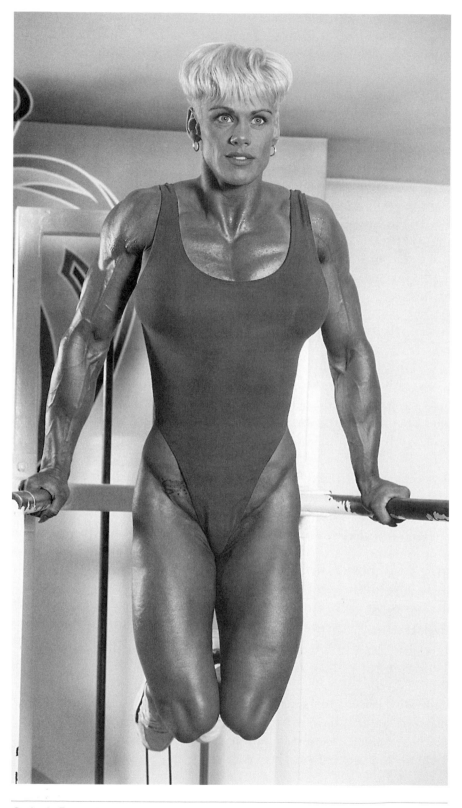

Cathy LaFrancois

intensity. The pectoralis emphasis is primarily on the lower and outer sections of the pecs. Secondary emphasis is on the medial deltoids and upper back muscles responsible for rotating the scapulae.

Starting Position. There are two different types of dipping bars. The first is a V-shaped design; the second is a parallel design. Regardless of the bars used, take a grip that will have your palms facing each other and jump up to support your body at arm's length above the bars. Bend your legs for body stability, place your chin on your chest, and incline your torso forward.

   Note: for more triceps development, perform your dips with the torso at a 90-degree angle to the floor without tipping the torso forward.

Movement Performance. Allowing your elbows to travel out to the sides, bend your arms and slowly lower yourself as far below the bars as possible. From the bottom point, slowly push yourself back up to where your arms are straight. Repeat for the required rep count.

Variations. Dips can be too difficult to perform for many novices because they cannot yet press their body weight. Cybex-type assisted or self-spotting machines provide a foot platform to stand on while performing the exercise. Instead of adding to the resistance, the foot platform acts as an adjustable counterbalance to your body weight. Some dipping machines have either a cable and waist-belt attachment or foot platform incorporated into their design.

   More advanced trainers who can perform too many dips with their body weight need to add to the level of resistance. Nautilus pioneered the use of a padded weight belt linked to an adjustable source of increased resistance. Even more elemental but also very effective is simply attaching a dumbbell to your lifting belt for more intensity.

Flat-Bench Dumbbell Flyes
Incline-Bench Dumbbell Flyes
Decline-Bench Dumbbell Flyes

Emphasis. When you perform flyes, you can isolate your triceps from the movement and place very direct stress on your pecs and anterior deltoids. Secondary stress is on your medial deltoids and triceps. You can select the area of your pectorals that you wish to stress by the angle of the bench you use for the exercise. When the bench is parallel to the floor there is slightly more work load on the lower pectorals. As the incline increases toward a 90-degree angle, the work load

Art Dykes

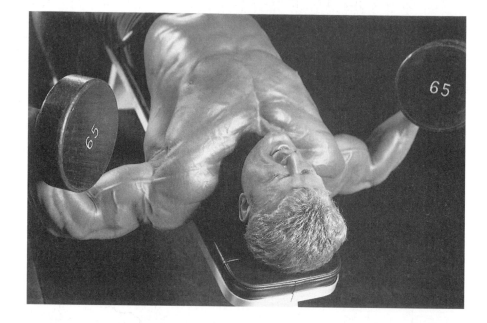

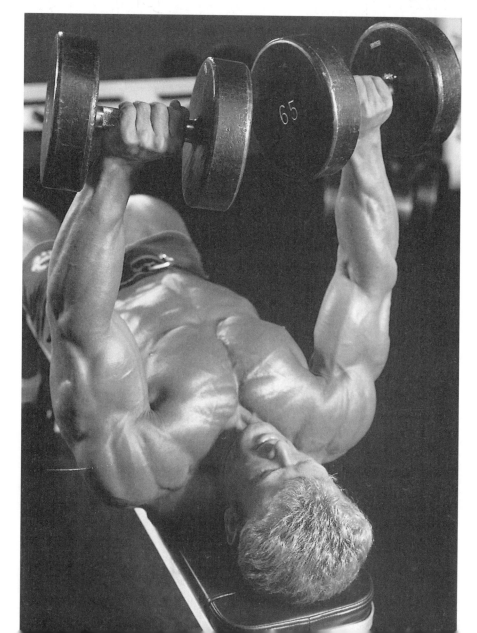

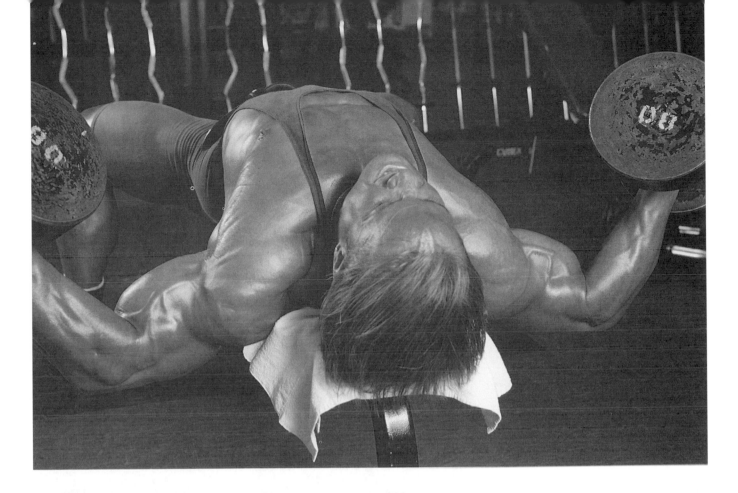

Craig Titus

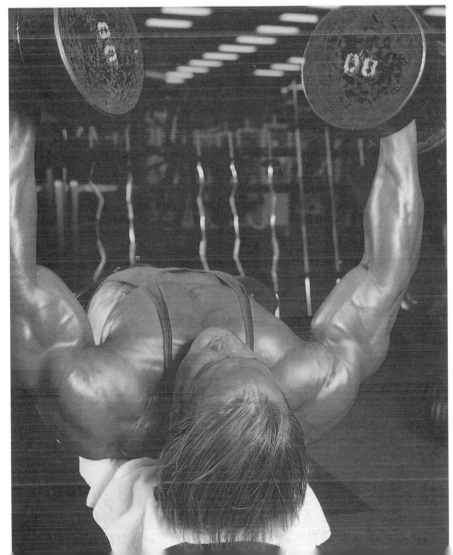

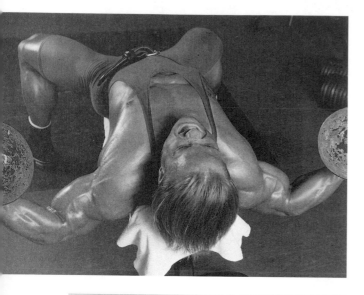

Craig Titus

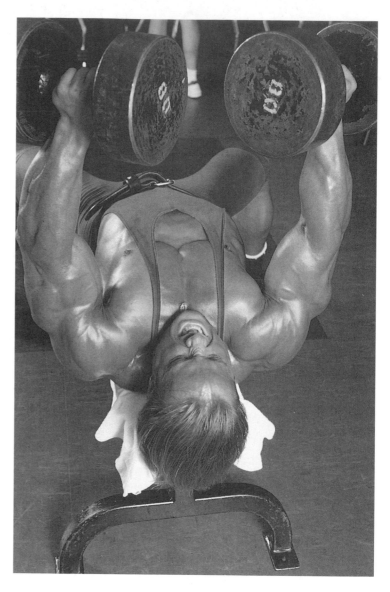

appropriately shifts to the upper chest and shoulder area. Likewise, as you lower the position of your head past parallel, the work is greatly increased in the lower pecs.

Starting Position. Grasp two appropriately heavy dumbbells and lie back on the bench. Bring the weights to straight-arm's length directly above your shoulder joints and rotate your wrists so your palms are facing each other. Bend your arms about 10 degrees and maintain this rounded-arm position throughout the movement.

Movement Performance. Being sure that your upper arms travel directly out to the sides, slowly lower the dumbbells in semicircular arcs to a low but comfortably stretched position. At the bottom level

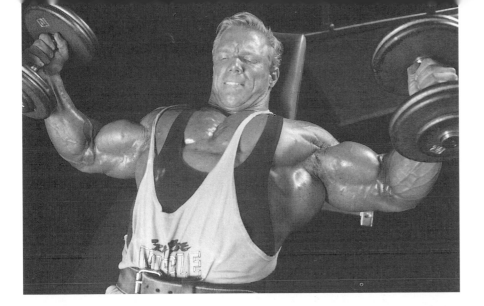

Dave Fisher

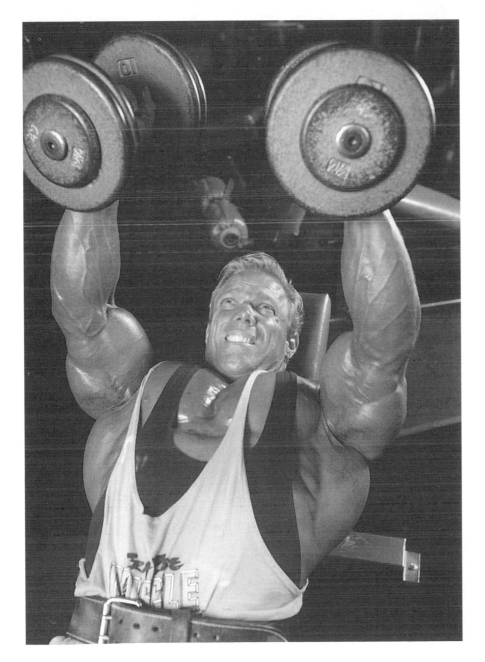

Laura Creavelle

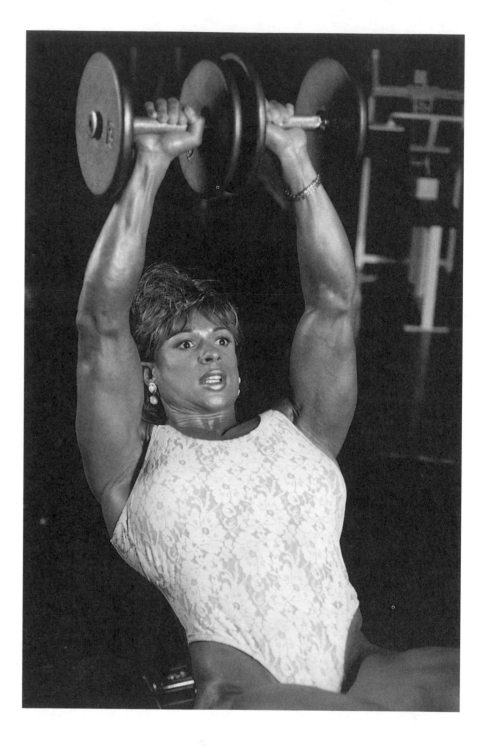

your elbows should be slightly below the level of your torso. Using just the power of your chest, slowly return the weights back along the same arc of travel to the starting point. Repeat for the targeted rep count.

Variations. As previously stated, elevating the incline of the bench you are using shifts the emphasis of work for the pecs. Additional variety and pec emphasis can be pursued with cable flyes or machine flyes.

Cable Crossovers

Comments. Many bodybuilders use crossovers to razor in deep grooves across the chest, especially right before contests.

Emphasis. Cable crossovers stress primarily the lower sections of the pectorals, plus the anterior deltoids.

Starting Position. Attach loop handles to the cables running through the high pulleys. Stand between the pulleys with your feet set about shoulder-width apart and grasp the two pulley handles. With your palms down throughout the movement, extend your arms upward at about a 45-degree angle in relation to the floor. Bend your arms slightly during the exercise.

Laura Creavelle

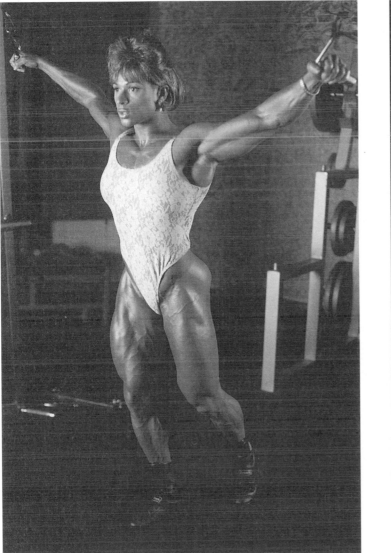

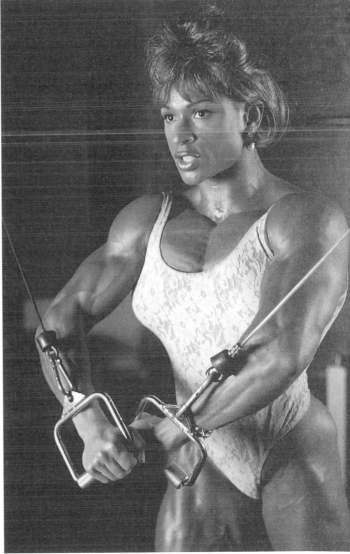

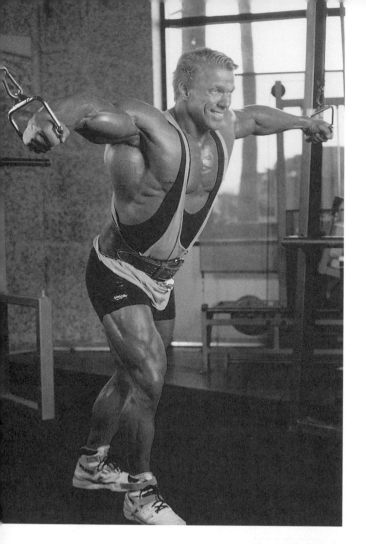
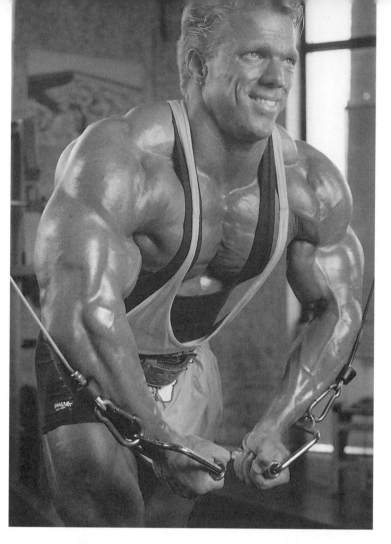
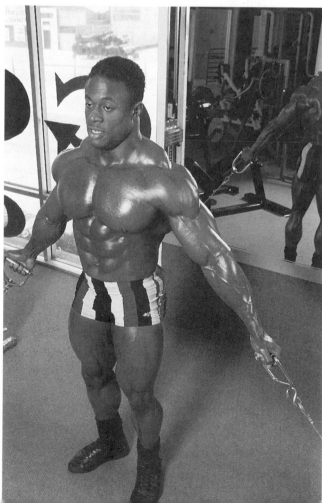
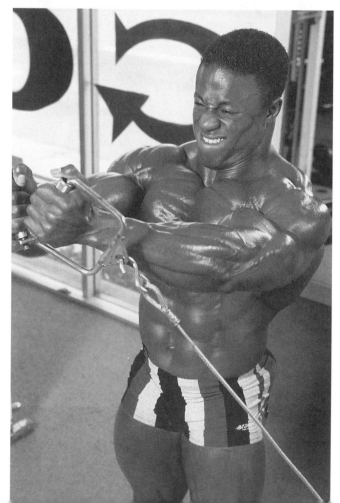

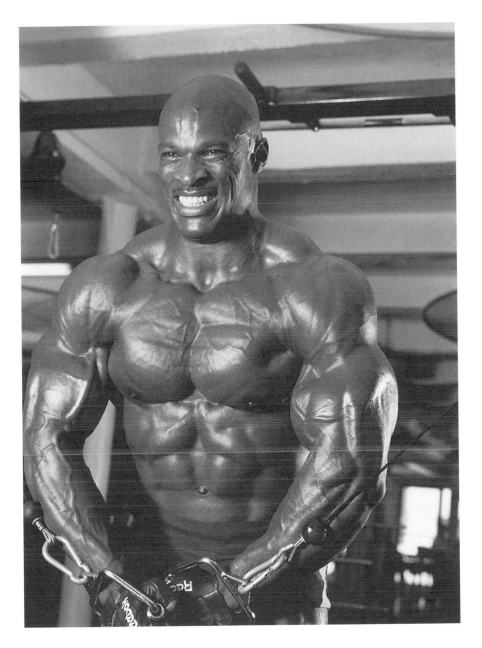

Dave Fisher (opposite page, top)
Garrett Downing (opposite page,
  bottom)
Ronnie Coleman (left)

Movement Performance. Use pec strength to move your hands downward and toward each other in semicircular arcs until they touch six to eight inches in front of your hips. Hold this position for a brief second, then allow your hands to slowly return to the starting point. Repeat for the desired number of reps.

Tips. Normally, your torso will be either erect or inclined slightly forward during this exercise, but it can also be performed in a standing position near parallel to the floor.

Pec Dec

Emphasis. This movement allows you to isolate stress on your pecs with only minimal involvement of the anterior deltoids. You'll find this movement particularly good for adding mass to the inner edges of the pectorals where they originate from the sternum.

Starting Position. Adjust the seat to a height that puts your upper arms parallel to the floor when you are sitting in the seat and have your hands resting over the top edge of the pads. Sit on the seat facing away from the weight stack and place your elbows against the padded surface, your forearms running straight up the pads, and your fingers curled over the top of the pads. Allow the weight to pull your elbow pads as far as comfortably possible to the rear.

Movement Performance. Use pec strength to push with your elbows against the pads, moving the pads forward until they touch each other directly in front of you. Hold this peak position for a split second, then allow the pads to slowly pull your elbows back to the initial starting point. Repeat for the desired rep count.

DB Across-Bench Pullovers

Emphasis. This movement strongly stresses the pectorals, latissimus dorsi, and serratus muscles.

Starting Position. Lay a moderately heavy dumbbell on its end about two feet from the center of a flat exercise bench. Lie crosswise on the center of the bench with just your upper torso in contact with the bench. Your feet should be about shoulder-width apart and placed flat on the floor to steady the body in position during the exercise. Reach over and place your palms flat against the inner sides of the top set of plates, with your thumbs around the dumbbell bar to keep the weight from slipping out of your hands. Pull the dumbbell up off the bench and bring it to a position supported at straight-arm's length directly above your chest.

Movement Performance. While maintaining your hips at a level slightly lower than the bench throughout the exercise, simultaneously lower the dumbbell downward in a semicircular arc behind your head and bend your arms at about 15 degrees. As soon as you have lowered the weight to as low a position as possible, return it back along the same arc to the starting position while straightening your arms. Repeat for the desired rep count.

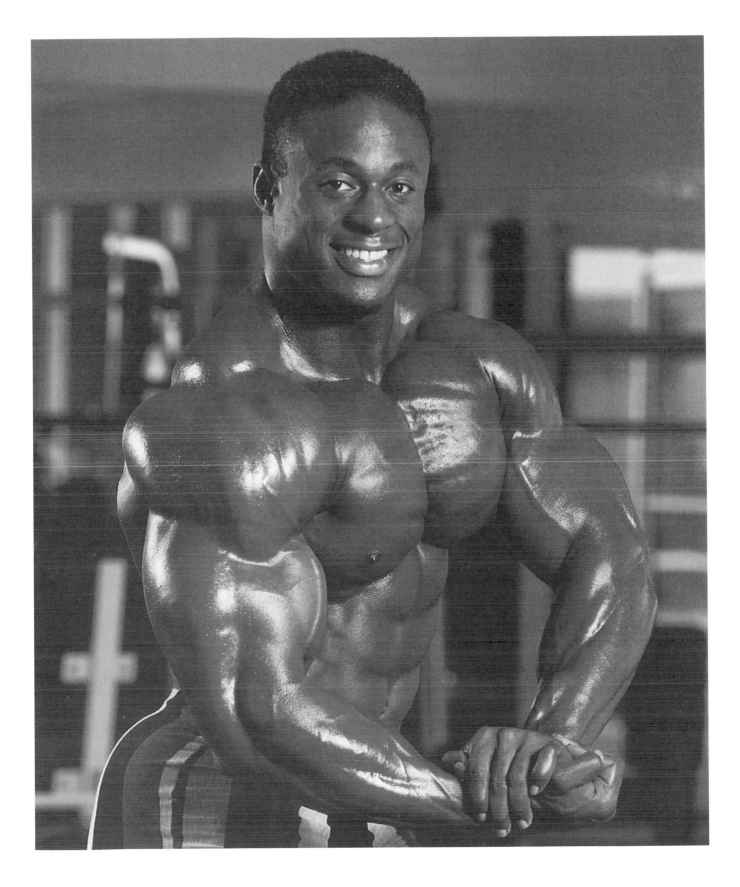

11

Biceps and Forearms

Standing Barbell Curls

Emphasis. The squat of biceps exercises, standing barbell curls are the most basic, and possibly the most effective, of all biceps movements. Not only do they strongly stress the biceps muscle but also the powerful flexor muscles on the inner sides of the forearm.

Starting Position. Take a shoulder-width undergrip on a moderately heavy barbell. In the starting position, this grip has the palms facing away from the body. With your lifting belt on and feet set about shoulder-width apart, stand erect with your arms hanging straight

Ronnie Coleman

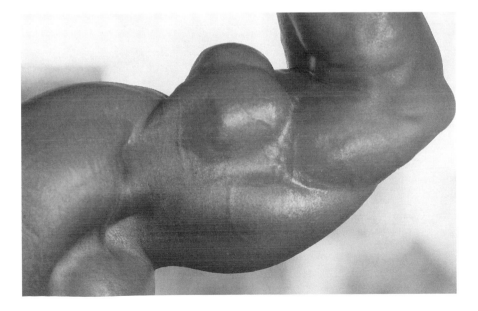

Drorit Kernes

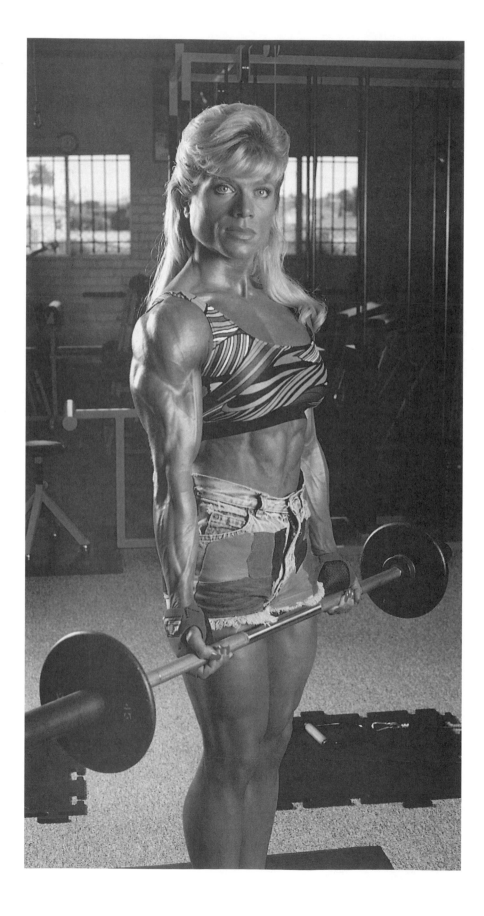

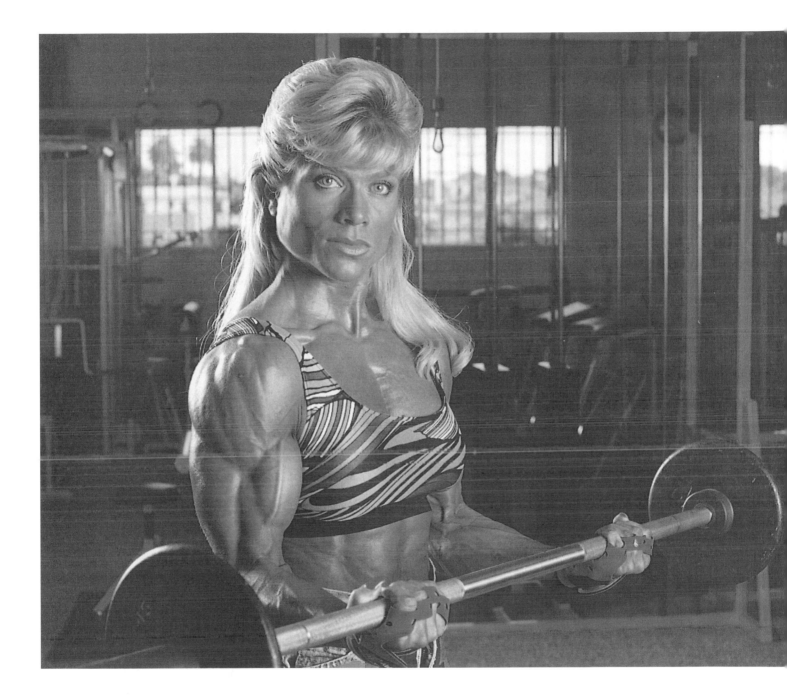

down at your sides and the barbell resting across your upper thighs. Press your upper arms against the sides of your torso and hold them in this position throughout the exercise.

Movement Performance. Moving only your forearms, use biceps strength to move the barbell across your upper thighs in a semicircular arc to a point just below your chin. For the entire movement, you should keep your wrists straight. Lower the weight slowly back to the starting point and repeat the movement.

Don Long

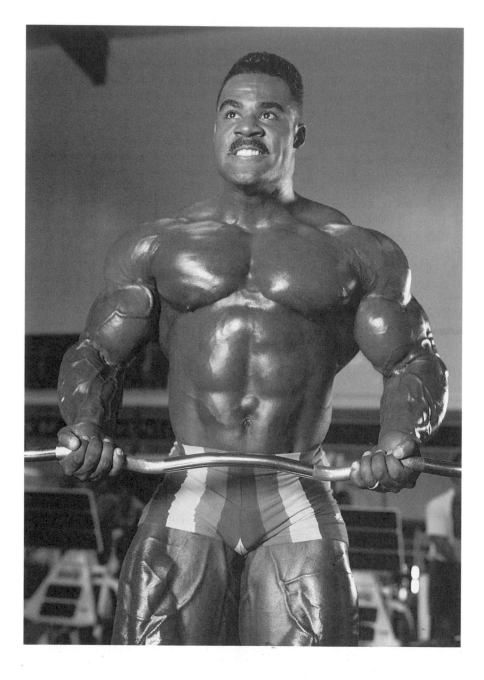

Tips. If there is any injury to the back, you may also perform the exercise while you lean against a sturdy pole or solid wall.

Variations. You can vary your grip over a wide range when doing standing barbell curls. You can use any width of grip from very narrow, with your hands actually touching at the bar's center, to one as wide as the bar allows.

There is also the EZ-curl bar, with its characteristic bends about shoulder width from the bar's center. The advantage to an EZ-curl bar is minimal discomfort for your wrists. The actual process of supinating your hands when curling can be somewhat troublesome if your wrists

Laura Bass

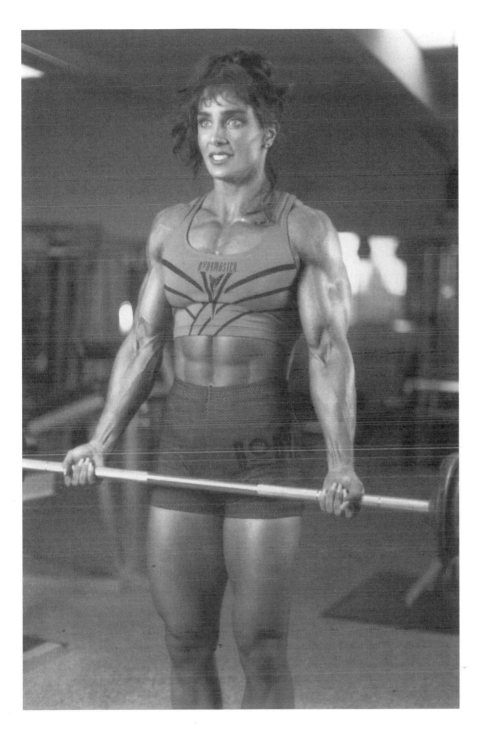

are sore or injured. The drawback to an EZ-curl bar is that, due to the lack of twisting to the wrists, there is no supination of the hand and hence far less potential for directly attacking the biceps. The odd-sounding exercise called drag curls involves the elbows being deliberately drawn backward and away from the sides of the torso. This is in contrast to the directions for regular curls, in which the elbows do not move. Finally, you may also choose to implement standing cable curls in place of barbell curls.

Machine Curls

Emphasis. The purpose of performing this movement is to take advantage of the high degree of biceps isolation machine curls yield. Minimal emphasis is placed on the brachialis and forearm flexors.

Starting Position. Adjust the seat so that when you have placed the backs of your upper arms against the pads, your arms hang comfortably on the area provided, with your hips and feet firmly secured in position. With a palms-up grip, grasp the handles so your arms are straight.

Movement Performance. Slowly curl the handles up toward your neck, contracting as fully as possible. Give a peak squeeze at the top of the movement, then slowly return down to the starting position. Repeat for the desired reps.

Tips. Be careful not to overextend (hyperextend) your elbows at the starting point or bottom of the movement.

Marika Johannson

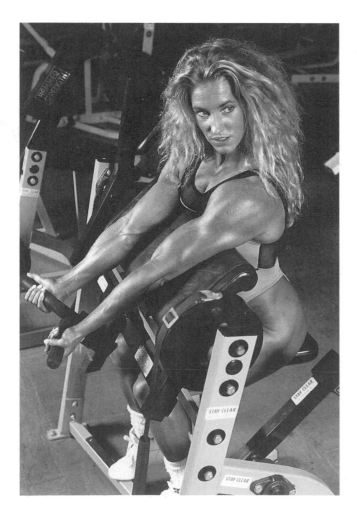
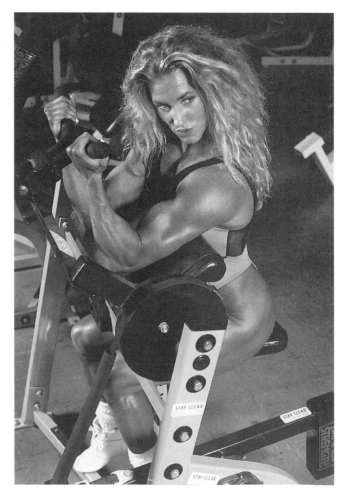

Dumbbell Concentration Curls

Emphasis. The entire biceps is stressed, with additional results seen in the center peak of the biceps.

Starting Position. Grasp a relatively light dumbbell in your left hand. Stand near a high, flat bench or dumbbell rack. Place your right hand on the bench or rack to brace your torso at about a 45-degree angle in relation to the floor. Hang your left arm directly down from your shoulder and straighten it completely. Be sure to keep your upper left arm completely motionless throughout the exercise.

Movement Performance. Being sure to fully supinate your hand, slowly curl the dumbbell up to your shoulder. Pause for a second in the peak contracted position. Lower the dumbbell back to the starting point, and repeat for the target rep count.

Variations. This exercise may be performed from a seated position, also known as seated concentration curls. For more variety, low cables may also be utilized with cable concentration curls.

Charles Clairmonte

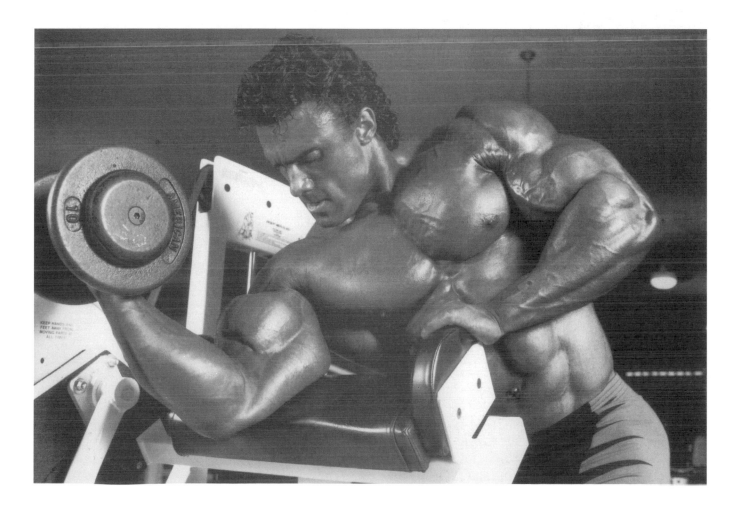

Overhead Cable Curls

Emphasis. This is a great movement for hitting the peak of your biceps as a primary target area. Second, work is performed by the brachialis and forearm flexors.

Starting Position. Attach a straight handlebar to an overhead lat machine and move a flat bench underneath. Position the bench so you can lie on your back under the pulley with your arms straight above the line of your shoulders. Take a narrow grip on the pulley bar and lie on your back on the bench, extending your arms directly upward toward the pulley. It's important to keep your arms motionless throughout the movement.

Movement Performance. Moving only your forearms, slowly curl the bar down to touch the base of your neck. Hold this peak contracted position for a moment, then allow the bar to slowly return to the starting point. Repeat for the desired number of reps.

Dave Hughes

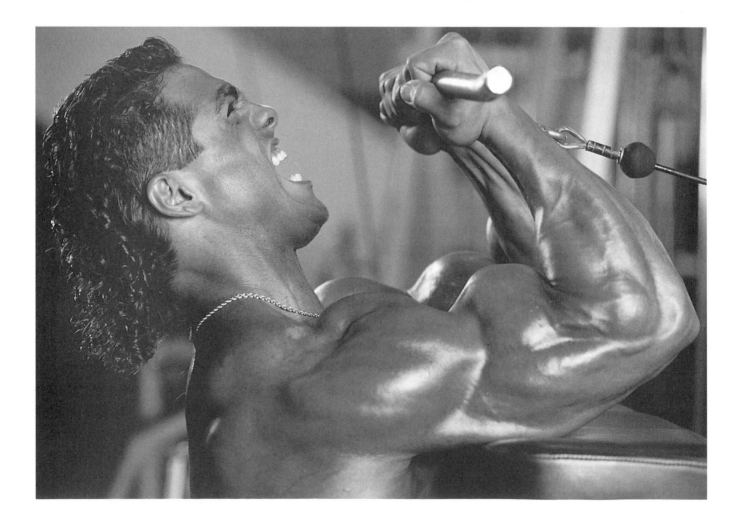

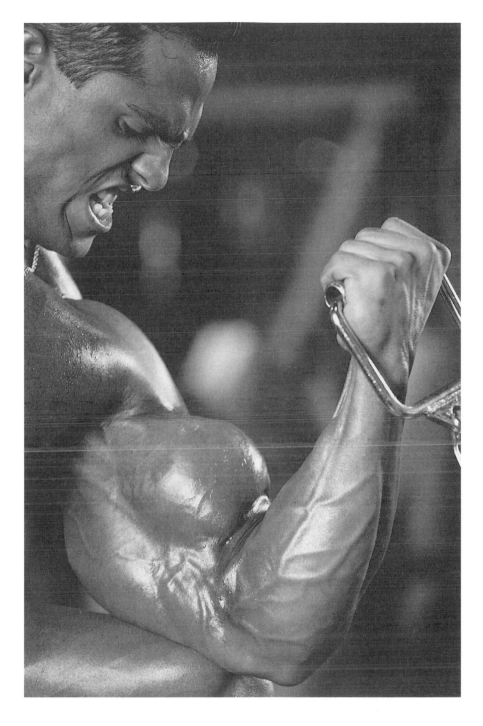

Variations. This may also be performed one arm at a time by using small single-hand cable handles.

Scott or Preacher Barbell Curls

Emphasis. All variations of this movement are tremendous for filling in the lower biceps. Secondary stress is felt by the brachialis and forearm flexors.

Darrin Lannaghan

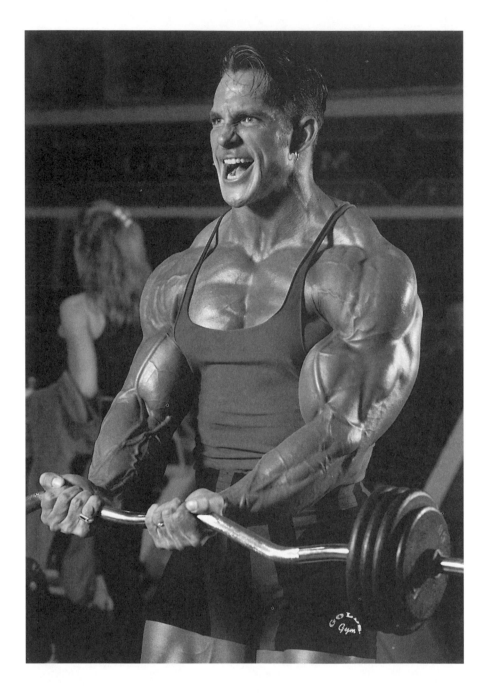

Starting Position. Take an undergrip on a barbell with your hands set slightly wider on each side than the width of your shoulders. Bend your arms fully, then lean over the top of a preacher bench and run your upper arms directly down the angled surface of the bench. Your forearms should be placed on the bench a little narrower than your width of grip on the bar. Slowly straighten your arms.

Movement Performance. Use your biceps strength to slowly curl the bar from the starting point to a position just at the base of your throat. Deliberately lower the weight back to the starting point and repeat for the desired rep count.

Ronnie Coleman

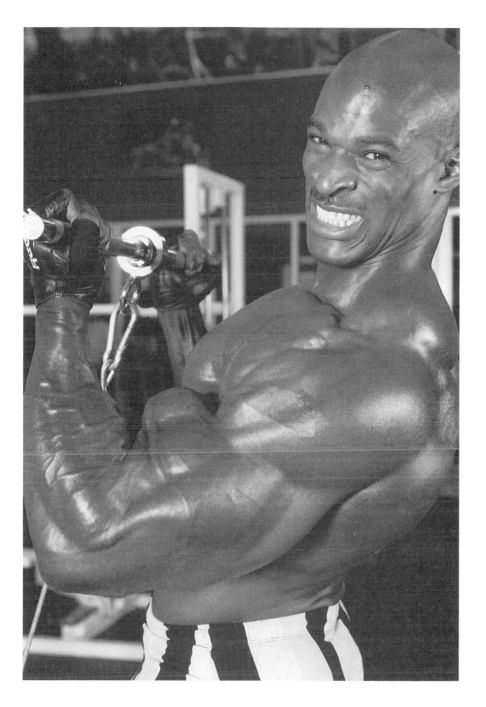

Tips. It is essential that you lower the bar back to the starting point in a slow, controlled, and deliberate manner. If you get sloppy and allow the bar to drop, you may be in for a blown bicep some day.

Variations. Many bodybuilders prefer to use an EZ-curl bar for this movement. Regardless of the bar used, you can vary the width of the grip considerably.

The reverse-grip Scott curl targets the brachialis and forearm flexors more than the biceps and may also be performed with dumbbells. Even cables can be incorporated when performing preacher curls.

Standing Dumbbell Curls

Emphasis. Dumbbell curls very effectively place major stress on the biceps muscle and secondary emphasis on the brachialis and forearm flexors.

Starting Position. Grasp two moderately heavy dumbbells, place your feet comfortably apart, and stand erect with your arms straight down at your sides and your wrists rotated so your palms are facing the sides of your legs. Keep your upper arms motionless throughout the entire movement.

Movement Performance. Slowly curl the dumbbells forward and up to your shoulders, simultaneously supinating your wrists so your palms face upward during at least the last half of the movement. Reverse the procedure to lower the dumbbells to the starting point and repeat.

Tips. You can curl one DB at a time, alternating one arm upward while the other is being lowered.

Seated Dumbbell Curls

Emphasis. This is essentially the same movement as standing dumbbell curls except for an even stricter isolation of the arms during the exercise.

Starting Position. You may choose to sit at the end of any sturdy flat bench. If you are without any shoulder injury, try assuming a position on the incline bench for even more radical impact on the arms.

Movement Performance. Follow basic sequence as in standing dumbbell curls.

FOREARMS

Barbell Wrist Curls with Hands Up and Down

Emphasis. Performing this exercise with your palms facing upward stresses the flexor muscles of your forearms. Alternatively, when the palms face downward, the extensor muscles come into primary play.

Starting Position. Take a shoulder-width undergrip on a moderately heavy barbell and sit at the end of a sturdy flat bench. Place your feet shoulder-width apart and run your forearms down your thighs so your

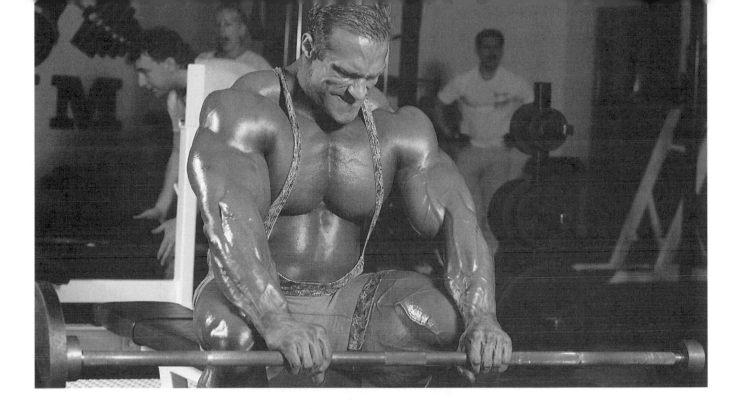

Mike Francois

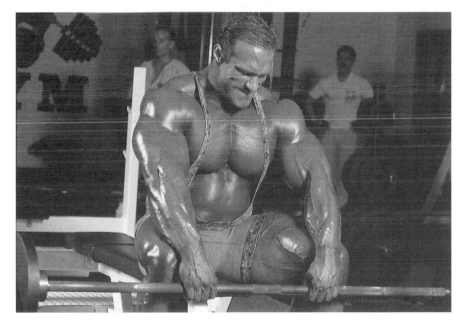

wrists and hands dangle off the ends of your knees. Allow the weight to pull your wrists downward as far as possible.

Movement Performance. Using forearm strength, flex your wrists and curl the barbell upward as high as possible in a small semicircular arc. Lower the weight back to the starting point and repeat the exercise for the target reps. Reverse the initial arm position to hit the other side of the forearm.

Variations. This exercise may also be performed with a dumbbell.

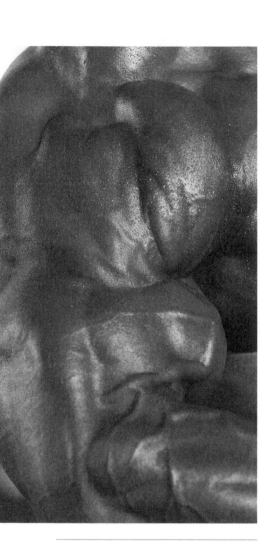

Ronnie Coleman

Standing Reverse Barbell Curls

Emphasis. Reverse curls place primary stress on the brachialis and supinator longus muscles. Secondary work is performed by the biceps.

Starting Position. Take a shoulder-width overgrip (opposite of regular barbell curls) on a barbell. Place your feet a comfortable distance apart and stand erect with your arms hanging straight down at your sides and the barbell resting across the front of your thighs. Press your upper arms against the sides of your torso and hold them in this position throughout the movement. You should also keep your wrists straight throughout the exercise.

Movement Performance. Moving only your forearms, slowly curl the barbell in a semicircular arc from the starting point to a position just beneath your chin. Slowly lower the barbell back along the same arc to the starting point and repeat the exercise for the desired rep count.

Variations. As in regular curls, you can utilize an EZ-curl bar.

Dumbbell Hammer Curls

Emphasis. This is a brachialis and forearm flexor stressing version of the conventional dumbbell curl.

Starting Position. Grasp two moderately heavy dumbbells, place your feet about shoulder-width apart, and stand erect with your arms running straight down at your sides. You should rotate your hands so your palms are facing the sides of your thighs. Keep your hands parallel to one another throughout the exercise.

Movement Performance. Slowly curl the dumbbells up to the level of the front delts, then lower back to the starting position. Repeat for your rep goal.

12

Triceps

The triceps brachii on the back of your upper arm is a three-headed muscle that contracts to straighten your arm from a bent position. You can direct more stress to the inner head, outer head, or medial head by holding your hands in different positions and doing specific triceps exercises that seem to stress one head more than the others. If you read this chapter, carefully noting the emphasis sections, you can selectively train your triceps heads to create any triceps development you want.

Close-Grip Bench Press

Emphasis. Close-grip bench presses stress the entire triceps brachii muscle complex in conjunction with the pectorals and anterior deltoids.

Starting Position. Load a bar lying on a bench-press rack with an appropriate poundage. Lie on your back with your shoulders about three inches ahead of the support uprights and place your feet flat on the floor to balance your body on the bench. Take a narrow overgrip on the bar—about six inches between thumbs. Straighten your arms and lift the bar off the rack to a supported position directly above your shoulder joints.

Movement Performance. Bend your arms and slowly lower the barbell down to touch the middle of your chest. Without bouncing the bar off your chest, slowly press it back to straight-arm's length. Repeat the movement for the rep goal.

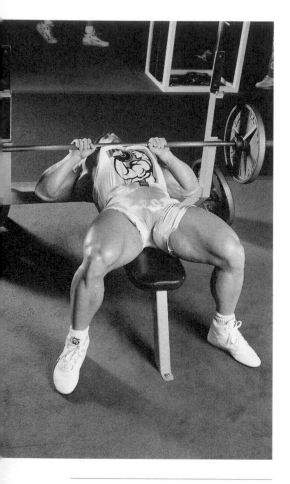

Phil Hernon

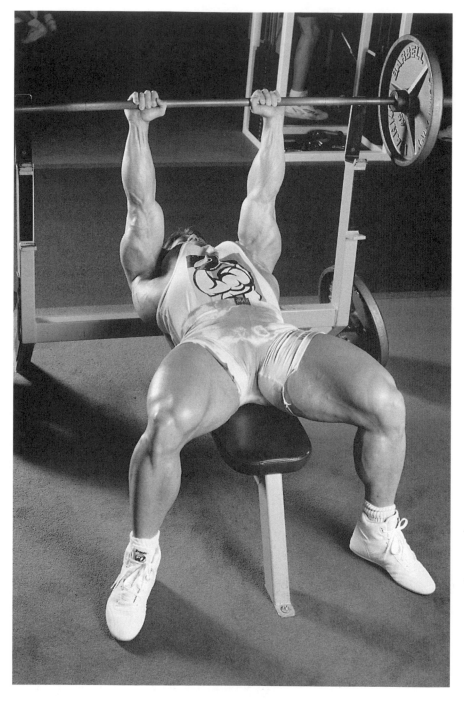

Tips. You can also use an EZ-curl bar to take some strain off the wrists.

Variations. The Clark reverse-grip bench press is an extreme form of triceps attack. The reversal to an undergrip, as if doing a barbell curl, seems to blast away at the triceps like nothing else. Anthony Clark, "The World's Strongest Man," regularly performs this movement with more than 700 pounds.

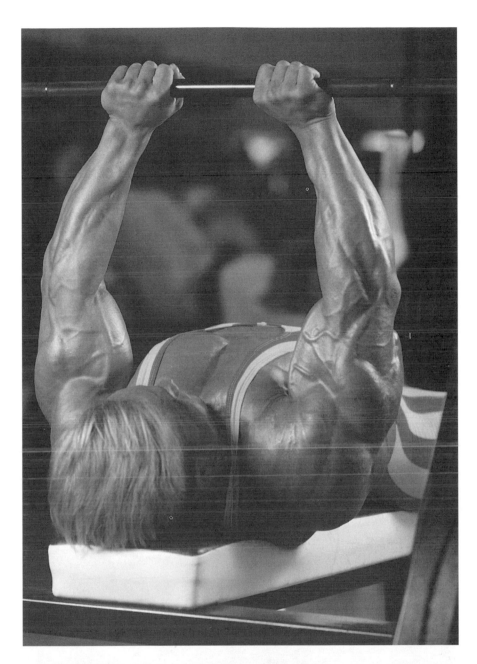

Craig Titus

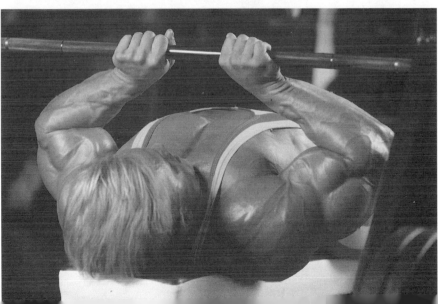

Triceps Bar Dips

Emphasis. When performed in the manner described in this section, parallel-bar dips place very strong stress on your triceps. Secondary work is performed by your pectoral and anterior deltoid muscles.

Starting Position. Jump or step up on a set of parallel bars with your palms facing inward and your arms straight to support your body. You can bend your legs slightly, but be very careful to keep your torso in as upright a position as possible throughout the movement. Allowing

Matt Cline

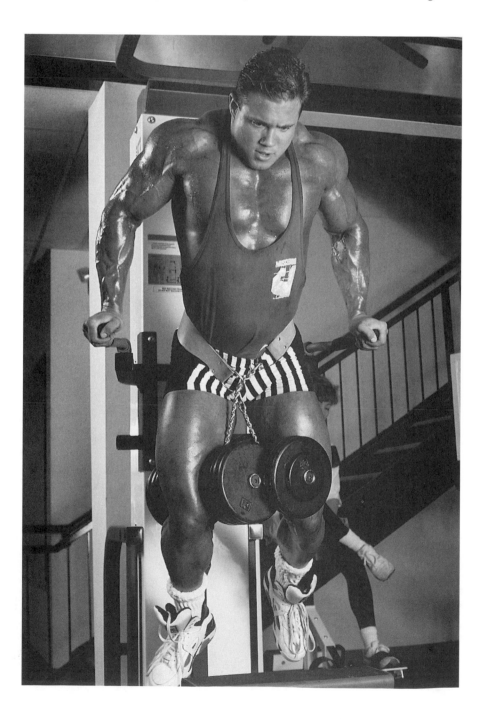

your torso to incline forward will shift too much emphasis to the pectorals.

Movement Performance. Keeping your upper arms close to your torso, slowly bend your arms and lower your body as far down as possible. Push yourself back up to the starting point. Repeat until desired reps are completed.

Variations. Variations include machine dips.

Bench Dips

Emphasis. This movement is great for working the outer and medial heads of the triceps, with secondary emphasis on the inner head.

Starting Position. Place two flat exercise benches about three feet apart. Put your feet on one bench and your hands on the other. Your hands should be about six inches apart, your fingers pointed toward your toes. Straighten your arms completely.

Edgar Fletcher

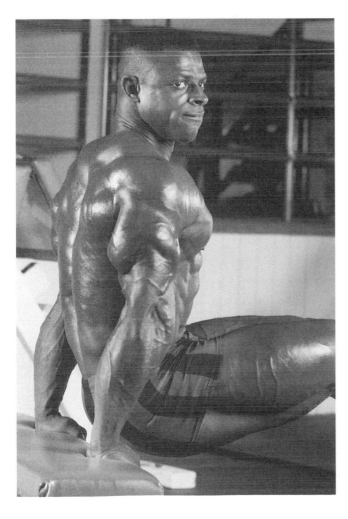
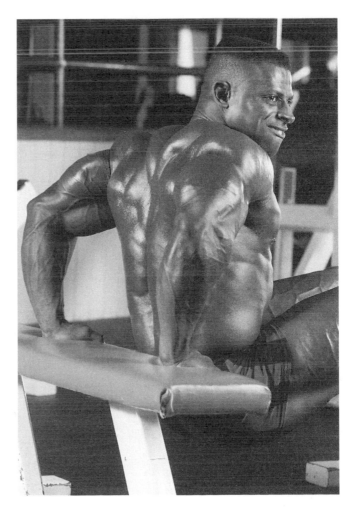

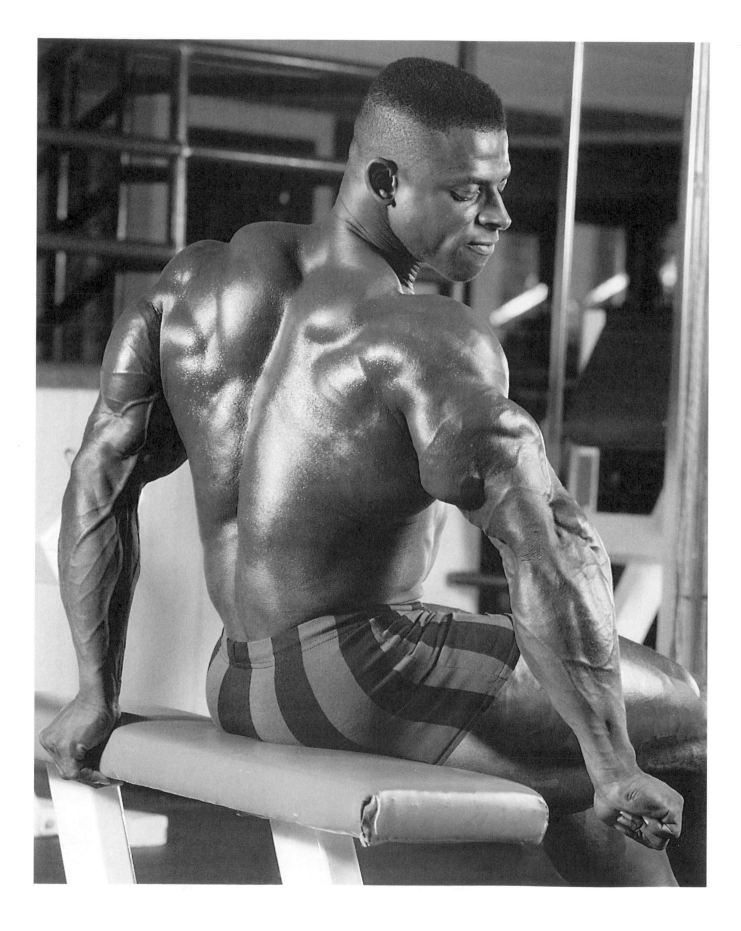

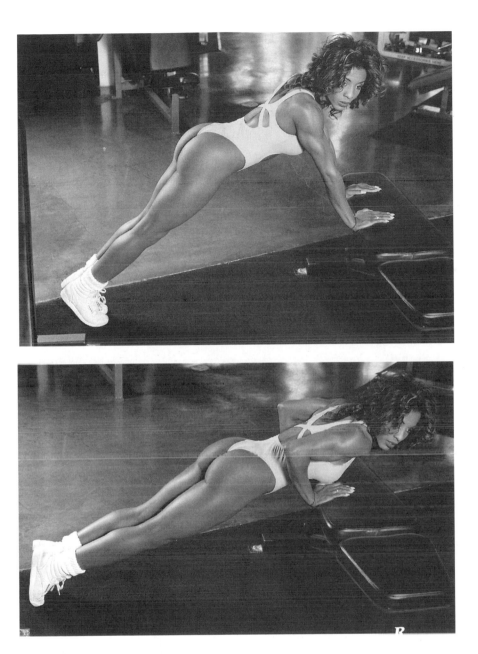

Movement Performance. Slowly bend your arms as far as possible, lowering your body down between the benches. Slowly push back up to the starting point and repeat for the desired reps.

Tips. You can add resistance to this exercise by having a spotter place a barbell plate across your lap.

Flat-Bench Barbell Extensions

Emphasis. This is a great triceps brachii isolation movement that primarily stresses the inner and medial triceps heads.

Note: due to the leverage factors of the elbow joint, you must always thoroughly warm up before training your tris with even moderate weights.

Starting Position. Take a narrow overgrip in the middle of a barbell handle (there should be about six inches between your index fingers). Lie back on a flat exercise bench, position your feet flat on the floor to balance your body in a secure position, and extend your arms straight up from your shoulders.

Movement Performance. Keeping your upper arms motionless, slowly bend your arms and lower the barbell in a semicircular arc from the starting point to your forehead. After lightly touching your forehead with the bar, use triceps strength to push it back along the same arc to the starting point. Repeat the movement for the desired rep scheme.

Variations. For a different attack plan on the triceps, you can make use of dumbbells or an EZ-curl bar. These are also known as skull crushers and French presses.

Incline or Decline Barbell Extensions

Emphasis. This movement is similar to flat-bench extensions but is performed on either an incline or a decline bench. Both variations of the exercise place primary stress on the inner and medial heads and secondary stress on the outer triceps brachii head.

Dave Hughes

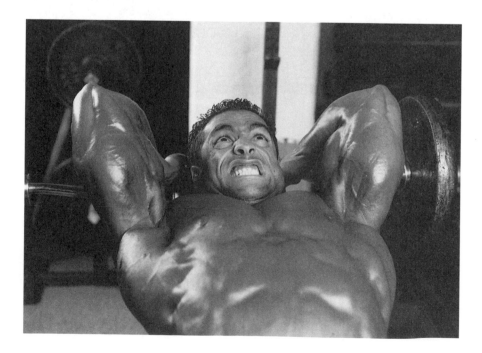

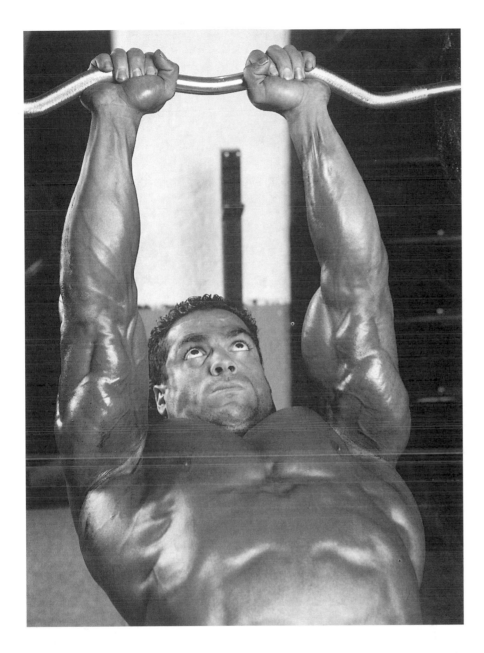

Starting Position. Take a narrow overgrip in the middle of a barbell handle (about six inches between index fingers). Lie back on the bench, extending your arms straight overhead until they are perpendicular to the floor.

Movement Performance. Keeping your upper arms motionless, slowly bend your arms and lower the barbell in a semicircular arc. Use triceps power to push the barbell back along the same arc to the starting point and repeat for the desired number of reps.

Variations. Pulley equipment allows you to perform the exercise as incline or decline cable extensions.

Standing Barbell Extensions

Emphasis. Standing triceps barbell extensions place primary stress on the inner and medial triceps brachii.

Starting Position. Take a narrow overgrip in the middle of a barbell handle (there should be about six inches between your index fingers). Place your feet a little wider than shoulder width, bring the barbell to a directly overhead straight-arm position, and stand erect.

Dinah Anderson

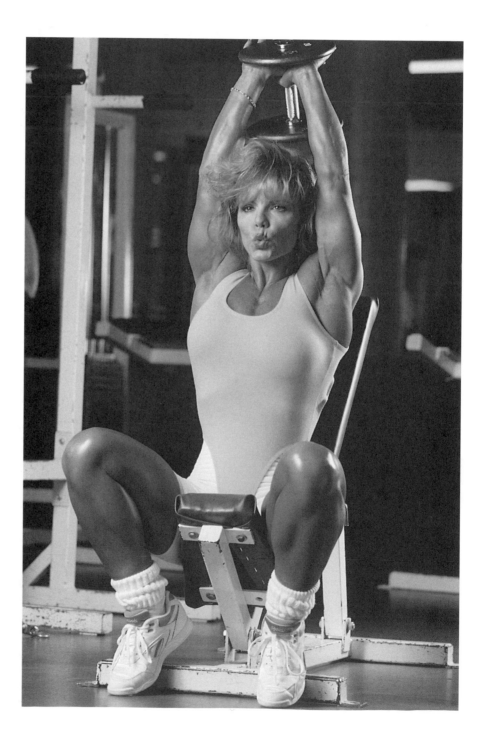

Movement Performance. Keeping your upper arms motionless and close to your ears, bend your arms and slowly lower the barbell downward in a semicircular arc behind your head until your arms are fully bent. Use triceps strength to return the barbell along the same arc to the starting position and repeat until reps are completed.

Variations. One particularly effective variation is dumbbell extensions, performed by placing your palms flat against the insides of the upper set of plates on a dumbbell. Circle your thumbs around the dumbbell's bar to prevent slipping. These may also be performed one arm at a time. You can perform standing cable extensions by attaching a long cable to a rope-type handle and bringing the ends of the rope handle to a point directly overhead, as in conventional barbell extensions.

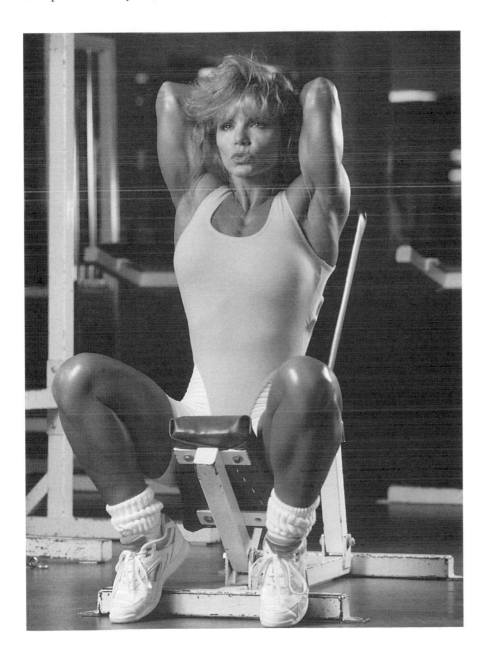

Dumbbell Kickbacks

Emphasis. Dumbbell kickbacks are an excellent outer- and medial-head developer of the triceps group.

Starting Position. Grasp a light dumbbell in your right hand with your palm toward your body throughout the entire movement. Split your left foot forward and right foot slightly to the rear. Bend over until your torso is parallel to the floor and place your left hand on a flat bench to maintain this torso position. Pin your right upper arm to the side of your torso with your upper arm parallel to the floor. Bend your right arm at a right angle.

Movement Performance. Slowly straighten your right arm, hold that position for a split second to intensify the peak contraction effect, lower back to the starting point, and repeat for the target rep goal.

Variations. You can also do this movement with two dumbbells. The low cable pulley allows for cable kickbacks.

Machine Extensions

Emphasis. The best-designed equipment provides tremendous targeted stress on all three heads of the triceps brachii.

Starting Position. Adjust the seat according to the manufacturer's instructions. Place your elbows securely against the pads provided. Place your wrists against the upper pads and sit with your back straight.

Aaron Maddron

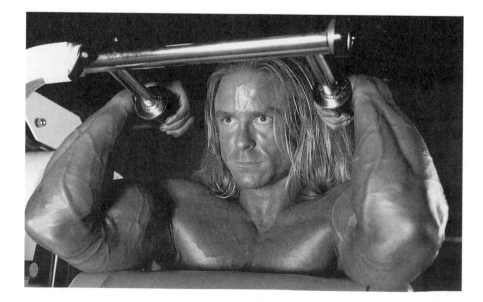

Movement Performance. Using your triceps power, slowly straighten your arms by pushing against the pads with your wrists. At full extension, begin to reverse the direction of travel while resisting with the strength of your triceps. Lower back to the starting point. Repeat for the targeted rep number.

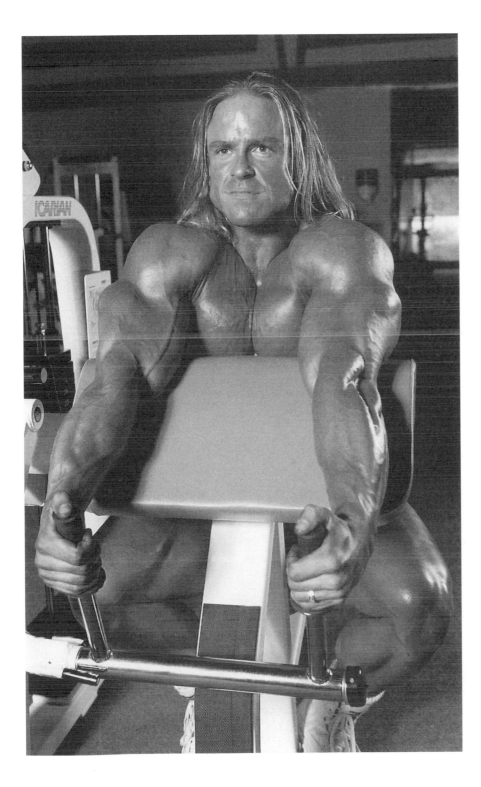

Triceps Cable Pushdowns

Emphasis. This is one of the best movements for developing the outer head of your triceps brachii. Secondary emphasis is placed on the medial and inner heads.

Starting Position. Attach a short-angled handle to the end of a cable running through an overhead pulley. Take an overgrip on the handle with your hands as close together as possible. Step back about a foot from the pulley, bend your arms fully, press your upper arms against your torso throughout the movement, and lean slightly toward the cable.

Ronnie Schweyher

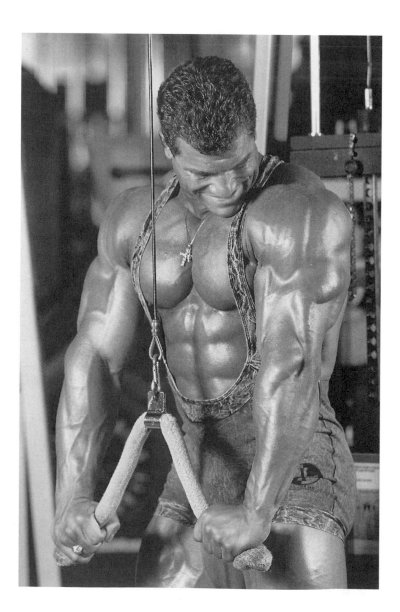

Movement Performance. Moving only your forearms, slowly push the handle downward in a semicircular arc until it rests across your upper thighs and your arms are locked straight out. Slowly return the handle to the starting position and repeat until satisfied with your reps.

Variations. A rope handle is sometimes used to do this exercise. The straight handle may be substituted for the angled one. Reversing your grip to an undergrip is called reverse cable pushdowns.

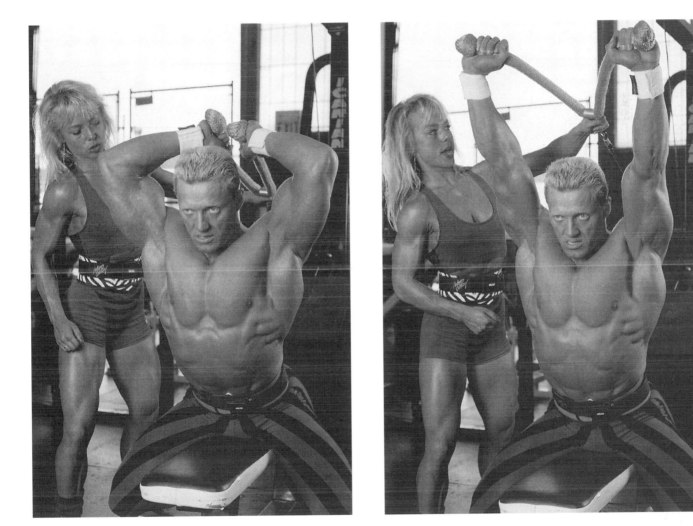

Nanna Bjone and Svend Karlson

13

Calves

There are two major muscle groups in your calves, plus one along the front of your shins. The largest lower-leg muscle is the gastrocnemius, which looks like an inverted heart on the upper part of your lower leg. The gastrocnemius contracts to extend your foot and toes. Beneath the gastrocnemius is a wide, flat muscle called the soleus, which also helps to extend the foot, but which can only be fully contracted when your leg is bent. And running over your shinbone is the tibialis anterior muscle, which contracts to flex your foot and toes toward your knee.

Standing Calf Raises

Emphasis. This movement allows you to very strongly stress the gastrocnemius muscles.

Starting Position. Wear your lifting belt. Stand up to the machine and bend your legs enough to solidly position yourself under the two pads that fit over your shoulders. Place your toes and the balls of your feet on the calf block or board with your feet set about a foot apart. Simultaneously stand erect while straightening your knees so the weight stack is supported by the pads on your shoulders. Now allow your heels to slowly descend into a fully stretched position.

Movement Performance. Pushing with your toes, rise up as high as possible on your toes, descend back to the starting point, and repeat for the target reps.

Tips. Do not bounce, thinking how cool you look with all that weight. In the long run, calf bouncers have bird legs. Always make certain to

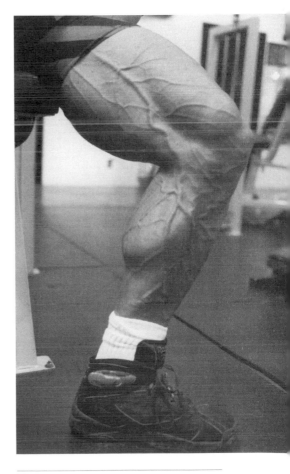

Jim Quinn

Sammy Iaonnidis

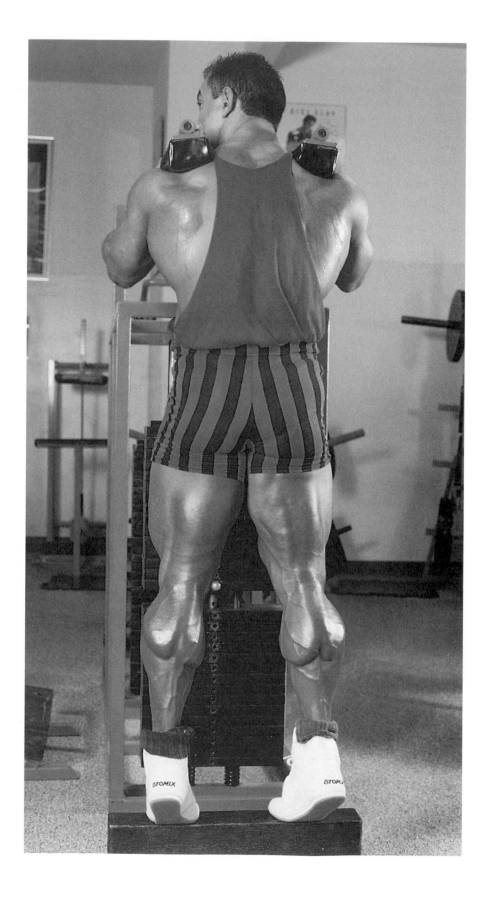

fully stretch all muscle groups, especially calves, with full-range training motions.

Variations. Be sure to vary both the width of your foot placement and the angle of your feet on the board or block.

Donkey Calf Raise with Partner

Emphasis. This is an excellent exercise for placing direct stress on the gastrocnemius muscles of your calves.

Starting Position. Wear your lifting belt. Place a calf block about two feet back from a flat exercise bench. Place your toes and the balls of your feet on the calf block and bend over to place your hands on the bench. This will maintain your torso in a position parallel to the floor as you work through this move. To provide the required stress for your calves, have a training partner sit just behind the point where your lifting belt fits and place his or her hands on the backs of your delts for balance. Now allow your heels to slowly drop down into a fully stretched position.

Movement Performance. Pushing with your toes, rise up as high as possible on your toes, descend back to the starting point, and repeat for the target reps.

Variations. Be sure to vary both the width of your foot placement and the angle of your feet on the board or block.

Hack-Machine Calf Raises

Emphasis. This is a tremendous move for your gastrocnemius, but it can be next to impossible if you are more than six feet tall.

Starting Position. This exercise is a little difficult to get the hang of. Stand on the angled foot platform of a hack squat machine, facing the padded back rest. Place your shoulders under the pads. Straighten your body and stand erect with a slight arch to your lower back. Move your feet back to the edge of the platform and slowly allow your heels to drop into a full stretch as in calf stretches.

Movement Performance. Pushing with your toes against the edge of the platform, rise up as far as possible to a point of peak contraction. Squeeze at the top and allow your feet to travel back into the full bottom stretch. Repeat for the targeted rep range.

Variations. Be sure to vary both the width of your foot placement and the angle of your feet on the board or block.

Machine Donkey Calf Raises

Emphasis. This is another excellent exercise for placing direct stress on the gastrocnemius muscles of your calves without the need for a training partner.

Starting Position. Adjust the machine's hip–lower-back pad to your frame. Assume a bent-over-at-the-waist position with your forearms resting on the higher set of pads in the front. The bottom edge of your lifting belt should be in contact with the hip–low-back pad. With a slight bend to your knees, rise up on your toes, which will lift the weight stack from a resting position. Maintain an arched lower back. Now slowly allow your heels to drop into a full stretch as in calf stretches.

Movement Performance. Push down with your toes to move the weight. Rise up as high as possible without bouncing and give a squeeze for peak contraction. Slowly reverse the movement and lower heels back to the starting position. Repeat for the target rep range.

Reverse Calf Raise on Block

Emphasis. This exercise hits the tibialis anterior muscle.

Starting Position. Place a calf board or block about two feet away from a pole or other sturdy upright. Stand with your heels on the board with your front toes straight ahead. Grab the pole firmly.

Movement Performance. Draw your toes as far toward your shins as possible, while balanced on your heels. Perform the movement slowly and deliberately, looking for a mental lock with the targeted muscles.

Leg Press Calf Raises

Emphasis. This move is performed on a 45-degree-angle, slide-type leg press machine. These are great for the gastrocnemius muscles.

Starting Position. Take your position as for regular leg presses but slide the balls of your feet and your toes to the bottom edge of the foot platform. Straighten your legs to raise the weight stacks along the slides.

Keep your knees slightly bent throughout the movement. Now slowly allow your heels to drop into a full stretch as in calf stretches.

Movement Performance. Extend your feet by pushing with your toes against the bottom edge of the platform. Push to a point of full extension for peak contraction. Slowly reverse the direction of movement, all the time pushing against the platform with your toes. It is important to take full advantage of the eccentric or negative portion of this exercise. Once a full bottom stretch has been reached, repeat for the target rep range.

Variations. Be sure to vary both the width of your foot placement and the angle of your feet on the platform edge.

One-Leg Dumbbell Calf Raises

Comments. Many consider this exercise the most phenomenal calf-stretching move.

Emphasis. This exercise provides tremendous movement for blasting away at your gastrocnemius muscles.

Starting Position Grasp an appropriately heavy dumbbell in your right hand, place the toes and ball of your right foot on a calf board or block, and with your left hand, grab a sturdy pole or upright for balance. Your left leg should be bent to keep it out of the movement. Now slowly allow your heel to drop into a full stretch as in calf stretches.

Movement Performance. Pushing with your toes, rise up as high as possible on your toes, descend back to the starting point, and repeat for the target reps. Do an equal amount of reps with your left leg, using your right arm to balance.

Tips. You can easily give yourself forced reps at the end of a set by pulling with your balancing arm.

Seated Calf Raises

Emphasis. This is one of the best soleus exercises.

Starting Position. Sit on the seat facing the knee pads. Place the ball of your foot and toes on the toe plate attached to the machine. Then place the pads over the top of your knees and adjust to a snug fit. Push down on your toes to raise up the weight and release the weight catch. Now slowly allow your heels to drop into a full stretch.

Movement Performance. Rise up on your toes as high as you can, then slowly return to the starting point. Repeat for the target rep range.

Variations. Be sure to vary both the width of your foot placement and the angle of your feet on the toe plate.

Sammy Iaonnidis

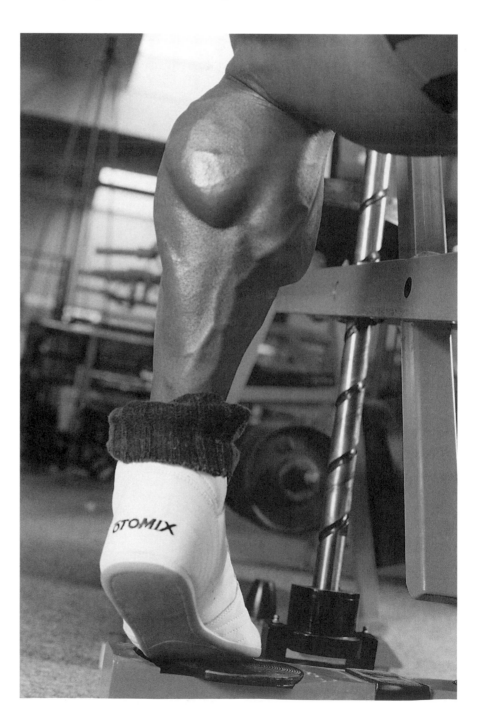

14

Abs

There are three muscle groups in the abdominals. The first of these is the rectus abdominis, the wall of muscle that covers the front of the abdomen and gives your abs a washboard appearance. The rectus abdominis helps flex your torso forward at the waist. When it contracts, it pulls your hips toward your shoulders.

The second important muscle group is the obliques at the sides of the hips. This group is usually called the external obliques, although there are really three layers of muscle, including the external, internal, and transverse oblique muscles. The obliques contract to bend your torso to the side and help you twist your torso in relation to your hips.

The final muscle group is the intercostals, which run diagonally across your sides above the obliques. Your intercostals run from the top of your obliques up to the serratus muscles of your chest, and they contract to help flex your body at the waist and twist your torso in relation to your hips and legs.

Leg Raises

Emphasis. All leg-raise movements stress the entire front abdominal wall, particularly the lower sections of the rectus abdominis.

Starting Position. Lie on your back on an adjustable abdominal board with your head toward the upper end of the board. Reach back and grasp either the roller pads or the edges of the board to secure your body in position as you do the exercise. Bend your legs slightly and keep them bent throughout your set in order to keep undue stress off your lower back.

Movement Performance. Use abdominal strength to move your feet in a semicircular arc from the bench to a point directly above your hips.

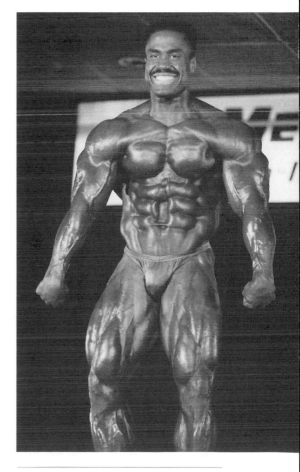

Mike Ashley

Return your feet slowly back to the starting point and repeat for the desired reps.

Tips. By not touching your heels to the board at the bottom of each rep, you have accomplished half your goal of keeping continuous tension on your front abdominals. The other half of the key to continuous tension is raising your legs only to the point where your thighs are at a 45-degree angle with the floor.

Variations. Bench leg raises are performed while lying back on a flat bench and holding the sides of the bench or support uprights to steady your torso in a secure position during the exercise. The advantage to bench leg raises is that you can lower your feet below the level of the rest of your body to increase the range of motion.

Reverse Crunches

Emphasis. Reverse crunches place tremendous stress on the entire front abdominal wall, but particularly the lower section of your abs.

Debbie Kruck and Lee Apperson

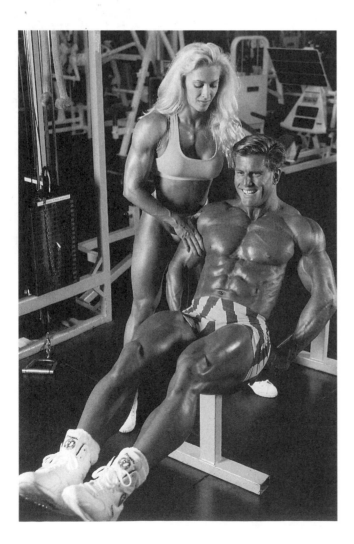
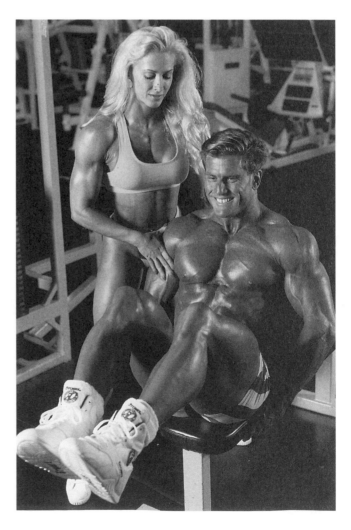

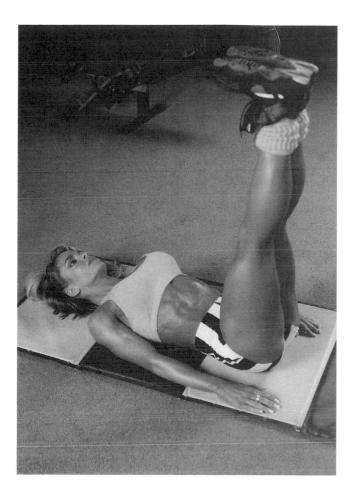 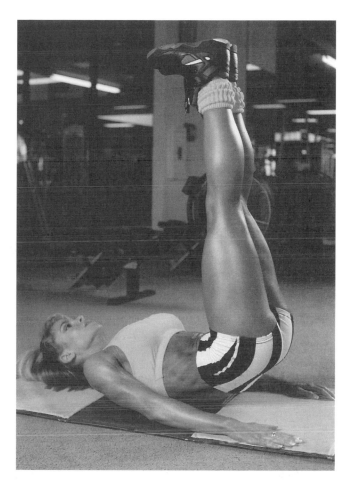

Starting Position. Lie back on the end of a flat bench as if performing a bench-press movement. Instead of reaching for the bar, grasp the uprights just below the rests for the bar. Your head should be about six inches from the uprights. Extend your legs straight out in front of you so they are parallel to the floor.

Amy Fadhli

Movement Performance. As if rolling into a ball, draw your knees toward the uprights while simultaneously rolling upward and back, with your hips following your knees. At the point of tightest contraction, hold for a split second, then reverse the direction and slowly return to the starting point. Repeat the sequence for the desired rep count.

Hanging Frog Kicks

Emphasis. Hanging frog kicks provide tremendous tension to your lower abdominals.

Starting Position. Use a stool or jump to grasp a chinning bar with a shoulder-width overgrip. Hang your body straight down from the bar.

Kim Nix

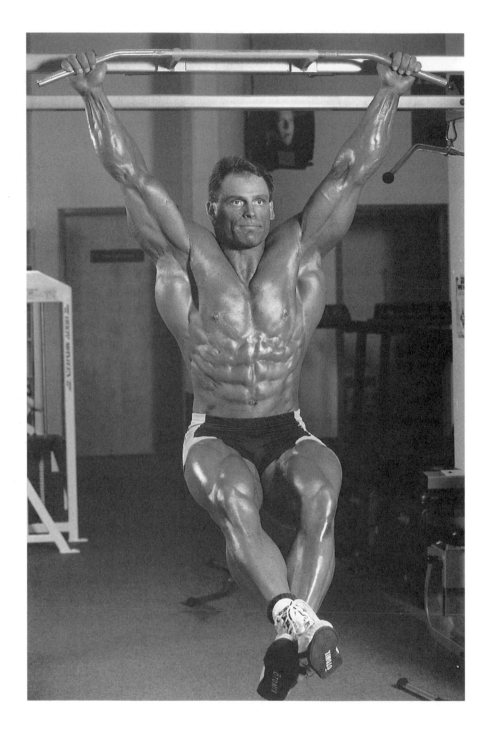

Movement Performance. Pull your knees toward your chest as far as possible, with your legs fully bent. Hold this top position for a second, lower back to the starting point, and repeat.

Tips. Lifting straps may be very useful here due to the need to maintain your grip while supporting your entire body weight. The straps will prevent your grip from giving out.

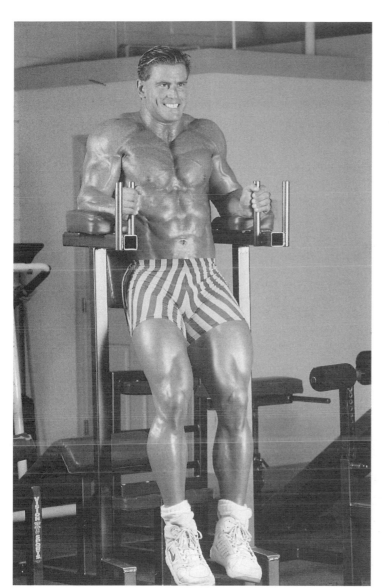

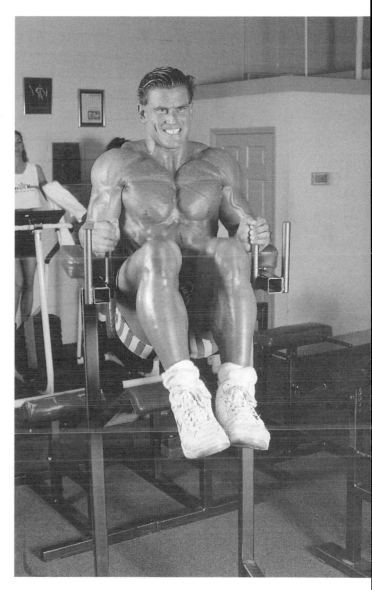

Lee Apperson

Variations. Additional work is forced on to your intercostals by twisting from side to side on successive reps. If your legs are strong in the hip-flexor area, try some reps with them held straight out in front of you as in leg raises.

Floor Crunches

Emphasis. Crunches of any type are some of the most direct exercises for stressing the front abdominal wall, particularly the upper section of your rectus abdominis.

Starting Position. Lie on your back on the floor with your lower legs over a flat bench, your thighs perpendicular to the floor. Place your hands behind your head and neck and hold them there.

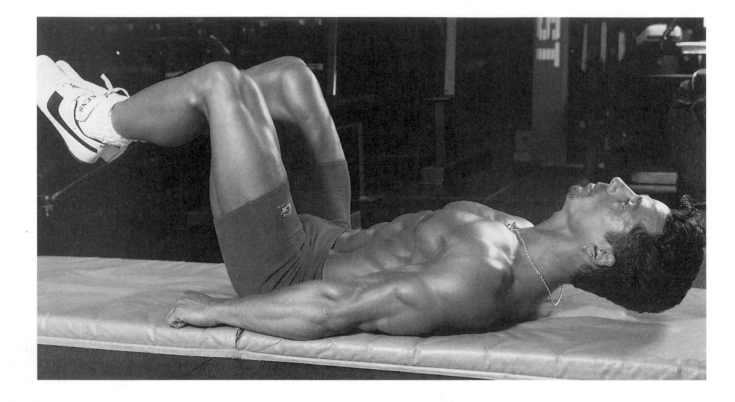

Larry Gonsalvez

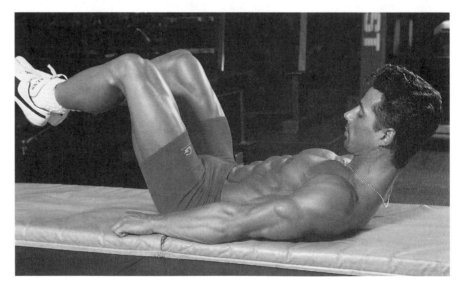

Movement Performance. You must do four things at once to perform crunches:

- Force your shoulders toward your hips.
- Use lower abdominal strength to raise your hips from the floor.
- Use upper abdominal strength to raise your head and shoulders off the floor.
- Forcefully blow out all your air.

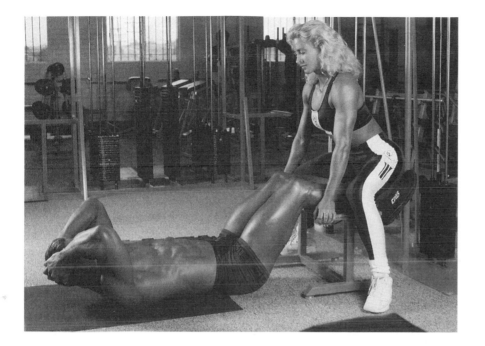

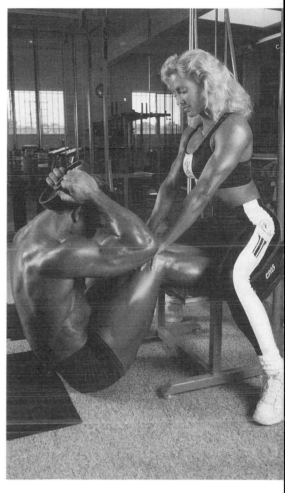

When you perform these four tasks, you will feel a very powerful contraction in your front abdominal wall. Hold this contraction for a brief moment, lower back to the starting point, and repeat the exercise.

Variations. You can perform wall crunches in which you lie on the floor with your glutes in the corner formed by the floor and wall, with your legs running straight up the wall. The many designs found in the generically termed "ab crunch rollers" offer advantages for both novices and experienced bodybuilders who need a change of pace.

Debbie Kruck and Lee Apperson

Rope-and-Cable Crunches

Emphasis. Rope-and-cable crunches stress the entire front abdominal wall, particularly the upper section of the rectus abdominis. Secondary work is performed by the serratus and intercostal muscles.

Starting Position. Attach a rope handle to an overhead cable and grasp the two ends of the rope extending down from the cable in your hands. Kneel down about a foot back from the weight stack and extend your body toward the pulley.

Movement Performance. You must simultaneously perform three tasks in order to do an effective rope-and-cable crunch:

- Bend over at the waist until your forehead touches the floor.
- Do a small, pullover movement to bring your arms from an

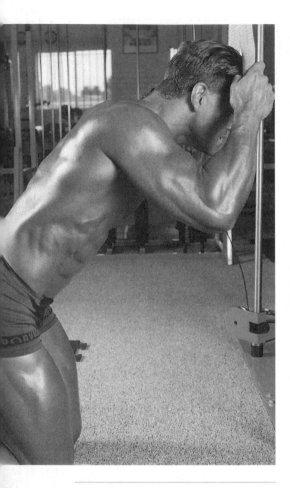

Lee Apperson

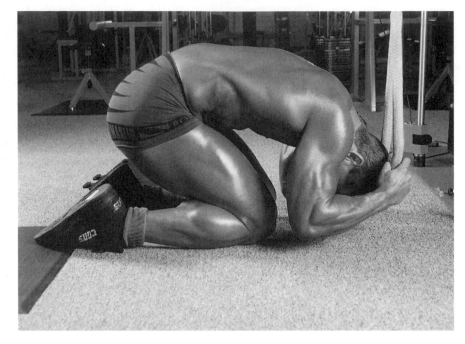

extended position to one in which they are bent at 90-degree angles and your hands are near the floor just in front of your head.

• Forcefully blow out all your air.

When you perform these three tasks, you will feel a strong contraction in your abs. Hold this contraction for a second, and return to the starting point. Repeat for the desired rep count.

Variations. This movement can be performed with one arm at a time, but be sure to keep the reps balanced on both sides.

Machine Crunches

Emphasis. Machine crunches allow for a convenient method of adding resistance to the exercise. As in crunches, the upper abs are stressed, but even more than with body weight alone.

Starting Position. Sit on the seat and adjust according to your frame. Hook your feet under the restraints as provided. Reach back and grasp the handles of the machine. Put your chin to your chest at the starting point of the movement.

Movement Performance. Perform the crunch movement as previously described, hold the point of peak contraction for a second, return to the starting point, and repeat.

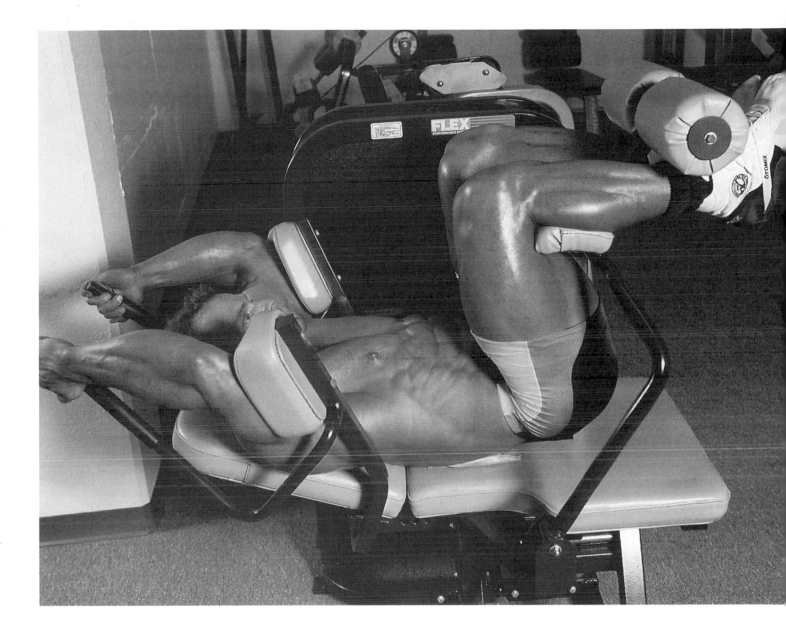

Variations. As opposed to grasping handles, some manufacturers utilize a set of upper-chest pads you place your chest against to provide a point of contact with the machine.

Kim Nix

Roman-Chair Sit-Ups

Emphasis. Roman-chair sit-ups stress the entire front abdominal wall, particularly the upper section of the rectus abdominis muscle group.

Starting Position. Sit on the bench facing the toe-restraint wedge and place the front portion under the pads. Cross your arms over your chest and keep them in this position throughout the movement.

Movement Performance. Recline backward with your torso until it is at approximately a 30-degree angle with the floor. Sit forward only until you feel tension come off your abs, then move back to the low position. Rock back and forth along this short range of motion for the desired rep count. Actually try to perform as if you were folding your torso around an imaginary bar halfway up the front of your abs.

Variations. This exercise may also be executed with a side-to-side twisting motion.

Laura Creavelle

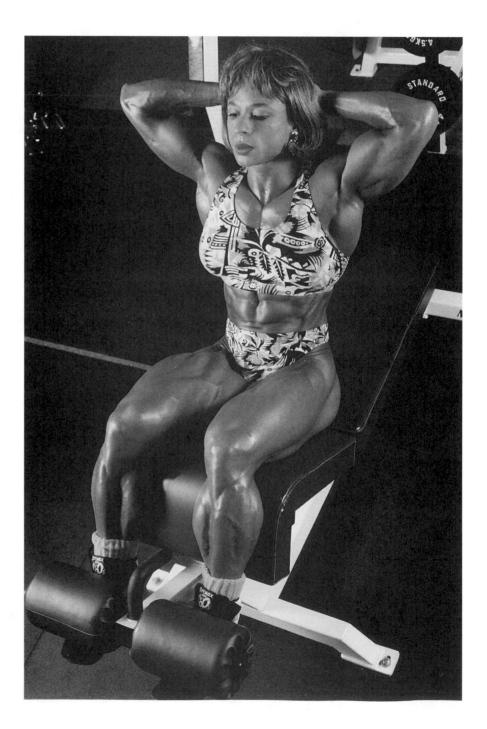

Side Twists with Pole

Emphasis. This movement is for the oblique muscles, although it is incorrect to believe that doing thousands will spot trim the sides of your waist.

Note: do not perform this exercise if you have any lower-back injury or weakness.

Starting Position. Stand erect with your feet set slightly wider than shoulder width. Place a stretching stick across your shoulders and behind your head. Wrap your forearms over and across the stick. Be certain not to move your hips and legs during this exercise or you will lose most of the desired effect.

Movement Performance. Twist as far as you can to the left and right in a moderately slow rhythm for equal reps per side.

Variations. Twists may also be performed while seated at the end of an exercise bench.

Lee Garroute

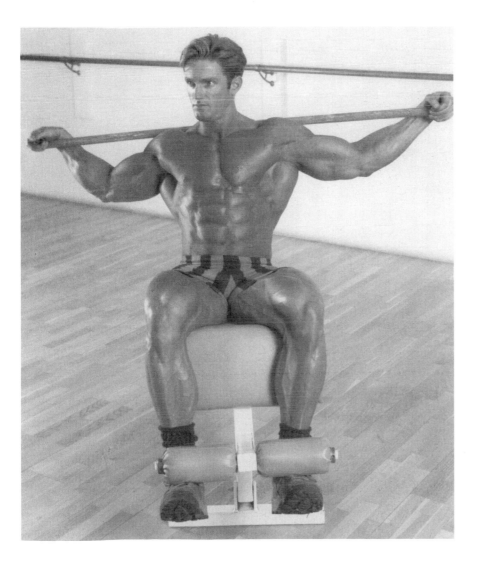

Side Bends with Dumbbell

Emphasis. This movement very directly stresses the obliques and serratus muscles.

Starting Position. Grasp a light dumbbell in your hands and stand erect with your feet set just slightly wider than shoulder width.

Movement Performance. Maintaining an erect posture throughout the exercise, alternately bend to the right and left as far as comfortable, with equal reps to each side.

Larry Gonsalvez

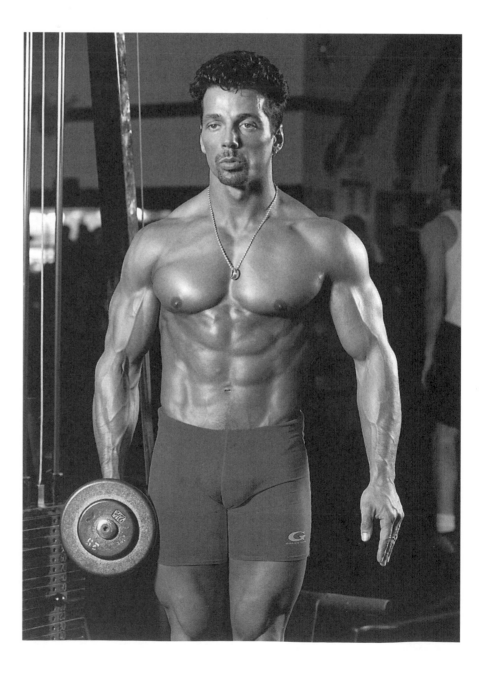

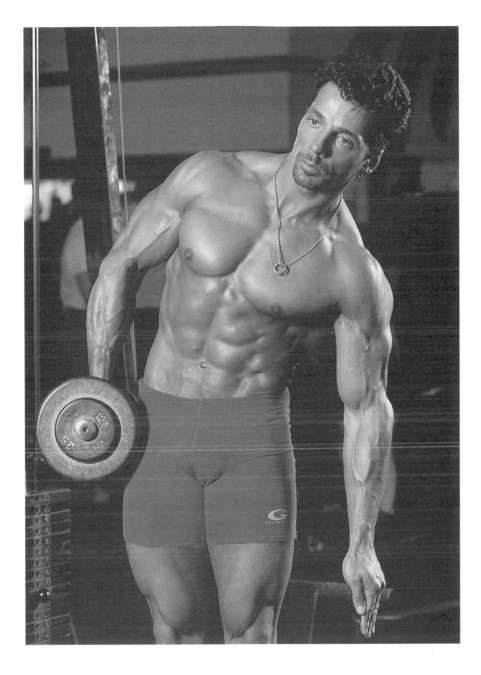

Tips. Do not perform this exercise if you are already thick through the midsection. This movement can add thickness to your waist. Only a few sets, maybe 2 or 3, are required for stimulation, so don't overdo this one.

Variations. One-arm side bends may also be performed using a handle and low-pulley setup.

15

Aerobics and Stretching

To the question of what aspect of their workouts gets skipped, many bodybuilders are heard to answer: "Sometimes I forget to stretch" or "I do my aerobics at home." Along these lines, we've taken the step of incorporating both stretching and aerobics into a single chapter. More than merely pumping iron, your success as a bodybuilder will involve flexibility, injury prevention, and the efficient transport and use of oxygen.

WARMING UP

In similar fashion to warming up the engine of a car on a cold winter's night, an exercise warm-up provides the initial movements within the body that produce heat and begin the transition from a resting state to one of active exertion. A thorough warm-up period goes a long way toward preventing injuries.

AEROBIC EXERCISE

Four definitions of the word *aerobic* are:

1. of or pertaining to the presence of air or oxygen

2. able to live and function in the presence of free oxygen

3. requiring oxygen for the maintenance of life

4. of or pertaining to aerobic exercise

In that bodybuilding is concerned with external appearance far

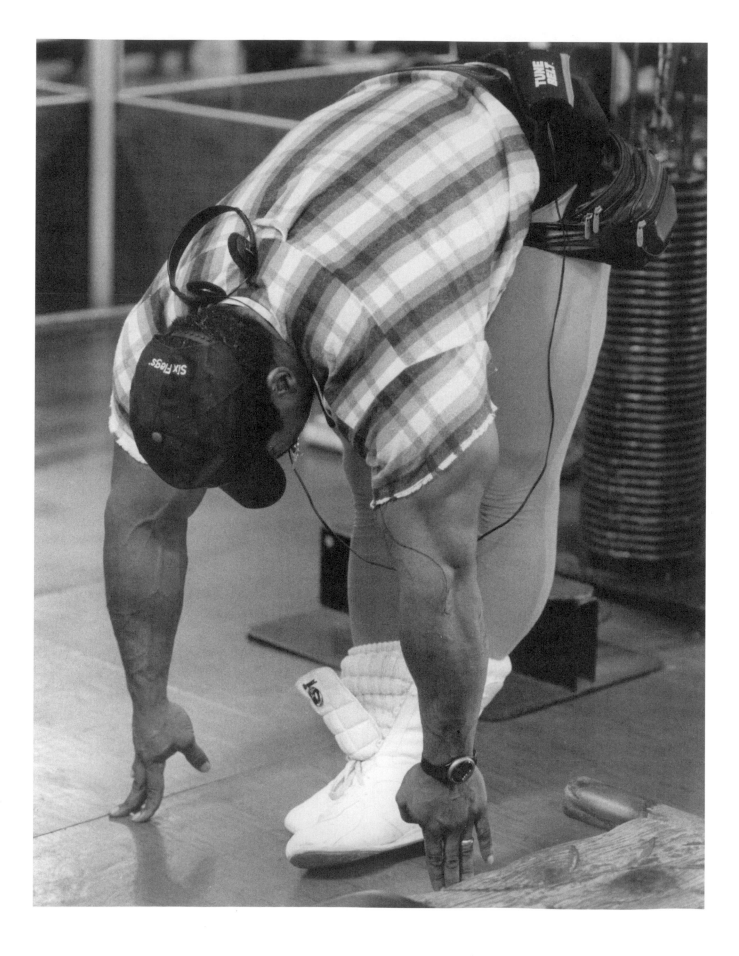

more than any health aspect, we will approach this topic from the bodybuilder's perspective of cuts.

First and foremost, bodybuilders want to understand how to remove as much of their external fat as possible, while simultaneously leaving the hard-won muscle tissue intact. Second, maximum health as it relates to aerobics is on the minds of bodybuilders, especially those under 30 years of age. If our general bits of advice and directions are followed without approaching extremes, there is every reason for you to feel confident of obtaining a fantastic state of energized personal health. So, implementing the knowledge contained in this book in a safe and prudent manner can also help you achieve the health and well-being in which the sport of bodybuilding has its historical roots.

To achieve the muscular appearance needed to win as a bodybuilder, you must be able to regularly increase your expenditure of calories above your intake. Here is where the impact of properly executed aerobic exercise becomes invaluable. Bodybuilding mandates the focus be on slabs of ripped beef with a maximum degree of deeply etched cuts and striations. Aerobics focuses on requiring additional effort by the heart and lungs to meet the increased demand by the skeletal muscles for oxygen. In the context of bodybuilding, aerobic exercise is close to being interchangeable with fat burning.

Aerobic Training

Going back a few years, it was accepted as factual that there was a mystical fat-burning zone in the area of 65 percent of an individual's maximum heart rate. The opinion was based on scientific observations of the different rates of energy substrate consumed during aerobic activity. Above the 65 percent range was considered to overly rely on carbohydrate stores rather than fat stores for energy consumption. This thinking has now been updated. A more current consensus is that both the intensity of exercise along with the duration are determining factors in the amount of total fats burned during aerobic exercise. The greater the intensity, the more calories burned; the higher the number of calories consumed, the higher the number of fat calories used. The focus is no longer on the ratio of substrates used to fuel the effort but on the total energy cost of the effort.

Bodybuilding aerobics have now become more effective but harder. To facilitate your understanding of terms used in relationship to aerobics, get a feel for the following:

▌ Maximum oxygen uptake or aerobic capacity, or VO_2 max, is the greatest amount of oxygen that can be transported from the lungs to the working muscle tissue.

Aaron Baker (opposite page)

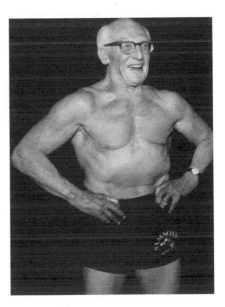

Gains come at any age. Eighty-seven-year-old Harry Otto shows what a consistent aerobics program provides: a great physique and, for Harry, a long life.

Amy Fadhli

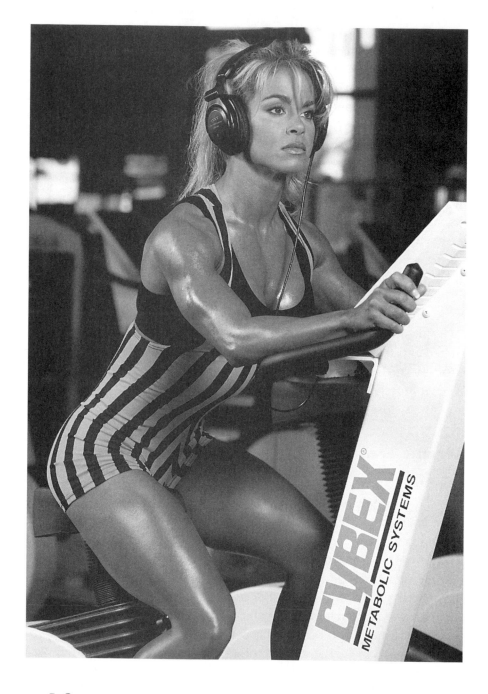

▌ Oxygen consumption is the amount of oxygen in milliliters per minute required by the body for normal aerobic metabolism, normally about 250 milliliters per minute.

▌ Oxygen debt or excess post-exercise oxygen consumption (EPOC) is the quantity of oxygen taken up by the lungs during recovery from a period of exercise that is in excess of the quantity needed for resting metabolism during the pre-exercise period.

▌ Oxygen debt represents repayment of oxygen and energy stores that were depleted during the time that oxygen uptake from the environment was inadequate for aerobic metabolism.

▌ Oxygen transport is the process by which oxygen is absorbed in the lungs by the hemoglobin in circulating deoxygenated red cells, and carried to the peripheral tissues. The process is made possible because hemoglobin has the ability to combine with oxygen present at a high concentration, such as in the lungs, and to release this oxygen when the concentration is low, such as in the peripheral tissues.

▌ Respiratory exchange ratio is the ratio of carbon dioxide product to that of oxygen consumption or uptake, expressed by the formula VCO_2/VO_2. (VO_2 is the symbol for oxygen uptake.)

AEROBIC TECHNIQUE

In that the total calories consumed during the activity are the best measure of fats consumed as energy, those bodybuilders attempting to get cut would benefit from aerobic training. If the period of 30 minutes is used as the relative baseline for time, then the factor to be measured and altered will be the target heart rate. The chart following indicates a wide range of maximum and target heart rates.

AEROBIC GUIDELINES			
Maximum heart rate = 220 − age			
Target heart rate = maximum heart rate × (%)			
Age	Max	Target of 80%	85%
15–20	200 bpm	160 bpm	170
20–25	195 bpm	156 bpm	166
25–30	190 bpm	152 bpm	162
30–35	185 bpm	148 bpm	158
35–40	180 bpm	144 bpm	153
40–45	175 bpm	140 bpm	149
45–50	170 bpm	136 bpm	145
50–55	165 bpm	132 bpm	140
55–60	160 bpm	128 bpm	136
60–65	155 bpm	124 bpm	132
65–70	150 bpm	120 bpm	128

To determine your training heart rate, follow these steps:

Step 1: Maximum heart rate is obtained by starting with 220 beats per minute, then subtracting your age. The number indicated by the 220 minus age formula is your maximum heart rate. At this level of exertion, all available energy stores are quickly depleted, while toxins from exercise metabolism rapidly accumulate. The end result is the inability to maintain the exercise long enough to impact the caloric balance within the body.

Step 2: Using your calculated maximum heart rate number, next decide at which level of intensity you will be performing the workout

Rod Corn

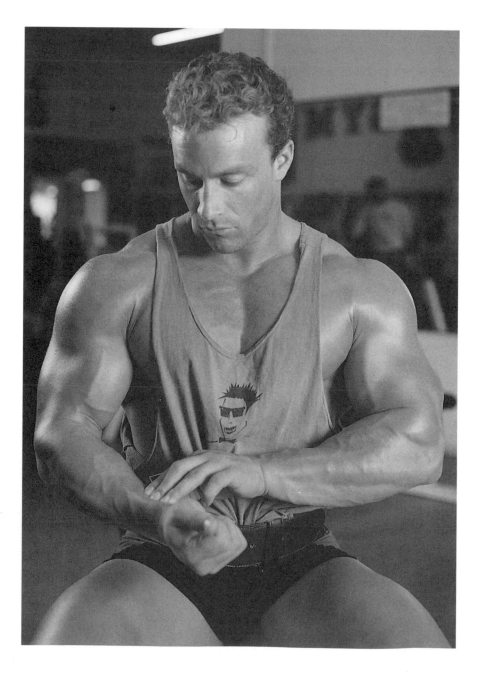

that day. If at 80 percent, then simply take the maximum heart rate and multiply by 80 percent for your calculated target heart rate. Bodybuilding aerobics can be approached one of two ways: lower intensity (less than 80 percent THR) for an extended time period or moderate to high intensity (85 percent THR effort) for a moderate to relatively short time period.

Upon the initiation of aerobic activity, a warm-up period of 10 minutes may be used to sufficiently elevate the heart rate. For a warm-up, 50 percent THR is good. After the warm-up, begin to increase the level of activity to the point where your heart rate reaches the desired THR. Increase at specific time intervals.

It becomes undeniable at this point: the harder you work, the more calories you burn; the more calories you burn, the more fats are consumed as fuel. The only way to lose the body fat you desire is through expending more calories than you take in.

EXCESS POST-EXERCISE OXYGEN CONSUMPTION (EPOC)

The EPOC phenomenon is associated with increased aerobic intensity. It is now indicated that the greater the amount of calories burned, the more increased caloric expenditure will occur at the end of the exercise period. EPOC is described in greater detail in the previous section on oxygen debt.

Studies have indicated that over a post-exercise period of 24 hours, the energy expenditure of high intensity versus low intensity is greater in the high-intensity groups. The increased release and subsequent oxidation-rate increase produce the characteristic deep cuts.

AEROBIC ACTIVITIES

There are many aerobic methods available to today's bodybuilders, such as:

stationary bike
jump rope
indoor skiing
rowing
spinning
walking
running
jogging
circuit resistance training
swimming
rock climbing

Ursula Sarcev

AEROBICS FOR MORE THAN JUST CONTEST TIME

Other areas of positive impact regular aerobic exercise is associated with are:

coronary health
pulmonary health
cardiovascular health
glucose management
stress reduction, which leads to shifting many metabolic parameters

Sarah Melton

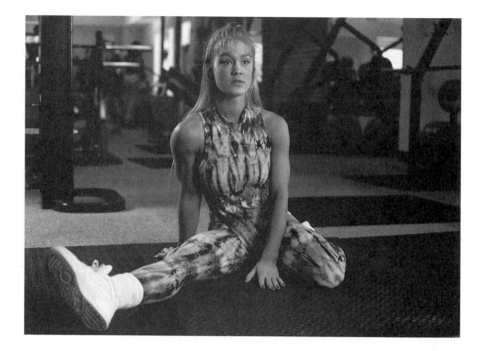

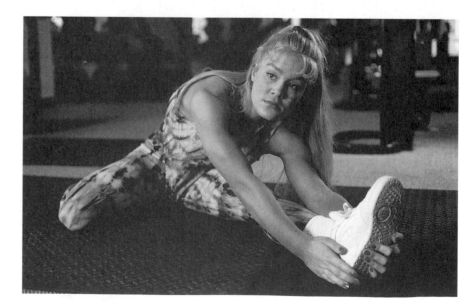

optimal immune system function

increased caloric expenditure

increased metabolic rate—to what degree or for exactly how long is still open for discussion

STRETCHING

Whether stretching sessions come before or after your resistance training, they are an important opportunity to provide your muscles with every possible opportunity to function at their highest level of performance. In addition to its commonly perceived role in injury protection, stretching is a good way to alleviate some minor soreness between workouts. It is a natural pain reliever and modifier. Studies have also indicated a role for stretching in the prevention and relief of certain types of muscle spasm.

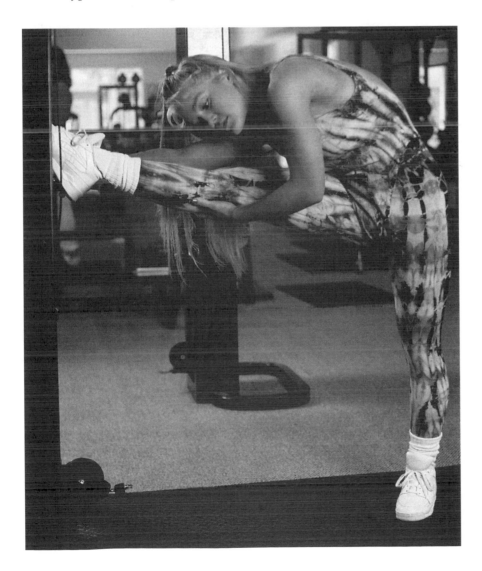

Sarah Melton

Dana Dodson

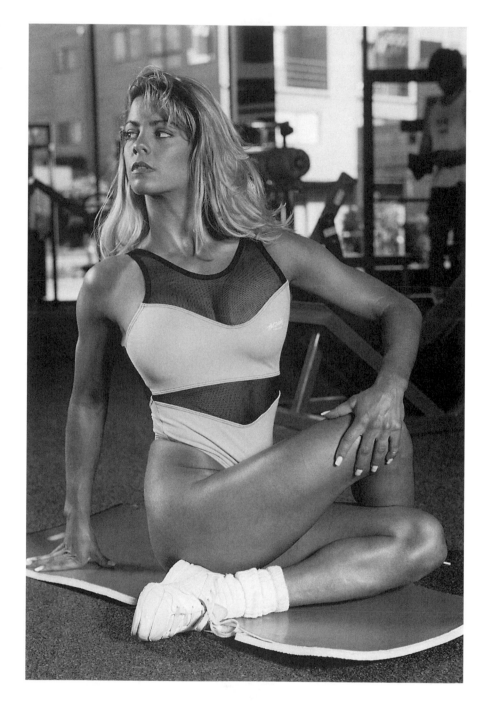

Before Training

As part of the warm-up protocol, stretching can be lightly performed in the time between light cardiovascular work and weight training.

After Training

If you prefer, the time immediately after you finish lifting is a great time for a full stretch, especially of the areas pumped to maximum fullness.

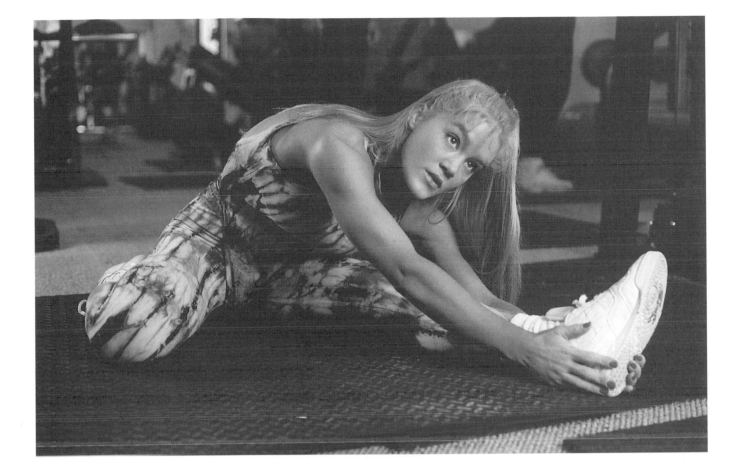

In the eccentric-focused manner of training, the shortened muscle fiber can take up to two full hours to return to its normal length. This is another good reason to gently and passively stretch the areas that have been trained and may be in a temporary state of shortened range of motion. A period of 5 to 10 minutes of stretching after your workout allows the shortened muscle to return to its normal length. The state of normal muscle-fiber length versus a temporary state (two hours is temporary in bodybuilding terms) is required for the release and uptake of the essential biochemical factors involved in the recovery and growth process.

Sarah Melton

Stretching Technique

While following the photos illustrating different positions in a stretching program, keep these ideas in mind as performance guidelines:

- Hold the stretch in the fullest position with gentle yet firm control.
- Exhale as you hold at the deepest position.
- Absolutely do not bounce or do ballistic stretching.
- Do not use weight or other means to increase pull on joints.

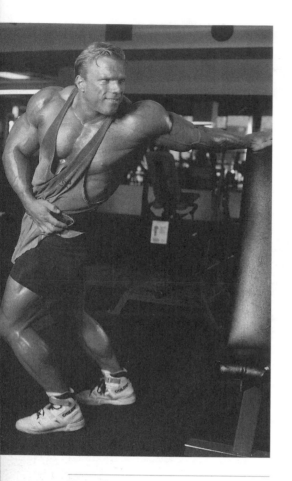

Dave Fisher

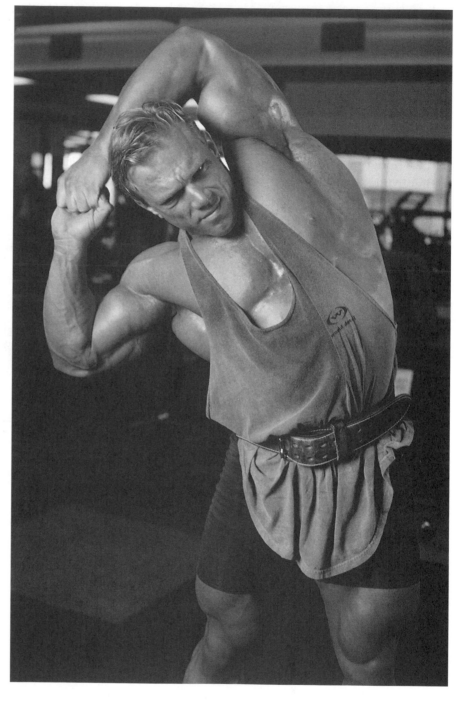

In the same manner as weight training, treat stretching as a progressive program of gradually increasing effort and results. Stretch in a progressive fashion.

As with all types of exercise the more exciting and fresh the program, the more likely it will be adhered to and followed. If your gym is fully equipped, there will be an exciting array of the latest generation of stretching machines or benches. You can also use a partner-assisted stretching arrangement.

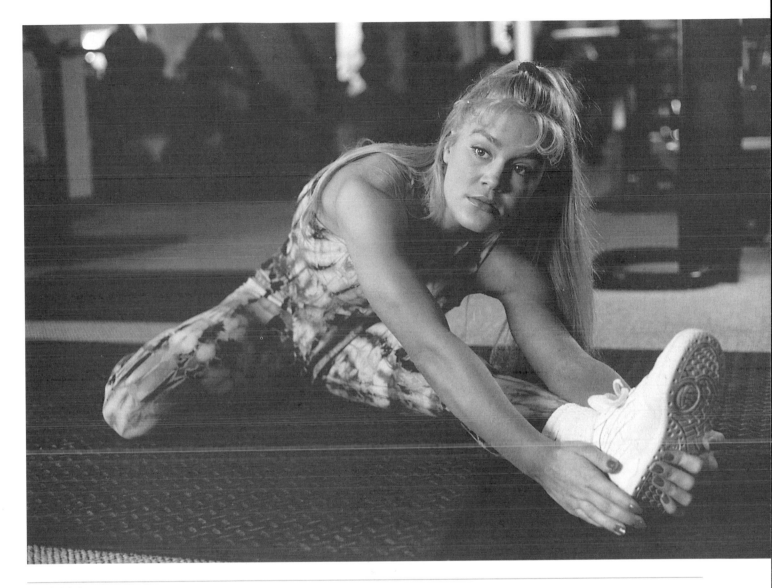

Sarah Melton

16

Gaining Lean Muscle

On a historical note, during the 1960s, a 200-pound bodybuilder was considered outrageously huge. In the 1970s, the biggest man to step onstage was Gold's president, Pete Grymkowski, who competed at 250-plus pounds. The decade of the 1980s saw other men of 250 pounds—although infrequently. Enter the 1990s and the envelope is stretched to a bursting 270 pounds or more. Does this indicate a slowing of the potential for growth beyond limits, or will the Mr. Olympia become a remote outpost for men of 300 pulsating peptide-packed pounds? It will take an absolutely staggering amount of food on a daily basis to hold this kind of size for any period of time. Talk about mass consumption of natural resources!

As you begin to become bigger, the first thing to go will be your shoelaces—not that they will break, but you won't need any due to the fact that you're always so stuffed with food you'll wear slip-ons or no shoes at all.

LBM EQUALS LEAN BODY MASS

When considering the laborious process of dropping fat pounds at contest time, it makes a strong argument for staying as lean as you can year-round. Weight gain should be a process of maximizing your lean body mass. LBM is the combination of cell solids, extracellular and intracellular water, and mineral mass of the body. It is essentially all the nonfat components in your body.

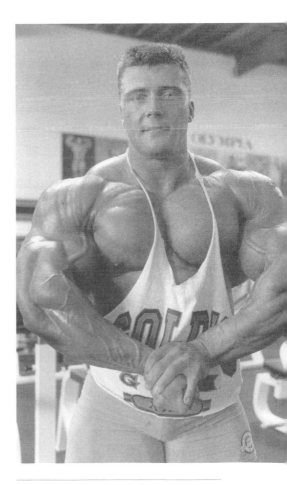

Jean-Pierre Fux

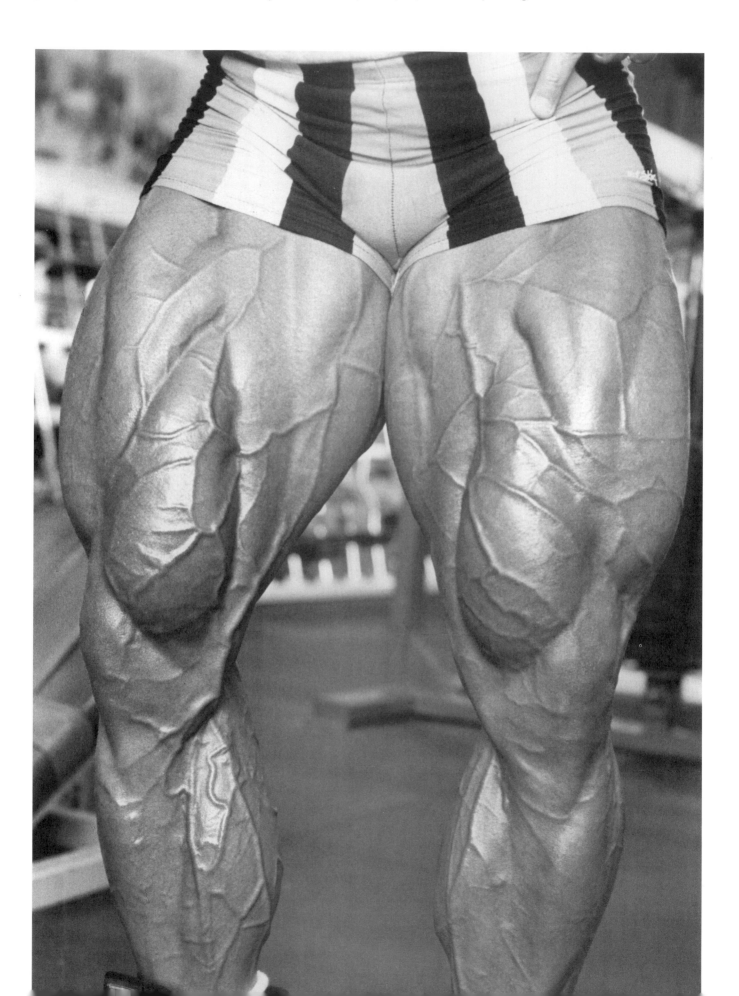

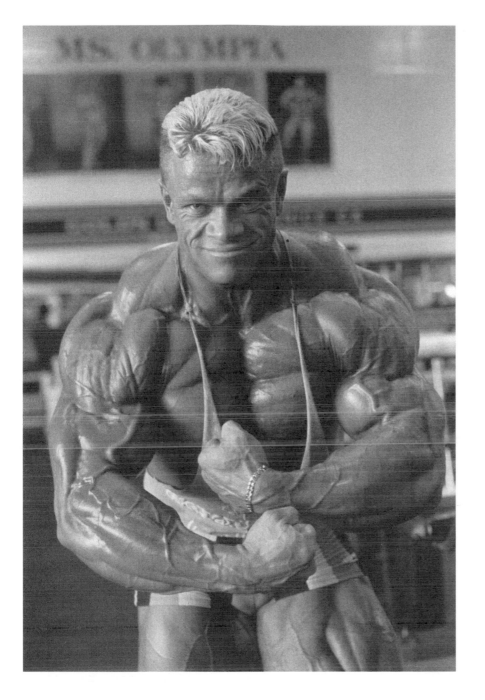

WHAT IS WEIGHT?

The vague concept of weight is more an unclear goal than a declaration of intent. The most readily accessible indicator of weight gained is the scale. So even though your real goal is to win a contest or prepare for a photo shoot, you'll be looking at the scale to monitor your mission. If an observed increase in body weight was achieved relatively fast and you weren't juiced, it is likely some chunky fat deposits were being made. If, on the other hand, the acquisition was a lesson in patience and determination, it is far more likely that the increase was mostly LBM.

DEFINE THE GOAL

Even though identifying the specific details of your weight-gain goal does not impact your physical self, goal clarity is central to your mental success pattern. Bodybuilding is a sport made up of countless minigoals continually set, accomplished, and revised in a cycle of progress. You need to be specific in the statements you form to describe your goals.

Ronnie Coleman

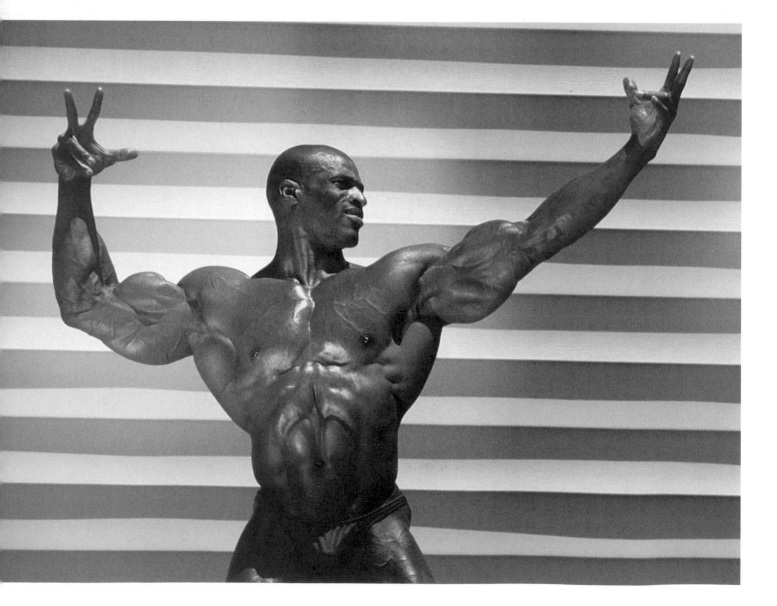

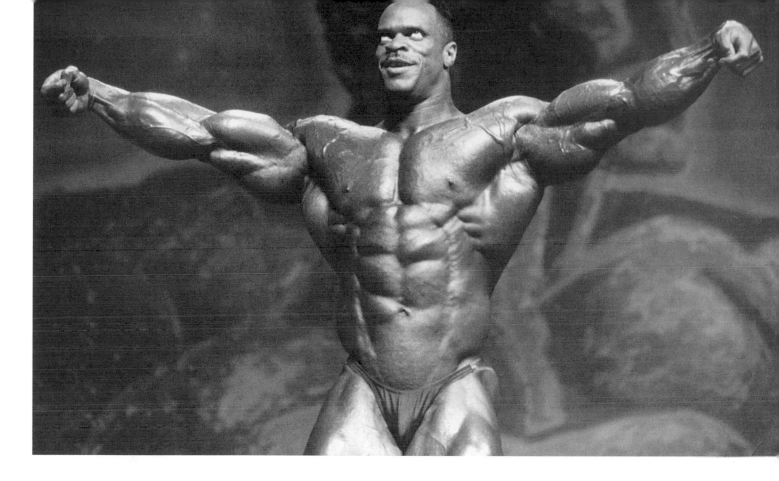

Paul Dillett

We hope you will value success highly enough to record these goals just as you record your training sessions. When committing the goal to paper, be clear and focused. Avoid phrases such as "gain some weight for summer" or "pack on a few pounds." Instead, make it something similar to "I want to gain 10 pounds in the next 90 days" or "I want to win my class and place no lower than second overall at the [whatever contest] 180 days from now." The more precise the goal statement, the easier it becomes to assess the status of your progress.

CALORIC ALLOCATIONS

Calculator and paper time—determining caloric allocations is a matter of math. For a 200-pound bodybuilder, the formula for increasing calorie intake is as follows.

First, the bodybuilder would calculate current daily calorie intake, then compare the number to the following chart:

15 kilocalories per pound
18 kilocalories per pound
21 kilocalories per pound
24 kilocalories per pound

Depending on where this number lands in the range of 15 to 24 kilocalories per pound, the next level of calorie intake will serve as a starting point for increasing the kilocalories.

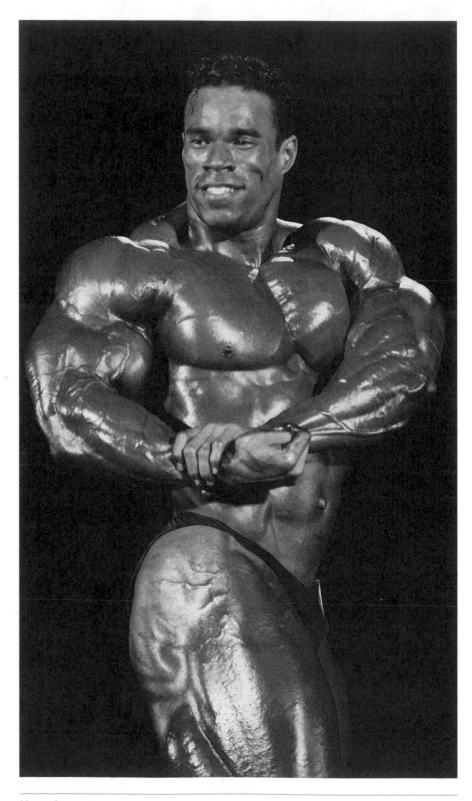

Kevin Levrone

If, for example, the calculated daily intake is 19 kilocalories per pound (or 3,800 kilocalories), the starting point for increasing caloric intake will be 21 kilocalories per pound (or 4,200 kilocalories) daily. This is a daily caloric increase of 400 kilocalories, which translates into about an 11 percent increase above the maintenance level for the original body weight of 200 pounds.

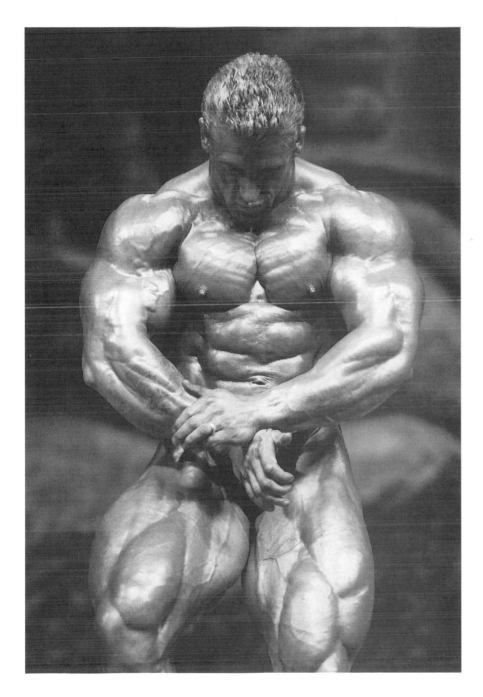

Mr. Olympia—Dorian Yates

NUTRIENT PROPORTIONING

The subject of nutrient proportioning is covered in-depth in chapter 4. Remember, the overriding goal of more muscle must come from protein.

Think of your body as a factory which produces muscle as the finished product. It becomes easy to understand that producing more of the product (weight gain in the form of LBM) mandates that more raw material (protein) be sent to the factory to meet the increased demand.

More muscle means more protein.

The remaining portion of dietary allocations holds relatively steady at 30 percent fat and 40 percent carbohydrate.

Guenther Schlierkamp

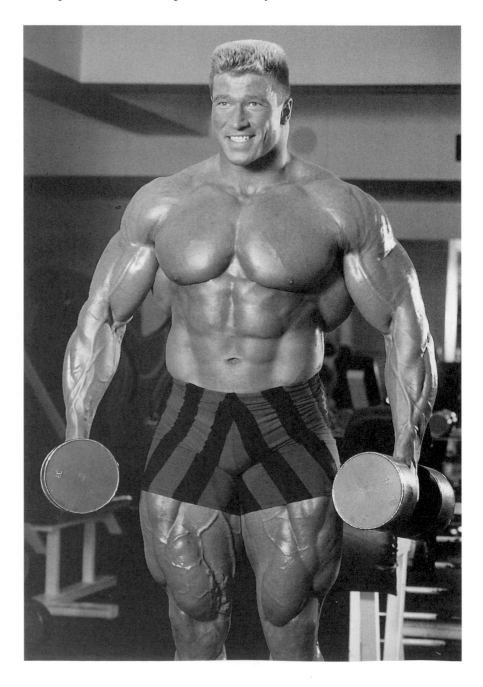

SUPPLEMENTS

Besides correct diet, there is a singular must-do in the quest to increase muscle mass: use supplemental protein powders. But a general rule of thumb is to avoid any product identifying itself as a "weight gainer." Almost always, these are a rocket ride to fat city. Skip them. Learn to eat food and then some more food. If, after you learn how to eat enough food for two people and drink a couple of protein shakes every day, you still haven't gained the muscle mass you're looking for, then maybe go check out the types of high-calorie protein combinations that make up weight-gain products.

If you want to legally feel some of the effects illegal steroids impart, then creatine monohydrate makes good sense. When used along with a sufficient quantity of water intake, the fullness is dramatic indeed. The muscles apparently superhydrate themselves into a state of engorgement. When taken to its fullest potential, creatine monohydrate gives the effect of a 24-hour-a-day total body pump. (You must be somewhat lean to see the change.)

Additionally, creatine bumps up your reps by giving your superhydrated muscles increased leverage advantages. The practical result from increased leverage advantages will be increased levels of strength. This increased strength actually begins a growth cycle. As the muscle fibers superhydrate or swell to full volume, the leverage increases in your training movements. This increased strength and the resulting increased weights lifted result in increased stress within the muscle.

Your muscle wants to grow in response to this increased stress load and will gladly do so if it is nourished and properly rested. The end result of these small bouts of muscle growth is increased pounds on the scale—lean permanent pounds. The only snafu that can derail this natural process is overtraining, or to a lesser degree, underfeeding.

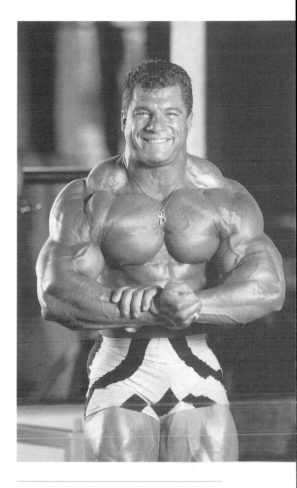

Ronnie Schweyher

Roland Cziurlok

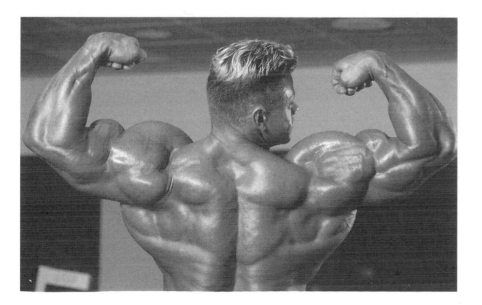

Aaron Maddron

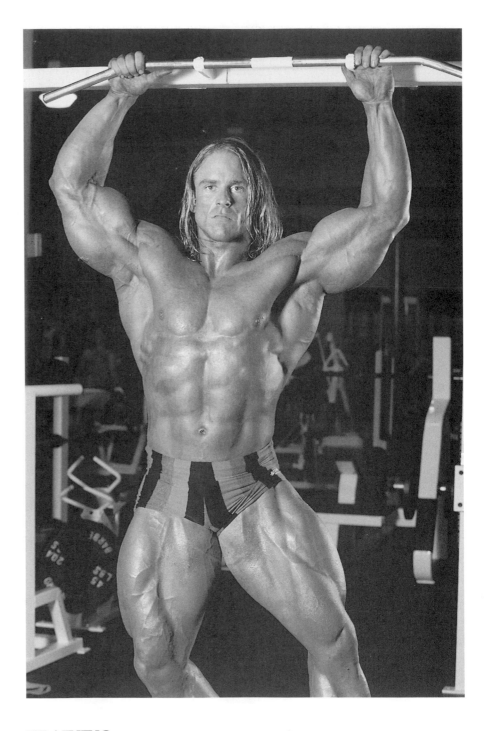

TRAINING

What more can be said about training than we've drummed on about throughout the book. Most bodybuilders need to combine less training volume and greater intensity with more food and rest. Less training volume performed in a harder method generally equals size increases, which of course register as weight increases.

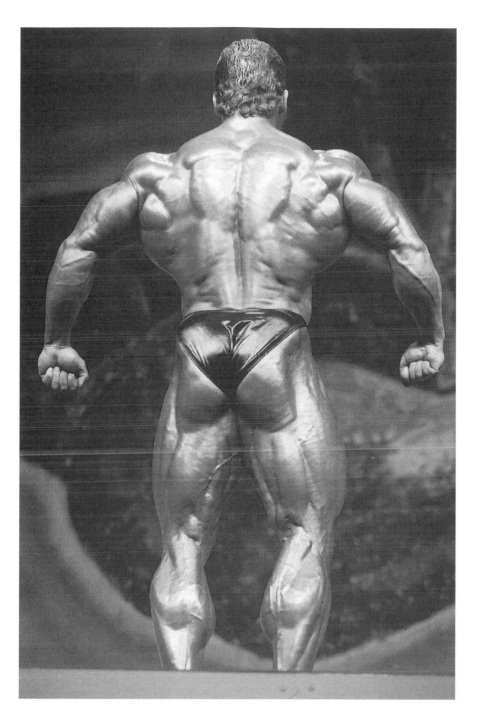

Mr. Olympia—Dorian Yates

CHAPTER 16 REFERENCES

Bompa, T. 1994. *Periodization of Strength: The New Wave in Strength Training.* Chandler, Arizona: Progenix.

Bucci, L., ed. 1993. *Nutrients as Ergogenic Aids for Sports and Exercise.* Boca Raton: CRC Press.

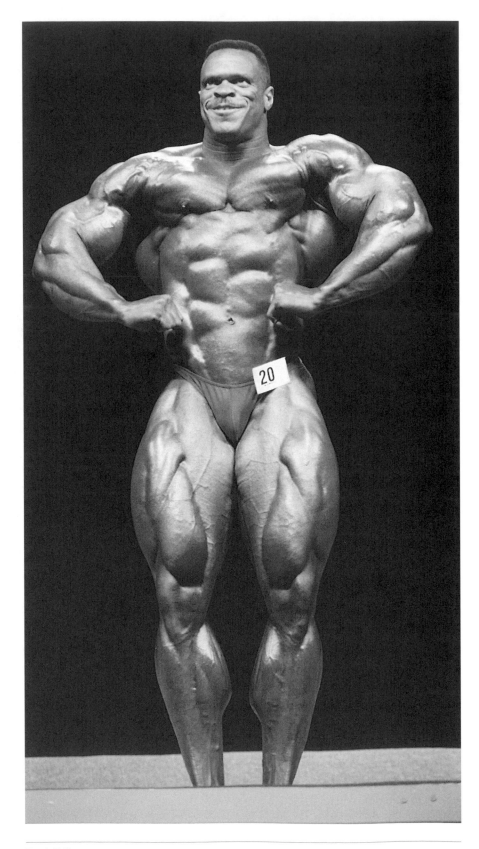

Paul Dillett

Ebbing, C., and P. Clarkson. 1989. "Exercise-Induced Muscle Damage and Adaptation." *Sports Medicine*: 7:207–234.

Ferrier, L. K., L. J. Caston, S. Leeson, J. Squires, B. J. Weaver, and B. J. Holub. 1995. "A-Linoleic Acid and Docosahexaenoic Acid–Enriched Eggs from Hens Fed Flaxseed: Influence on Blood Lipids and Platelet Phospholipid Fatty Acids in Humans." *American Journal of Clinical Nutrition*: 62:81–6.

Friedman, M., ed. 1989. *Absorption and Utilization of Amino Acids*, Vol. 1. Boca Raton: CRC Press.

Komi, P. V., and E. R. Buskirk. 1972. "Effect of Eccentric and Concentric Muscle Conditioning on Tension and Electrical Activity in Human Muscle." *Ergonomics*: 15:8.

Latifi, L., ed. 1994. *Amino Acids in Critical Care and Cancer*. Austin: R. G. Landes.

Talag, T. S. 1973. "Residual Muscular Soreness as Influenced by Concentric, Eccentric, and Static Contractions." *Research Quarterly*: 44:458–469.

Wolinsky, I., and J. F. Hickson, eds. 1994. *Nutrition in Exercise and Sport*, 2nd ed. Boca Raton. CRC Press.

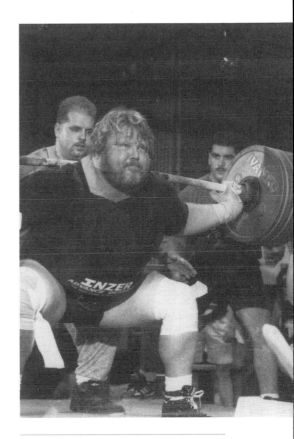

Matt Dimmel—Larger than life, Matt Dimmel makes this 1,000-pound squat look easy!

17

Successful Competition

The list of requirements for successful competitors looks something like discipline first, desire second, and talent third. There is everything to gain by competing and essentially nothing to lose. The condition you achieve, regardless of the contest's outcome, can be used to build for the next set of goals.

Use this chapter to ascertain the best protocol for off-season body-fat–reduction periods—the material is not only for competing. Details on nutrition and training are covered in prior chapters. This chapter will tie these loose ends together into a practical pattern for you.

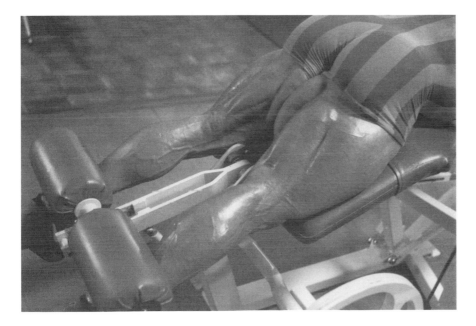

Dave Palumbo

IT'S CONTEST TIME

We hope once you've checked the calendar, it will show you have about 20 weeks until the day of your show. As a general rule of thumb, the more time you have spent in the sport, the closer to contest time you can begin your preparations. You will have by this time become more familiar with how your particular metabolism reacts to different combinations of foods. This self-awareness is invaluable and cannot be purchased from any outside source.

Jean-Pierre Fux

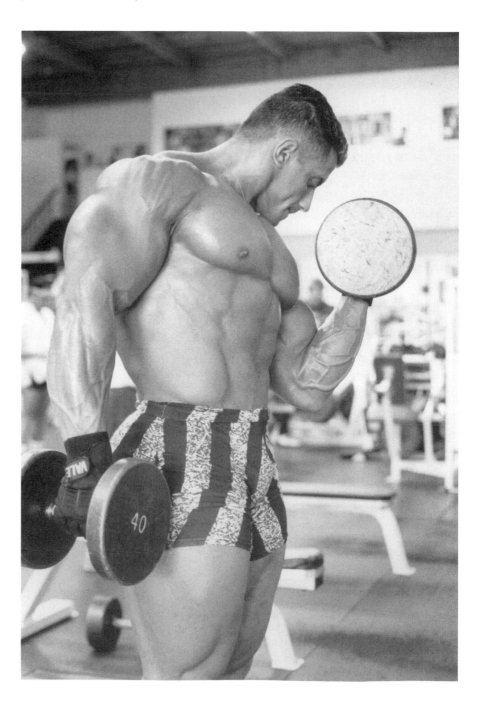

The range of contest prep times, as far as dieting is concerned, is six to 24 weeks. The person who is ready to go onstage after six weeks of dieting was in very good condition before starting a deliberate contest attack. Twenty-four weeks is indicated for those bodybuilders who are not in great condition. The longer contest prep times also serve those cautious individuals who simply wish to take the process as slowly as possible. Remember though—the longer the diet period is stretched out, the more difficult it becomes.

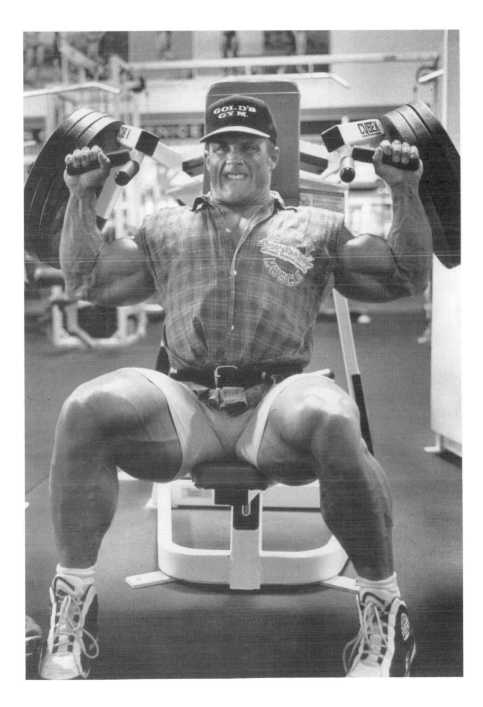

Craig Titus

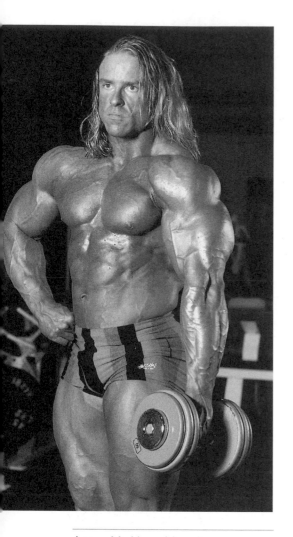

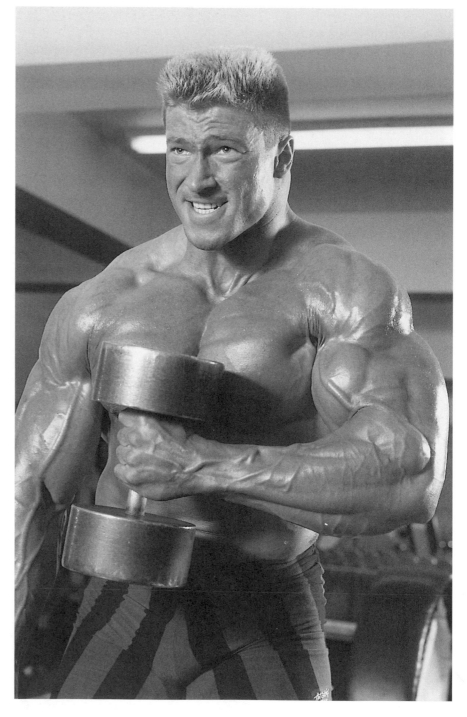

Aaron Maddron (above)
Guenther Schlierkamp (right)

DIET

The space required to delve into the fascinating world of a body-builder's contest diet would fill an entire book. So we'll boil this down to its most essential point: calorie deficit. There are a number of ways to achieve a caloric deficit, but it is the common denominator to all contest diet approaches.

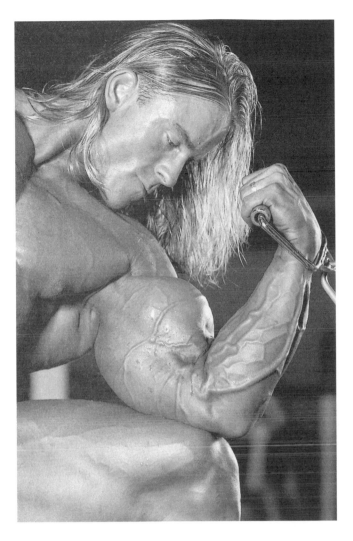

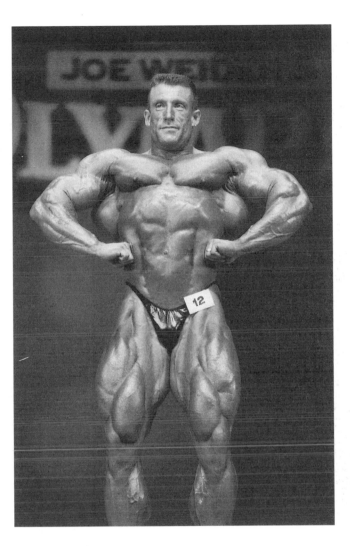

We recommend a sensible approach to nutrition as set forth in Chapter 4. To utilize this dietary formula for a contest prep, simply follow these steps to achieve your specific caloric numbers:

- Calculate the average daily calorie intake for your maintenance weight.
- Depending on where this number lands in range of 27 to 18 kilocalories per pound, the next lower level of calorie intake will serve as the starting point for the diet.

  27 kilocalories per pound
  24 kilocalories per pound
  21 kilocalories per pound
  18 kilocalories per pound

- Allocate the nutrients as called for in your plan (see chapter 4).
- Using 200 pounds as an example, calculated daily intake is 25 kilocalories per pound or 5,000 kilocalories. The starting point will be 24 kilocalories per pound or 4,800 kilocalories daily. This

Aaron Maddron
Mr. Olympia—Dorian Yates

Garrett Downing

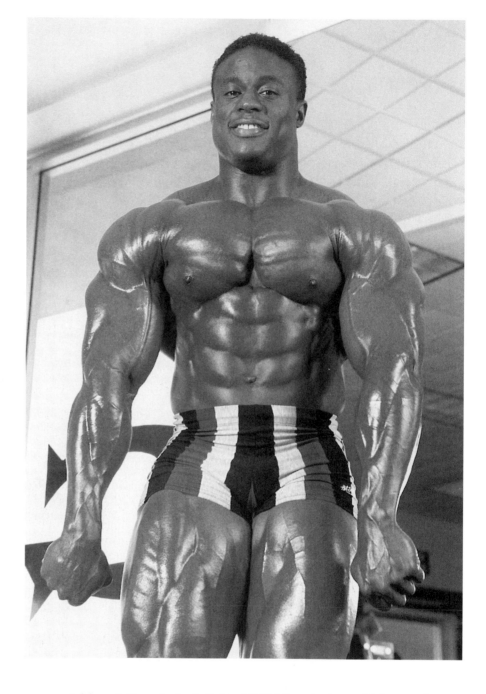

yields a daily caloric deficit of 200 kilocalories, which translates into about a 4 percent decrease below the maintenance level for the original body weight of 200 pounds.

- Repeat this next level of calorie-intake pattern until you see the cuts come in. It won't take too long.

Also, stay far away from food or snack items blaring their FAT-FREE status—especially processed foods. Numerous studies have indicated that diets which included free selection of regular or fat-free foods found that the fat-free groups ate more calories and tended to increase body weight due to insulin response and glucagon shutdown. This is exactly the opposite of what you are looking for.

WATER

For a healthy individual, for every 20 to 25 pounds of body weight, you should attempt to drink eight ounces of pure water. So a 200-pounder should get at least 10 cups (one cup equals eight ounces) of clear water every day. There is room for much more and it's not at all unheard of for this amount to be doubled.

Your water requirement increases under the following conditions:

- during hot, humid weather
- when doing outdoor work or physical labor

Mr. Olympia—Dorian Yates

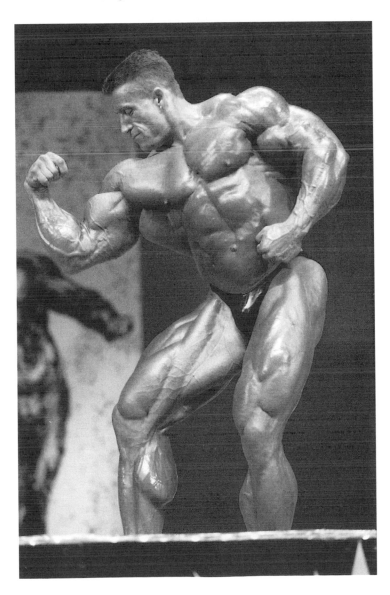
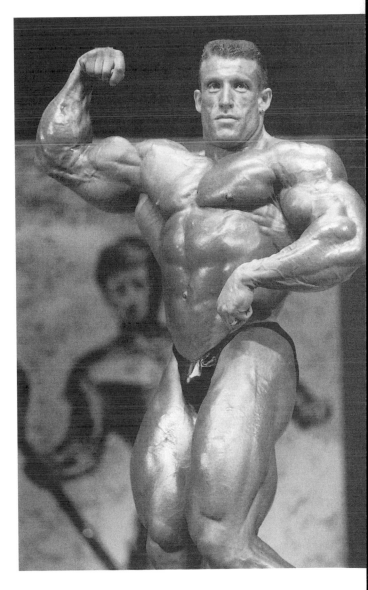

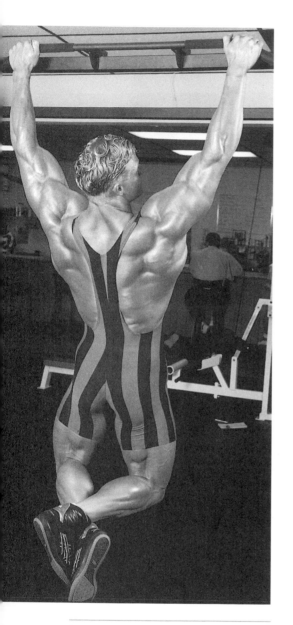

- on low-carb diets—as you near ketosis, the lower the percentage of carbs, the more important water becomes for staying healthy
- when eating high levels of dietary protein, or the average body-builder's diet
- during illness, especially fever

SUPPLEMENTS

Although not as essential to success as during times of increasing your LBM, there are good supplements that assist the cutting and prepping process.

Along with your daily multivitamin-mineral product, vitamin C, and probably some form of supplemental protein, the list of open can-

Jeremy Freeman (above)
Kevin Levrone (right)

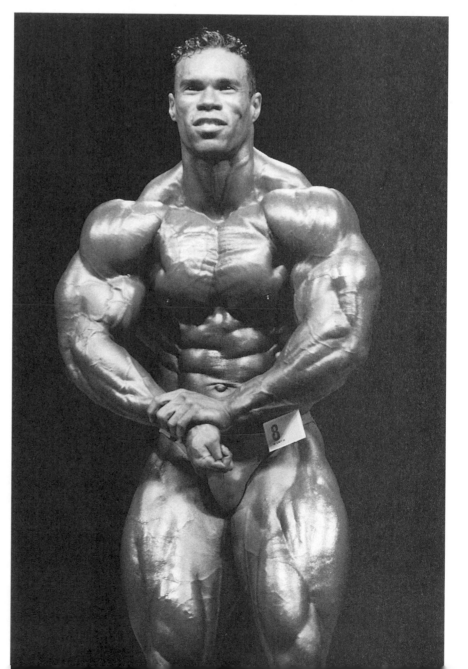

didates for blasting your way into phenomenal condition on contest day includes: creatine monohydrate, chromium picolinate, vanadyl sulfate, and other similar insulinogenic agents (during the time when your dietary level of carbs is above 25 percent). Depending on where you live, a number of tremendously effective thermogenic herbs and over-the-counter drugs are available to increase the body's use of fat substrates for fuel. Specifically, some of the more well known are ephedra, guarana, white willow bark, ephedrine HCL, caffeine, and aspirin.

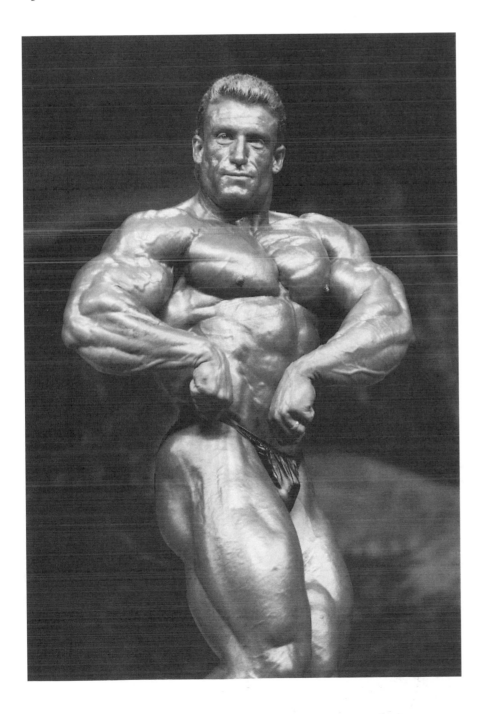

Mr. Olympia—Dorian Yates

AEROBICS

A simple rule is to leave yourself some room for a burst of aerobic activity the week or so before your show. If you start out your prep period with 60 minutes of biking six days per week and the plan is for 12 weeks of prep time, then where do you go to increase the activity? You won't hold up too well under two hours of aerobic anything. The idea is to *coax* the fat off, not to attempt to somehow rip or melt it off. An extreme approach to any aspect of contest prep is certain to backfire in the end. There are no shortcuts to good condition through discipline!

Sue Price

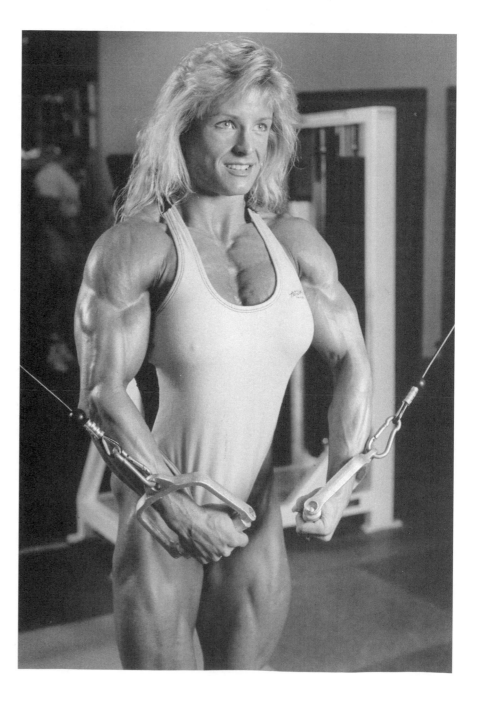

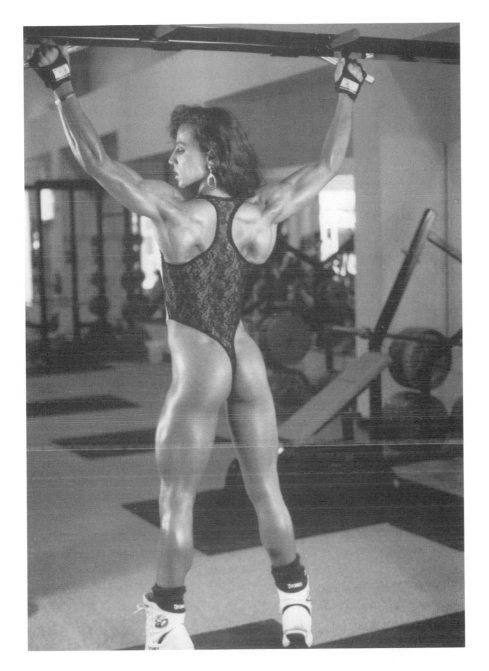

Sherilyn Godreau

If you've never competed before, you might do well to start out at moderate-intensity aerobics for 25 minutes three days per week (if you aren't already at this level). See chapter 15 for further information. The progression from this point is your call—just stay focused on your goal and be consistent!

Some consideration should be given to the time of day you perform the aerobic session. Early morning upon rising and before eating is tremendous for fat loss—though tough. If your diet calls for the body to go on low carbs (less than 205 of the total calories), then the time of day becomes less of a priority. Evening workouts are good for depleting stored carbs and gaining quick access to fats to ensure the deepest cuts.

Shawn Ray

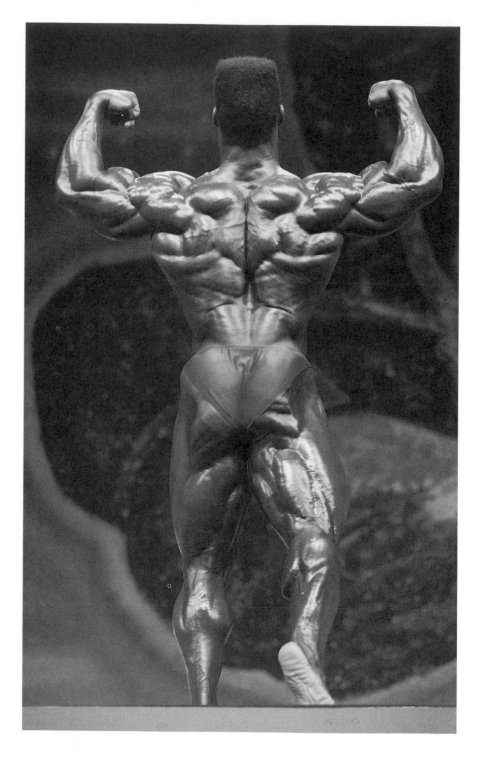

TRAINING

Face the fact: if you're not as big as you want to be by the time you begin to trim down, then it's too late. You cannot get bigger at the last minute. Your actual training approach doesn't need to shift that significantly. The fact that you will not grow while dieting and your need to

Cathy LaFrancois

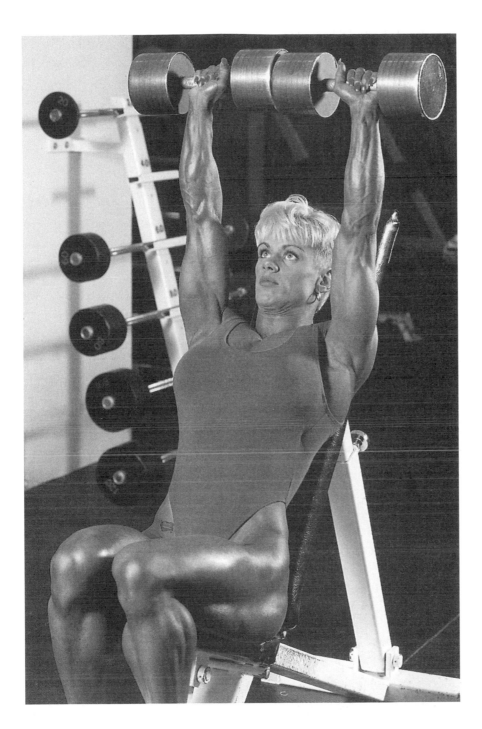

avoid injury dictate that your intensity drop off somewhat. The fierce-
ness you used to train to grow might work against you now. So put the
excess energy into keeping track of your diet and aerobics program.

Delete any forced reps or other means utilized to elevate intensity.
There is strong likelihood that your strength level will drop off a bit—
this is not a vital concern. Other than yourself no one will know how

Cathy LaFrancois

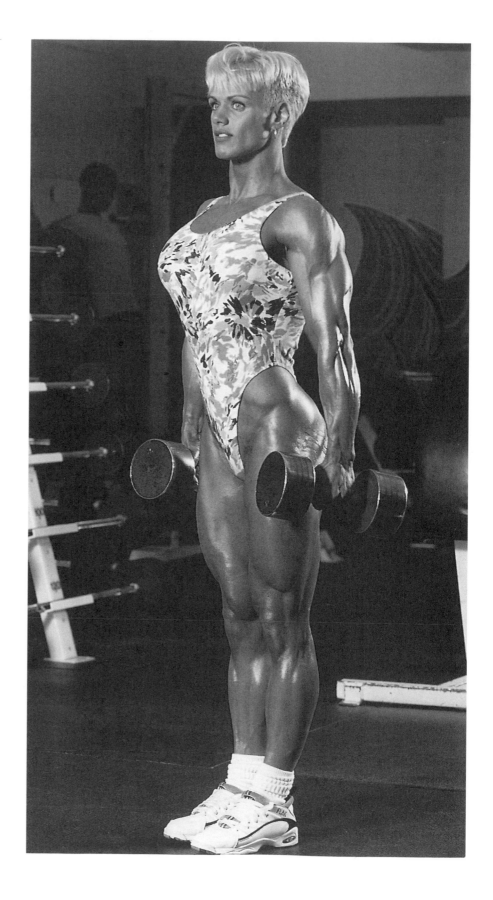

heavy or light you trained for a show. No awards are given for strongest *losing* bodybuilder.

THERMOGENICS

Thermogenics is literally the generation of heat. In bodybuilding terms it is associated with the process of fat loss. Various herbs, drugs, and other substances which elevate the body's core temperature through numerous mechanisms are responsible for this effect. For details of these agents, check your local statutes regarding their legal over-the-counter or prescription status in your community. For most of us, coffee and some form of ephedra will do a great job of notching up the thermostat. A single aspirin added to this creates an increased response.

GOALS

This chapter is of interest to you because you are going to fully complete the bodybuilding cycle by entering a competition. This is indicative of an individual with goals. Competition requires the utmost in self-discipline and is a line of demarcation between boys and men. Write down your goals!

OUTLOOK

Stay clear and focused. Always maintain a state of prudent patience. This is not an activity to rush into. The result of spontaneous reactions during prep time is failure. Relax, you're gonna look great.

CAUTION—BAD DRUGS!

The period of contest preparation is the most dangerous for a bodybuilding chemical catastrophe. It's petrifying to think of those few very insecure, nervous bodybuilders who will go to any length to win having free run in a pharmacy. There are hundreds of powerful and extremely effective drugs that almost automate the contest-prep process. If this is a particular interest to you, so be it. Good luck. But there isn't any more that can ethically be said about this complex and risky aspect of bodybuilding. The most injurious agents in use are dinitrophenol, creosol, and other oxidative uncouplers—bastardized biochemistry at its worst.

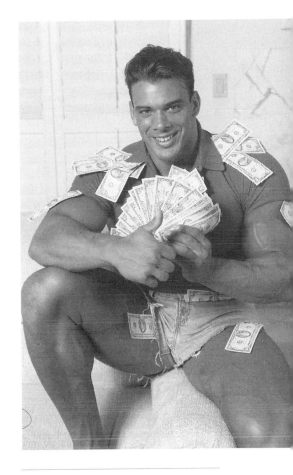

Frank Sepe

Chris Aceto and Mike Francois

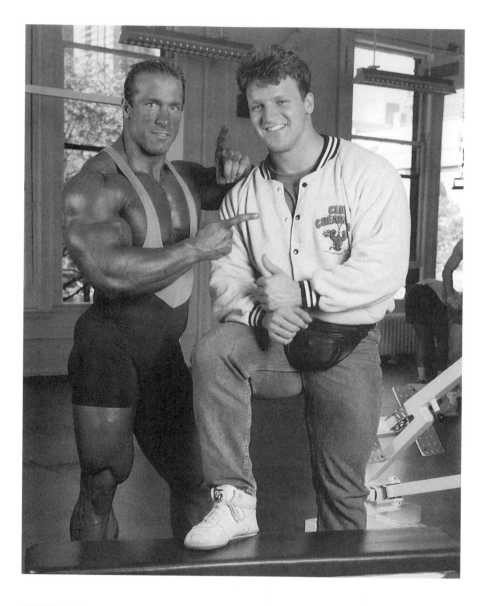

DIURETICS

Diuretics are extremely dangerous and banned in competition. Questions?

CHAPTER 17 REFERENCES

Dullo, A. G. 1993. "Ephedrine, Xanthines and Prostaglandin Inhibitors: Actions and Interactions in the Stimulation of Thermogenesis." *International Journal of Obesity*: 17 [Suppl. 1]:S35–S40.

Dullo, A. G. 1993. "Strategies to Counteract Re-Adjustments Towards Lower Metabolic Rates During Obesity Management." *Nutrition*: 9:366–372.

Appendix A
Guide to Further Reading

There is an incredible information explosion in today's muscle magazines. Pages of complex bio-medical technology research fill issue after issue. We believe many bodybuilders would serve their cause well if they spent as much time reading as training.

No longer solely the domain of wimpy wannabes, reading difficult and even boring material can be the sword with which the best of the best sever the chains that hold them in mortal status. Imagine 100 bodybuilders with similar structures and genetics have qualified to compete in the Olympia. All of them train in the same high-intensity manner with the same weights. But there is only one champion. In

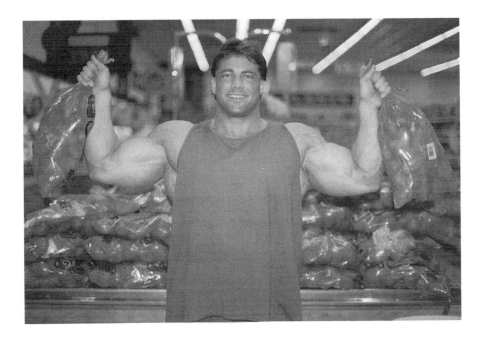

Phil Hernon

Chris Faildo

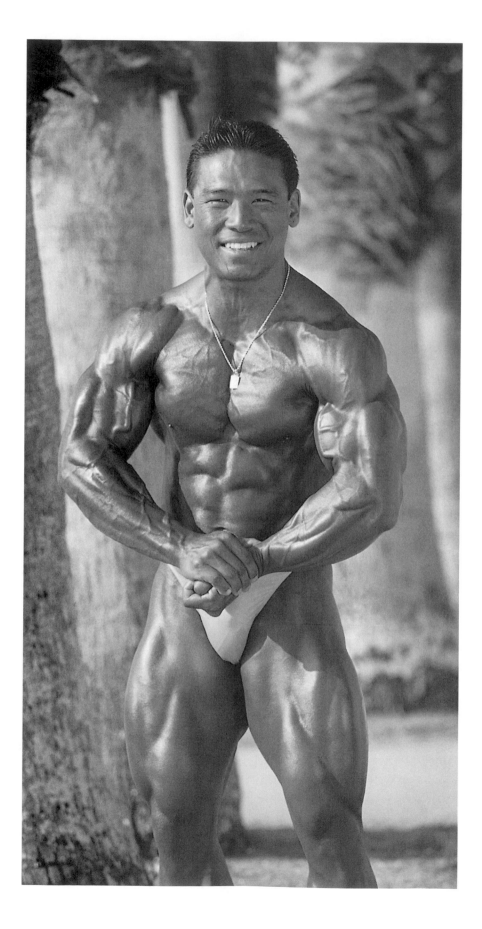

Sue Price

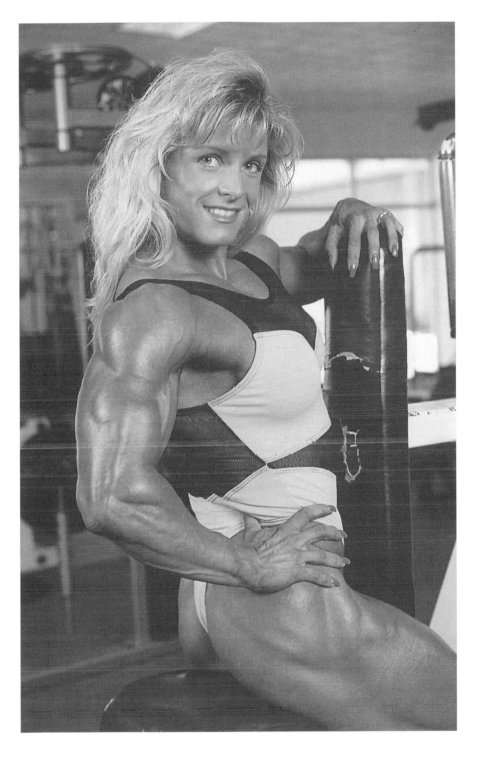

other words, if potential variables are held constant, the difference between first or second ($100,000 versus $50,000) will be based on knowledge.

This appendix is intended to provide you some ideas on where to go for more bodybuilding-related material. These sources could provide the edge for your first-place win!

Edgar Fletcher

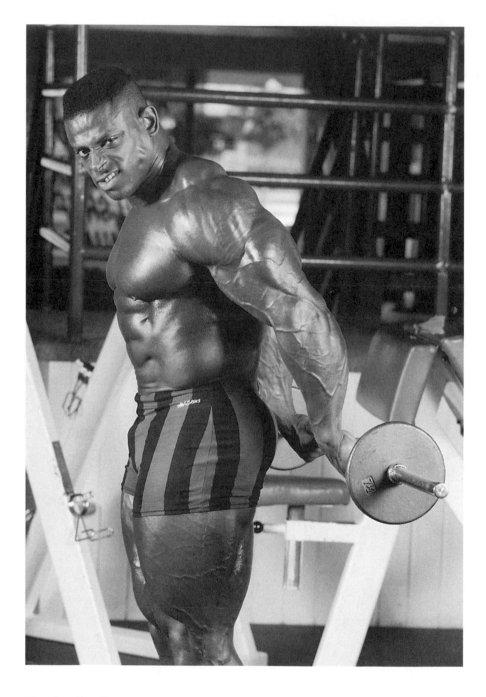

Periodicals

Smart Drug News
Information newsletter focusing on the areas of personal cognitive-function optimization and health enhancement.

> Cognitive Enhancement Research Institute (CERI)
> P.O. Box 4029
> Menlo Park, CA 94026
> (415) 321-CERI
> www.CERI.com

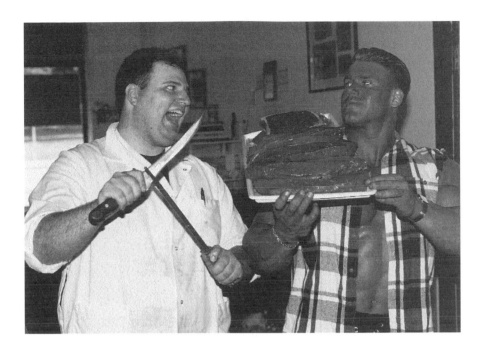

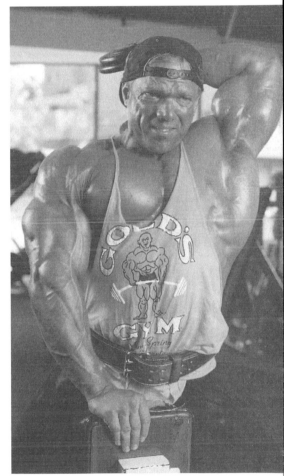

Jay Cutler

Hard Core Muscle
A high-quality, honest newsletter produced by Dante. Focuses on training techniques and ultra-intense routines.

> Hard Core Muscle
> 3529 Cannon Rd.
> Suite #2B-416
> Oceanside, CA 92056
> (760) 414-1025

Powerlifting USA
The powerlifter's lifeblood—all you'll ever need to know about those 700-pound benches and 1,000-pound squats.

> Powerlifting USA
> P.O. Box 467
> Camarillo, CA 93011

CP (Clinical Pearls) News
Monthly newsletter reviewing thousands of the most current articles from the world of health research. Focus is on nutritional and other alternative therapies outside the scope of mainstream healthcare. Each issue comes with addresses for free reprints of full research articles. Incredibly good value for the subscription price.

> I.T. Services
> 3301 Alta Arden #2
> Sacramento, CA 95825

Dave Fisher

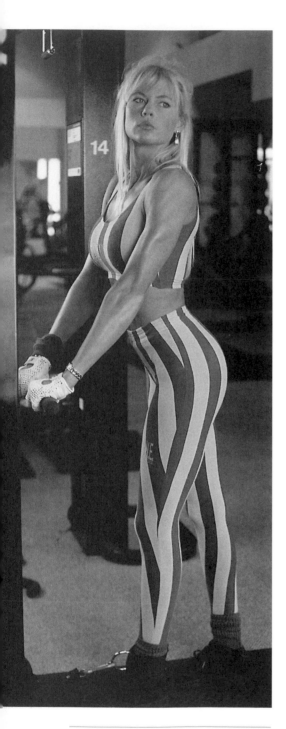

Tracy Smith

Books

Cynober, L. A., (eds.). *Amino Acid Metabolism and Therapy in Health and Nutritional Disease.* Boca Raton: CRC Press, 1995.

Gilman, A., T. Rall, A. Nies, and P. Taylor, (eds.). *The Pharmacological Basis of Therapeutics.* Oxford: Pergamon Press, 1990.

Hochachka, P. W., (eds.). *Muscles as Molecular and Metabolic Machines.* Boca Raton: CRC Press, 1994.

Jayde, N. *Super Vixen.* Chicago: Contemporary Books, 1994.

Kochakian, C. D., (eds.). *Anabolic-Androgenic Steroids in the Handbook of Experimental Pharmacology*, Vol. 48. Springer-Verlag, 1976.

Kruskemper, H. I. *Anabolic Steroids.* New York and London: Academic Press, 1968.

Miller, J. F., and W. B. Saunders. *Encyclopedia and Dictionary of Medicine, Nursing, and Allied Health.* Philadelphia, 1992.

Pennington, J. E. *Food Values of Portions Commonly Used.* New York: HarperCollins, 1989.

Reynolds, B., and N. Jayde. *Sliced: State-of-the-Art Nutrition for Building Lean Body Mass.* Chicago: Contemporary Books, 1991.

Reynolds, J. E., (ed.). *Martindale—The Extra Pharmacopoeia 30th Edition.* London: The Pharmaceutical Press, 1994.

Steinke. *New Protein Foods in Human Health: Nutrition, Prevention and Therapy.* Boca Raton: CRC Press, 1996.

Viru, A. *Adaption in Sports Training.* Boca Raton: CRC Press, 1995.

Special Interest

Quantum Resources

Your ability to focus and master your mental and emotional state is just as critically important as training and nutrition are for achieving true success. Imagine having the secrets that countless other bodybuilders have used to skyrocket their progress! Well, you no longer have to imagine because now you can develop these "state management" secrets that will launch your training intensity and your progress into the stratosphere.

David Young is simply the best there is at developing a personal battle plan for achieving your goals. He is a wizard at getting you to master the most valuable goal-achieving techniques used by the most successful athletes of all time.

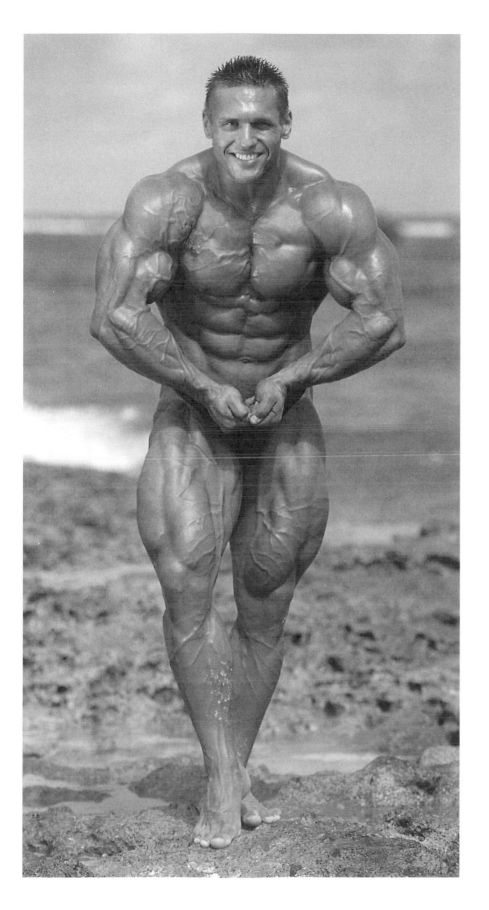

Jeno Kiss

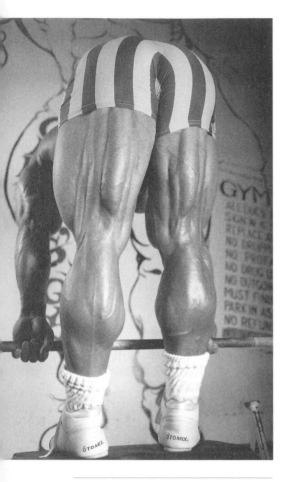

Mike Francois

Whether you are a beginner, advanced, natural, enhanced, or whatever, you will easily acquire the skills that only a few athletes at the elite levels of our sport utilize. And you'll learn how to perform your absolute best during those crucial "make it or break it" workouts that determine the achievement of your long-sought-after goals.

Quantum Resources
Attn: David Young
21008 Victor Street, Suite #36
Torrance, CA 90503

Infomed Services

This brainchild of Will Block and John Morgenthaler offers specialized-literature searches of the world's medical libraries. For a fee, Infomed will research any topic of interest and produce a set of abstracts. If there is anything about the human machine you want to know more about, or if you want to learn how to access such information, drop these guys a line. For details on both custom and completed searches, write Will Block at:

Life Enhancement Products, Inc.
P.O. Box 751390
Petaluma, CA 94975-1390

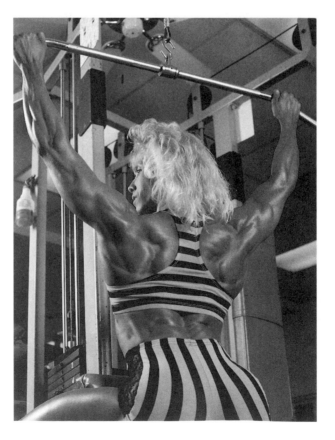

Debbie Muggli

Appendix B
Drugs

For better or worse, drugs and the take-a-pill-for-a-quick-fix mentality have arrived to stay in the sport of bodybuilding. By definition, bodybuilding conveys a vastly increased amount of muscle. Unfortunately, drugs can effect this process quite efficiently. Drug use in bodybuilding is an immense and controversial issue beyond the scope of this appendix.

We do not advise, suggest, or support anyone's use of illegal substances. Consider the following: if steroids were as dangerous as their reputation indicates, there would be many dead bodybuilders, football players, wrestlers, track athletes, cyclists, etc. However, the implied lack of outright danger does not convey safety by default. On the other hand, if steroids worked as magically as alleged, there would be thousands of 300-pound bodybuilders lumbering around.

The fact is that steroids or any other drug would not need to be banned if no one thought they worked. They are not a fountain of size, but they do allow increased rates of recovery. You still have to train intensely and eat correctly to grow.

The dangers of drug use become dramatically apparent with polypharmacy—the use of many different drugs in order to achieve a specific condition. Generally this is done in the period prior to a contest. There are untold reactions and cross-reactions possible when drugs are combined. At the very least, these multilayered drug programs will severely strain the liver and kidneys.

Ask yourself: Since these drugs cost incredible amounts of money, is there a payoff to using them? Certainly, for perhaps five top pros. The others must do whatever is required to obtain the drugs. If a drug cycle costs you $5,500 and you go through a minimum of three cycles per year for five years, the total cost is in excess of $80,000 for five years. Therefore, you must earn around $23,000 (gross pay) as a bodybuilder before you break even.

Ask yourself: How many bodybuilders earn even $100 every year from the sport? There aren't any figures on the $100 amount, but as for the $23,000 amount, there may be 20 or 30 in the entire world. You have a better chance of becoming pope or president. Since it is extremely unlikely you will ever make $10 as a bodybuilder, why risk going to jail (with small testicles— facts are facts)?

The choice to use drugs is purely personal, but we hope some thought will prompt a desire to remain or get drug free and be involved in the pure sport of bodybuilding.

The following categories and lists demonstrate the vast range of drugs used by bodybuilders or other athletes. It is not complete—there are too many drugs and too little space.

Category of Medical Indications

thermogenic agents

beta 1, 2, and 3 agonists

insulin

insulinogenics

insulinmimetics

glucagonogenics

glucagonmimetics

antigout drugs

antihistamines

nootropics

phosphodiesterase inhibitors

cortisol antagonists

antiestrogens

gonadatropins

somatotropins

somatomedians

androgens

progestins

thyroid agents

thyroidmimetics

lipolytics

anorexics

nonsteroidal anti-inflammatories

opiate analgesics

opiate agonists

growth factors

cytokines

diuretics

blood-viscosity modulators

anxiolytics

antiparkinson agents

hypoglycemics

erythropoetins

calcium channel modulators

antiarrhythmics

antidiuretics

hypothalamic-releasing agents

Substances in Use: Past or Present

cathine

chlorphentermine

clobenzorex

cloforex

clortemine

temazepam

oxazepam

triazolam

dexamphetamine sulphate

diethylpropion or amfepramone

ethylamphetamine HCL

fencamfamin HCL

methylamphetamine HCL

mephenterine/mephetedrine

modafinal

oxazimedrine

phenatine

phenbutrazate

phendimetrazine

phenmetrazine

phentermine

pipradol

prolintane HCL

pyrovalerone

anileridine

adinazolam

medazepam

midazolam

temazepam

bezitramide

brifentanil HCL

conorphone HCL

dextromoramide tartrate

dihydrocodeine

zatosetron

etoformin

EGF epidermal growth factor

NG-29 FDA

difluanine HCL

seglitide sodium

epimestrol

doliracetam

pioglitazone HCL

dipipanone HCL

eptazocine

ethoheptazine

papaveretum

pethidine HCL or meperidine

phenazocine

phenoperidine HCL

piritramide

adrafinal

amphetamine

amfecloral

amfenpentorex

amfonelic acid

aminorex/aminoxaphen

ampyzine

azabon

benfluorex

benzephetamine

propiram fumarate

tilidate HCL

tramadol

sermorelin acetate GEREF

difemetorex

l-692-429

etolorex

dopamantine

palmoxirate sodium

a-FGF acidic fibroblast growth factor

elryptamine acetate

dupracetam

nosiheptide

glypinamide

b-FGF basic fibroblast growth factor

oxitriptan

fenethylline

oxiracetam

glyparamide

fenfluramine

aniracetam

glycotamide

fenisorex

pramiracetam

glymidine sodium

fenproporex

linopirdine

leucovorin calcium

glymidine sodium

PDGF-AA platelet-derived
   growth factor

FG-4963

flucetorex

cyprodenate

triklate

glyhexylamide

PDGF-BB platelet-derived
   growth factor

phosphatidylserine

thyromedan HCL

glyhexamide

flumimorex

bromocryptine

suloxifen oxalate

glyburide

glibencamide

formetorex

minaprine

sermorelin acetate

glipicide

mefenorex

vinpocetine

deslorelin

etoformin

phendimetrazine tartrate

desmopressin

gonadarelin

nisterime acetate

phentermine HCL

centrophenoxine

prodifen HCL

phenmetrazine HCL

adrafinal

posatirelin

fenethylline HCL

fenozolone

fenproporex

fipexide

flutiorex/tiflorex

mazindol

mefenorex HCL

mefaxamide

dimoxamine

etamivan

triflubazam

vincamine

tirilazad mesylate

glucagon

flurothyl

acetyl-L-carnitine

orotic acid

NGF beta–nerve growth factor

etryptamine

idebenone

glycerol

fenproporex

nimopidine

alprazolam

bentazepam

lurazepam

lorazepam

lormetazepam

ozolinone

xanthinol nicotinate

oxypurinol

gamma-vinyl GABA (vigabatrin)

fenozolone

flerobuterol

fenodolpam

montirelin

CRF corticotropin-releasing factor

fenobam

mobecarb

formoterol

fengabine

etiracetam

histrelin

flerobuterol

formoterol

fargan

flubanilate HCL

pergolide mesylate

pareptide sulfate.

nebracetam

toremifene citrate

nitromifene citrate

idopamine

mefexamide

enclomifene

talopram

tirilazad mesylate

raloxifen HCL

mefenidil fumarate

montirelin

nitromifene citrate

isosuprine HCL

pyrovalerone HCL

viloxaxine HCL

FGF fibroblast growth factor

CSF colony-stimulating factor

ethylmorphine HCL

hydrocodone

ketobemidone

levophanol tartrate

nicomorphine HCL

normethadone

oxycodone HCL

FSLA fibroblast somatomedin-like activity

GEF gonadotropin-enhancing factor

GHRF, GH-RF growth hormone–releasing factor

HSGF hematopoietic stem-cell growth factor

LIF leukemia inhibitory factor

NGF nerve growth factor

PDGF platelet-derived growth factor

PDWHF platelet-derived wound-healing factor

SM-C/IGF somatomedin C/insulin-like growth factor

SRF somatotropin-releasing factor

Anabolic Androgenic Steroids (AAS)

androstanolone/stanolone

dihydrotestosterone: valerionate, propionate, enantate, benzoate

androsterone

bolasterone (7,17-dimethyl-testosterone)

bolazine

boldenone undecanoate

boldenone undecylenate

bolenol

bolmantalate

calustcrone

caproate

chloroandrostenolone

chloroxodienone

chloromethandienone

chlordrolone

chloromesterone

methyltestosterone

chloroxydienone

clostebol

clostebol acetate

chlorotestosterone

dehydroepiandrosterone

dihydrolone

dimethylandrostanolone

dimethandrostanolone

dimethazine

dromastanolone/drostanolone: propionate

enestebol

ethyloestrenol

formebolone/formyldienone

furazabol

hexoymestrol

hydroxystenozol

mebolazine

mesobolone

mestanolone

methylandrostanolone

mesterolone

methandienione

methylandrostenolone

methandriandrostenediol: bisenanthoyl, acetate, dipropionate

methenolone: enanthate, acetate

methylandrostanolisoazole

methyldiazirinol

methylclostebol

methylestrenolone

methylnortestosterone

methyltestosterone

mesterone

methyltrienolone

metribolone

mezabolone

mibolerone

nandrolone caproate

nandrolone: cyclohexylpropionate,
    cyclopentyl-propionate, cyclotate,
    decanoate, furylpropionate,
    hexahydrobenzoate,
    hydrogensuccinate,
    hexahydrophenylpropionate,
    laurate, phenylpropionate,
    propionate, and undecylate

nistermine acetate

norclostebol-acetate-17

norbolethone

normethandrolone

oxabolone cypionate

oxandrolone

oxymesterone

oxymetholone

penmestrol

prasterone

prometholone

propetandrol

renanolone

rosterolone

roxibolone

silandrone

stanazolol

stenbolone acetate

testolactone

testosterone acetate

testosterone propionate

APPENDIX B REFERENCES

Arnold, A., G. O. Potts, and A. L. Beyler. 1963. "Evaluation of the Protein Anabolic Properties of Certain Orally Active Anabolic Agents Based on Nitrogen Balance Studies in Rats." *Endocrinology*: 72:408.

Buttey, P. J., and P. A. Sinneff-Smith. 1984. "The Mode of Action of Anabolic Agents with Special Reference to Their Effects on Protein Metabolism—Some Speculations." *Current Topics in Veterinary Medicine and Animal Science*: 26:211.

Rogozkin, V. A. 1991. *Metabolism of Anabolic Androgenic Steroids*. Boca Raton: CRC Press.

Appendix C

Locations of Gold's Gyms Worldwide

UNITED STATES

Alabama
Anniston
Auburn
Birmingham
Dothan
Enterprise
Gadsden
Huntsville
Jasper
Mobile
Montgomery
Prattville
Roebuck
Sheffield
Tuscaloosa

Alaska
Anchorage

Arkansas
Fayetteville
Fort Smith

California
Antioch
Berkeley
Campbell
Chico
Citrus Heights

Crescenta Valley
El Cerrito
Escondido
Fairfield
Fresno
Goleta/UCSB
Hollywood
Huntington Beach
Long Beach
Marin
Merced
Modesto
Monterey
Mountain View
N. Hollywood
Northridge
Oakland
Oceanside
Palm Desert
Palm Springs
Petaluma
Redondo Beach
Redwood City
Riverside
San Clemente
San Diego
San Francisco/
    Brannan St.
    Valencia St.
San Jose

Santa Barbara
   Downtown
   Uptown
Santa Clara
Santa Clarita
Santa Cruz
Santa Maria
Santa Rosa
Scripps Mesa
Simi Valley
Sylmar
Temecula
Thousand Oaks
Vallejo
Venice
Victorville
Walnut Creek
Whittier

Colorado
Boulder/East
Colorado Springs

Connecticut
Bloomfield
Bristol
Danbury
Enfield
Manchester
New Haven
Norwalk
Shelton
Stamford
Waterford

Delaware
Newark

District of Columbia
Washington, DC/
   Capitol Hill
   Van Ness

Florida
Boca Raton
   East
   West
Bonita Springs
Bradenton
   East
   West
Brandon
Clearwater
Deerfield Beach
Fort Lauderdale
Fort Myers
Fort Walton Beach
Gainesville
Hollywood
Jacksonville (N.)
Jacksonville (S.)
Lakeland
Lake Mary
Largo
Melbourne
Miami
   South
Miami Beach
   North
   South
Miami Lakes
Naples
New Port Richey
Orange City
Orange Park
Ormond Beach
Palm Beach
Palm Beach Gardens
Palm Harbor
Panama City
Pembroke Pines
Pensacola
   North
Port Charlotte
Port Orange
Sarasota
Spring Hill

St. Petersburg
  South
Stuart
Sunrise
Tallahassee/
  Downtown
  North
Tampa
  Central
  Palms
  South
Venice
Winter Springs

Georgia
Albany
Athens
Augusta
Buckhead
Calhoun
Carrollton
Cartersville
Clarkesville
Columbus
Conyers
Douglasville
Gainesville
Kennesaw
La Grange
Lawrenceville
Lilburn
Macon
Marietta
Roswell
Sandy Springs
Statesboro
Valdosta
Warner Robins

Hawaii
Kailua-Kona
Maui
  Kihei
  Lahaina

  Wailuku
Oahu

Idaho
Boise

Illinois
Addison
Aurora
Bloomington
Bradley
Orland Park
Peoria

Indiana
Fort Wayne
Greenwood
Indianapolis (N.E.)
Merrillville
Mishawaka

Kansas
Merriam
Olathe
Wichita

Kentucky
Bowling Green
Paducah

Maine
Bangor
Portland

Maryland
Annapolis
Frederick
Gaithersburg
Glen Burnie
Greenbelt
Ocean City
Timonium
Towson
Wheaton

Massachusetts
Arlington
Attleboro
Boston
Braintree
Concord
Danvers
E. Bridgewater
Everett
Hyannis
Marlboro
Methuen
Milford
Natick
Needham
New Bedford
Plymouth
Salem
Salisbury
Springfield
Stoughton
Tewksbury
Westboro
W. Roxbury
W. Springfield
Woburn
Worcester

Michigan
Canton
Garden City
Harbor Country
Livonia
Royal Oak
Whitmore Lake
Wixom

Minnesota
Duluth
White Bear Lake

Mississippi
Columbus
Hattiesburg
Jackson
Ocean Springs
Starkville

Missouri
Cape Girardeau
Columbia
Festus
Independence
Kansas City
   North
   Downtown
Lees Summit
Manchester
Springfield
Westport

Montana
Missoula

Nebraska
Lincoln
Omaha
   North
   South

Nevada
Las Vegas
   East
   Northwest
   West

New Hampshire
Keene
Manchester
Merrimack
Nashua
Portsmouth

New Jersey
Belleville
Cranford
Delran
Flemington
Fort Lee
Green Brook
Hoboken
Howell
Laurel Springs
Lawrenceville
Mahwah

Middletown
Paramus
Princeton
Riverdale
Totowa
Washington Twnshp.
Whippany
Woodbridge
Woodbury

New Mexico
Albuquerque
Rio Rancho

New York
Albany
Astoria/Queens
Bellmore
Binghamton
Broadway/NYC
Bronx
  East
  N.W.
Brooklyn Heights
Brooklyn (West)
Buffalo
  North
  South
Chili
Croton On Hudson
Deer Park
DeWitt
E. Northport
Howard Beach
Latham
Liverpool
Lynbrook
Middletown
Monroe
Nanuet
Newburgh
North Shore
Rochester
Smithtown
South Shore
Staten Island
  North

Syosset
Wappingers Falls
Watertown
White Plains
Whitestone
Woodside
Woodstock
Yonkers

North Carolina
Cary
  West
Chapel Hill
Charlotte
  North
Concord/
  Kannapolis
Durham
  North
  South
Fayetteville
Garner
Gastonia
Greensboro
Pinehurst
Pineville
Raleigh
Salisbury
Wilmington
  North
Winston Salem
  West

Ohio
Columbus
Rocky River
Toledo

Oklahoma
Lawton
Oklahoma City
  North
  N.W.
Tulsa

Oregon
Albany

Bend
Corvallis
Eugene
McMinnville
Medford
Newburg
Portland
  Beaverton/Tigard
  Cedar Hills
  Downtown
  East
  Milwaukie
  Tualatin
Roseburg
Salem/
  Downtown
  South

Pennsylvania
Altoona
Elkins Park
Harrisburg
  East
  West
Kingston
Lancaster
Philadelphia/
  Downtown
  Northeast
Pittsburgh
  North Hills
  South
  West
Plymouth Meeting
Reading
Scranton
Southampton
State College
Thorndale
York
  North
  South

Rhode Island
Cranston

Providence
Smithfield
Warwick
Westerly

South Carolina
Aiken
Charleston
Columbia
  Harbison
  St. Andrews
Greenville
  E. North St.
  McAlister Sq.
Hilton Head
Myrtle Beach
Rock Hill
Spartanburg

Tennessee
Clarksville
Memphis
Murfreesboro
Nashville/South
Sevierville

Texas
Abilene
Amarillo
College Station
Conroe
Corpus Christi
Denton
El Paso
  East
  West
Galveston
Lake Jackson
San Antonio
Waco
Wichita Falls

Utah
American Fork
Bountiful

Draper
Layton
Ogden
Provo
West Valley

Virginia
Alexandria
Arlington
Baileys-Crossroads
Chantilly
Charlottesville
Fairfax (East)
Lynchburg
Manassas
Reston
Richmond
   South
Rosslyn
Springfield
Stafford
Tysons Corner
Virginia Beach
Winchester
Woodbridge

Washington
Bellevue
Bellingham
Bothell
Everett
Kirkland
Marysville
Olympia
Renton
Seattle
   Downtown
   West
Spokane
Tacoma
Tri Cities
Wenatchee
Yakima

West Virginia
Morgantown

Wisconsin
Green Bay
Kenosha
Madison

INTERNATIONAL
Argentina
Buenos Aires
Australia
Adelaide
Bahamas
Nassau
Canada
Edmonton, AB
Kelowna, BC
London, ON
Mississauga, ON
Vancouver (North), BC
Victoria, BC
Cyprus
   Nicosia
Ecuador
Cumbaya
Egypt
Cairo
England
Birmingham
London
   Hanwell
   N. Finchley
   Sutton
   Walworth
Finland
Helsinki
French West Indies
Guadeloupe
Germany
Berlin
Dortmund
Heidelberg

Langenhahn
Mannheim
Soest
Guam
Agana
Honduras
Tegucigalpa
Hungary
Budapest
Italy
Bari
Japan
Tokyo/East
  North
Korea
Seoul
  East
  West
Mariana Islands
Saipan
Mexico
Cuernavaca

Culiacan
Guadalajara
Hermosillo
Juarez
Leon
Los Mochis
Mexico City/Polanco
Queretaro
Netherlands
Amersfoort
Netherlands Antilles
Curacao
Peru
Lima
Qatar
Doha
Russia
Moscow (North)
Switzerland
Basel
U.S. Virgin Islands
St. Thomas

Glossary

actin. A protein found in muscle fibers that acts with myosin to bring about contraction and relaxation.

adenosine. A compound derived from nucleic acid, composed of adenine and a sugar, D-ribose. Adenosine is the major molecular component of the nucleotides adenosine monophosphate, adenosine diphosphate, and adenosine triphosphate and of the nucleic acids deoxyribonucleic acid and ribonucleic acid.

adenosine diphosphate. A product of the hydrolysis of adenosine triphosphate.

adenosine monophosphate (AMP). An ester, composed of adenine, D-ribose, and phosphoric acid, that affects energy release in work done by a muscle.

adenosine phosphate. A compound consisting of the nucleotide adenosine attached through its ribose group to one, two, or three phosphoric acid molecules. Kinds of adenosine phosphate, all of which are interconvertible, are adenosine diphosphate, adenosine monophosphate, and adenosine triphosphate.

adenosine triphosphatase (ATPase). An enzyme in skeletal muscle that catalyzes the hydrolysis of adenosine triphosphate to adenosine diphosphate and inorganic phosphate. Among various enzymes in this group associated with cell membranes and intracellular structures, mitochondrial ATPase is involved in obtaining energy for cellular metabolism, and myosin ATPase is involved in muscle contraction.

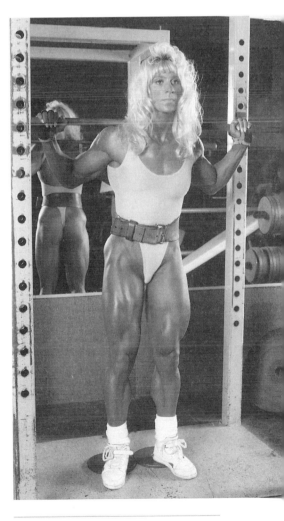

Ms. Olympia—Kim Chizevsky

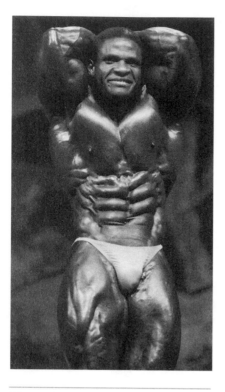

Thierry Pastel

adenosine triphosphate (ATP). A compound consisting of the nucleotide adenosine attached through its ribose group to three phosphoric acid molecules. It serves to store energy in muscles, which is released when it is hydrolyzed to adenosine diphosphate.

adrenal. Pertains to the adrenal or suprarenal glands located atop the kidneys.

adrenal cortex. The outer and larger section of the adrenal gland, which produces mineralocorticoids, androgens, and glucocorticoids—hormones essential to homeostasis.

adrenal gland. Either of two secretory organs located on top of the kidneys and surrounded by the protective fat capsule of the kidneys. Each consists of two parts having independent functions: the cortex and the medulla. The adrenal cortex, in response to adrenocorticotropic hormone secreted by the anterior pituitary, secretes cortisol and androgens. Adrenal androgens serve as precursors that are converted by the liver to testosterone and estrogens. Renin from the kidney controls adrenal cortical production of aldosterone. The adrenal medulla manufactures the catecholamines, epinephrine and norepinephrine.

adrenal medulla. The inner portion of the adrenal gland. Adrenal medulla cells secrete epinephrine and norepinephrine.

adrenocorticotropic hormone (ACTH). A hormone of the anterior pituitary gland that stimulates the growth of the adrenal gland cortex and the secretion of corticosteroids. ACTH secretion, regulated by corticotropin releasing factor (CRF) from the hypothalamus, increases in response to a low level of circulating cortisol and to stress, fever, acute hypoglycemia, and major surgery. Under normal conditions there is a diurnal rhythm in ACTH secretion, with an increase beginning after the first few hours of sleep and reaching a peak at the time a person awakens.

adrenocorticotropin. The adrenocorticotropic hormone (ACTH) secreted by the anterior pituitary gland that stimulates secretion of other hormones by the adrenal cortex.

amino acid. An organic chemical compound composed of one or more basic amino groups and one or more acidic carboxyl groups. Twenty of the more than 100 amino acids that occur in nature are the building blocks of peptides, polypeptides, and proteins.

The eight essential amino acids are isoleucine, leucine, lysine, methionine, phenylalanine, threonine, tryptophan, and valine. Arginine and histidine are essential in infants. Cysteine and tyrosine are quasiessential because they may be synthesized from methionine and phenylalanine, respectively.

The main nonessential amino acids are alanine, asparagine, aspartic acid, glutamine, glutamic acid, glycine, proline, and serine. From their structures, the amino acids can be classified as neutral, basic, or acidic, each group being transported across cell membranes by different carrier mechanisms. Arginine, histidine, and lysine are basic amino acids, aspartic acid and glutamic acid are acidic, and the remainder are neutral.

anabolic steroid. Any one of several compounds derived from testosterone or prepared synthetically to promote general body growth, to oppose the effects of endogenous estrogen, or to promote masculinizing effects. All such compounds cause a mixed androgenic-anabolic effect. Anabolic steroids are prescribed in the treatment of aplastic anemia, red-cell aplasia, and hemolytic anemia and in anemias associated with renal failure, myeloid metaplasia, and leukemia. Some common compounds used in such therapies are oxandrolone and nandrolone.

anabolism. Constructive metabolism characterized by the conversion of simpler compounds into more complex ones.

anaerobic catabolism. The breakdown of complex chemical substances into simpler compounds, with the release of energy, in the absence of oxygen.

anaerobic exercise. Muscular exertion sufficient to result in metabolic acidosis because of accumulation of lactic acid as a product of muscle metabolism.

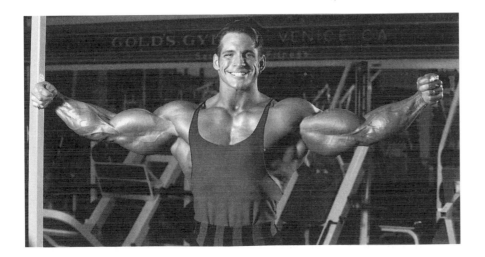

Darrin Lannaghan

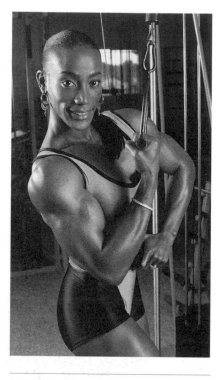

Ms. Olympia—Lenda Murray

anaphylactic shock. A severe and sometimes fatal systemic hypersensitivity reaction to a sensitizing substance, such as a drug, vaccine, food, serum, allergen extract, insect venom, or chemical. This condition may occur within seconds from the time of exposure to the sensitizing factor and is commonly marked by respiratory distress and vascular collapse.

anecdotal evidence. Pertains to knowledge based on isolated observations and not yet verified by controlled scientific studies.

anorexia. Lack or loss of appetite, resulting in the inability to eat. The condition may result from poorly prepared or unattractive food or surroundings, unfavorable company, or various physical and psychologic causes.

anorexia nervosa. A disorder characterized by a prolonged refusal to eat, resulting in emaciation, amenorrhea, emotional disturbance concerning body image, and an abnormal fear of becoming obese. The condition is seen primarily in adolescents, predominantly in girls, and is usually associated with emotional stress or conflict, such as anxiety, irritation, anger, and fear, which may accompany a major change in the person's life. Treatment consists of measures to improve nourishment, followed by therapy to overcome the underlying emotional conflicts.

anorexiant. A drug or other agent that suppresses the appetite, such as amphetamine, phentermine, diethylpropion, fenfluramine, or dexfenfluramine.

cachexia. General ill health and malnutrition, marked by weakness and emaciation, usually associated with serious disease.

carbohydrate. Any of a group of organic compounds, the most important being the saccharides, starch, cellulose, and gum. They are classified according to molecular structure as mono-, di-, tri-, poly-, and heterosaccharides. Carbohydrates constitute the main source of energy for all body functions, particularly brain functions, and are necessary for the metabolism of other nutrients. They are synthesized by all green plants and once in the body are either absorbed immediately or stored in the form of glycogen. Cereals, vegetables, fruits, rice, potatoes, legumes, and flour products are the major sources of carbohydrates. They can also be manufactured in the body from some amino acids and the glycerol component of fats.

cardiac muscle. A special type of striated muscle of the heart. Cardiac muscle is an exception among involuntary muscles, which are characteristically smooth. Its contractile fibers resemble those of skeletal muscle but are not as large in diameter. The connective tissue of cardiac muscle is sparser than that of skeletal muscle.

catabolic. A complex, metabolic process in which energy is liberated for use in work, energy storage, or heat production by the destruction of complex substances by living cells to form simple compounds. Carbon dioxide and water are produced, as well as energy.

concentric contraction. A common form of muscle contraction that occurs in rhythmic activities when the muscle fibers shorten as tension develops. At the onset of the movement, the actin and myosin filaments have tremendous pulling force and as such you will be stronger in the initial phase of most movements. Toward the end or near peak contraction the ability of the filaments to slide toward each other reaches a limit and strength weakens.

creatine. An important nitrogenous compound produced by metabolic processes in the body. Combined with phosphorus, it forms high-energy phosphate. In normal metabolic reactions the phosphorus is yielded to combine with a molecule of adenosine diphosphate to produce a molecule of the very-high-energy adenosine triphosphate.

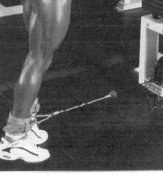

Cathy LaFrancois

creatine kinase. An enzyme in muscle, brain, and other tissues that catalyzes the transfer of a phosphate group from adenosine triphosphate to creatine, producing adenosine diphosphate and phosphocreatine.

eccentric contraction. Muscle contraction that involves lengthening the muscle fibers, such as when a weight is lowered through a range of motion. The muscle yields to the resistance, allowing itself to be stretched. It is the movement returning to the starting position of the exercise. Here the contractile filaments, actin and myosin, slide away from each other. Due to the added friction, the level of force generated is much higher in the eccentric phase as opposed to the concentric phase.

endocrine system. The network of ductless glands and other structures that elaborate and secrete hormones directly into the bloodstream, affecting the function of specific target organs. Glands of the endocrine system include the thyroid and the parathyroid, the anterior pituitary, the posterior pituitary, the pancreas, the suprarenal glands, and the gonads.

endogenous. Originating from within the body or produced from internal causes, such as a disease caused by the structural or functional failure of an organ or system.

epinephrine. An endogenous adrenal hormone and synthetic adrenergic vasoconstrictor.

estrogen. One of a group of hormonal steroid compounds that promote the development of female secondary sex characteristics.

exocrine. Of or pertaining to the process of secreting outwardly through a duct to the surface of an organ or tissue or into a vessel, such as a gland that secretes through a duct.

exocrine gland. Any of the multicellular glands that open onto the skin surface through ducts in the epithelium, such as the sweat glands and the sebaceous glands.

exogenous. Originating outside the body or an organ of the body or produced from external causes, such as a disease caused by a bacterial or viral agent foreign to the body.

extracellular fluid. The fluid filling the spaces between most cells of the body, providing a substantial percentage of the liquid within the body. Created by filtration through the blood capillaries, it drains away as lymph.

gluconeogenesis. The formation of glycogen from fatty acids and proteins rather than carbohydrates.

glucose. A simple sugar found in certain foods, especially fruits, and a major source of energy occurring in human and animal body fluids. Glucose, when ingested or produced by the digestive hydrolysis of double sugars and starches, is absorbed into the blood from the intestines. Excess glucose in circulation is normally polymerized and stored in the liver and muscles as glycogen, which is depolymerized to glucose and liberated as needed.

glycogen. A polysaccharide that is the major carbohydrate stored in animal cells. It is formed from glucose and stored chiefly in the liver, and to a lesser extent, in muscle cells. Glycogen is depolymerized to glucose and released into circulation as needed by the body.

glycolysis. A series of enzymatically catalyzed reactions, occurring within cells, by which glucose and other sugars are broken down to yield lactic acid or pyruvic acid, releasing energy in the form of adenosine triphosphate. Aerobic glycolysis yields pyruvic acid in the presence of adequate oxygen. Anaerobic glycolysis yields lactic acid.

Sue Price

hormone. Complex chemical substance produced in one part or organ of the body that initiates or regulates the activity of an organ or a group of cells in another part of the body. Hormones secreted by the endocrine glands are carried through the bloodstream to the target organ. Secretion of these hormones is regulated by other hormones, by neurotransmitters, and by a negative-feedback system in which an excess of target organ activity signals a decreased need for the stimulating hormone.

hypothalamic hormones. A group of hormones secreted by the hypothalamus, including vasopressin, oxytocin, and the thyrotropin-releasing and gonadotropin-releasing hormones.

hypothalamic-pituitary-adrenal axis. The combined system of neuroendocrine units that in a negative-feedback network regulate the body's hormonal activities.

hypothalamus. A portion of the brain that activates, controls, and integrates the peripheral autonomic nervous system, endocrine processes, and many somatic functions, such as body temperature, sleep, and appetite.

intracellular fluid. A fluid within cell membranes throughout most of the body, containing dissolved solutes that are essential to electrolytic balance and healthy metabolism.

Krebs cycle. A sequence of enzymatic reactions involving the metabolism of carbon chains of sugars, fatty acids, and amino acids to yield carbon dioxide, water, and high-energy phosphate bonds.

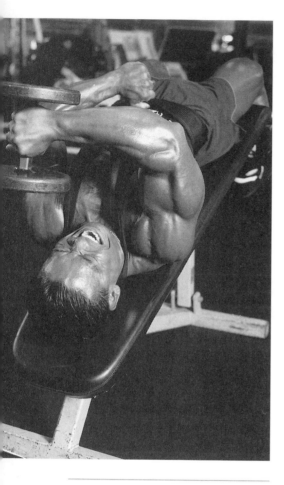

Chris Faildo

The cycle is initiated when pyruvate combines with coenzyme A (CoA) to form a two-carbon unit, acetyl-CoA, which enters the cycle by combining with four-carbon oxaloacetic acid to form six-carbon citric acid. In subsequent steps isocitric acid, produced from citric acid, is oxidized to oxalosuccinic acid, which loses carbon dioxide to form alpha-ketoglutaric acid. Succinic acid, resulting from the oxidative decarboxylation of alpha-ketoglutaric acid, is oxidized to fumaric acid, and its oxidation regenerates oxaloacetic acid, which condenses with acetyl-CoA, closing the cycle.

The Krebs cycle provides a major source of adenosine triphosphate energy and also produces intermediate molecules that are starting points for a number of vital metabolic pathways, including amino acid synthesis.

lipolysis. The breakdown or destruction of lipids or fats.

lipolytic. The chemical breakdown of fat.

lymph. A thin opalescent fluid originating in organs and tissues of the body that circulates through the lymphatic vessels and is filtered by the lymph nodes. Lymph enters the bloodstream at the junction of the internal jugular and subclavian veins.

mitochondrion. Small rodlike, threadlike, or granular organelle within the cytoplasm that functions in cellular metabolism and respiration and occurs in varying numbers in all living cells except bacteria, viruses, blue-green algae, and mature erythrocytes.

myosin. The skeletal muscle protein that makes up close to one half of the proteins that occur in muscle tissue.

nitrogen. A gaseous, nonmetallic element. Its atomic number is 7; its atomic weight is 14.008. Nitrogen constitutes approximately 78 percent of the earth's atmosphere and is a component of all proteins.

Compounds of nitrogen are essential constituents of all living organisms, the proteins and the nucleic acids being especially basic to all life forms. Nitrogen forms a series of oxides and oxyacids, the most important of which is nitric acid. It also unites with hydrogen to form ammonia and with many metallic elements to form nitrides.

Nitrogen is essential to the synthesis of proteins the body must have, particularly nitrogen-containing compounds or amino acids derived directly or indirectly from plant food. During a 24-hour period in a healthy individual, the nitrogen excreted in the urine, feces, and perspiration, together with the nitrogen retained in dermal structures, such as the skin and hair, equals the nitrogen consumed in food and drink.

The process of protein metabolism accounts for this nitrogen balance. When protein catabolism exceeds protein anabolism, the amount of nitrogen in the urine exceeds the amount of nitrogen consumed in foods, producing a negative nitrogen balance or a state of tissue wasting. A positive nitrogen balance exists in the body when the nitrogen intake in foods is greater than that excreted in urine.

nitrogen balance. The relationship between the nitrogen taken into the body, usually as food, and the nitrogen excreted from the body in urine and feces. Most of the body's nitrogen is incorporated into protein.

Positive nitrogen balance, which occurs when the intake of nitrogen is greater than its excretion, implies tissue formation. Negative nitrogen balance, which occurs when more nitrogen is excreted than is taken in, indicates wasting or destruction of tissue.

oxidation. Any process in which the oxygen content of a compound is increased.

oxidation-reduction reaction. A chemical change in which electrons are removed (oxidation) from an atom or molecule, accompanied by a simultaneous transfer of electrons (reduction) to another.

oxidative phosphorylation. An ATP-generating process in which oxygen serves as the final electron acceptor. The process occurs in mitochondria and is the major source of ATP generation in aerobic organisms.

peptide. A molecular chain compound composed of two or more amino acids joined by peptide bonds.

phosphate. A salt of phosphoric acid. Phosphates are extremely important in living cells, particularly in the storage and use of energy and the transmission of genetic information within a cell and from one cell to another.

pituitary gland. An endocrine gland suspended beneath the brain related to the production of seven hormones. The hormones, controlled by hypothalamic-releasing factors, include growth hormone (somatotropin), prolactin, thyroid-stimulating hormone, follicle-stimulating hormone (FSH), luteinizing hormone (LH), adrenocorticotropic hormone (ACTH), and melanocyte-stimulating hormone.

polypeptide. A chain of amino acids joined by peptide bonds. A polypeptide has a larger molecular weight than a peptide but a smaller molecular weight than a protein. Polypeptides are formed by partial hydrolysis of proteins or by synthesis of amino acids into chains.

prone. Being in a horizontal position when lying facedown.

protein. Any of a large group of naturally occurring, complex, organic nitrogenous compounds. Each is composed of large combinations of amino acids containing the elements carbon, hydrogen, nitrogen, oxygen, usually sulfur, and occasionally, phosphorus, iron, iodine, or other essential constituents of living cells.

Twenty-two amino acids have been identified as vital for proper growth, development, and health maintenance. The body can synthesize 14 of these amino acids, called nonessential, whereas the remaining eight must be obtained from dietary sources and are termed essential.

Protein is the major source of building material for muscles, blood, skin, hair, nails, and the internal organs. It is necessary for the formation of hormones, enzymes, and antibodies, may act as a source of heat and energy, and functions as an essential element in proper elimination of waste materials.

Rich dietary sources are meat, poultry, fish, eggs, milk, and cheese, which are classified as complete proteins because they contain the eight essential amino acids. Nuts and legumes, including navy beans, chick-peas, soybeans, and split peas are also good sources but are incomplete proteins because they do not contain all the essential amino acids.

protein metabolism. The processes whereby protein foodstuffs are used by the body to make tissue proteins, together with the processes of breakdown of tissue proteins in the production of energy. Food proteins are first broken down into amino acids, then absorbed into the bloodstream, and finally used in body cells to form new proteins.

Amino acids in excess of the body's needs may be converted by liver enzymes into keto acids and urea. The keto acids may be used as sources of energy via the Krebs citric acid cycle, or they may be converted into glucose or fat for storage. Urea is excreted in urine and sweat.

proteolysis. A process in which water added to the peptide bonds of proteins breaks down the protein molecule. Numerous enzymes may catalyze this process. The action of mineral acids and heat also may induce proteolysis.

proteolytic. Of or pertaining to any substance that promotes the breakdown of protein.

redox. An abbreviation for reduction-oxidation reaction.

sarcomere. The smallest functional unit of a myofibril. Within each sarcomere are thick filaments of myosin and thinner filaments that consist of actin.

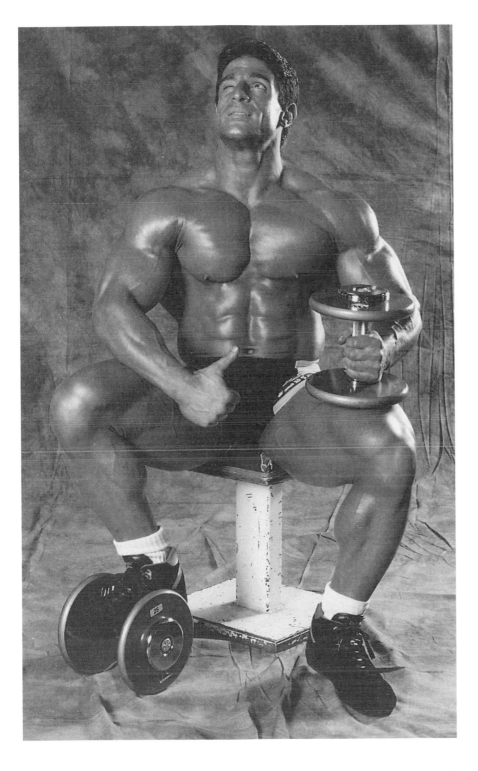

Franco Santoriello consults the ultimate training partner.

smooth muscle. One of two kinds of muscle, composed of elongated, spindle-shaped cells in muscles not under voluntary control, such as the smooth muscle of the intestines, stomach, and other visceral organs. The heart muscle is an exception because it is a striated involuntary muscle. Smooth muscle fibers are shorter than striated muscle fibers and are smooth in appearance. Known also as involuntary muscle or unstriated muscle.

somatotype. The classification of individuals according to body build based on certain physical characteristics. The primary types are ectomorph, endomorph, and mesomorph.

splanchnic. Of or pertaining to the visceral internal organs.

steroid. Any of a large number of hormonal substances with a similar basic chemical structure, produced mainly in the adrenal cortex and gonads.

steroid hormones. Any of the ductless gland secretions that contain the basic steroid nucleus in their chemical formulae. The natural steroid hormones include the androgens, estrogens, and adrenal cortex secretions.

striated muscle. Muscle tissue, including all the skeletal muscles, that consists of myofibrils. Striated muscles are composed of bundles of parallel, striated fibers. Each striated muscle is covered by a thin connective epimysium and divided into bundles of sheathed fibers containing smaller myofibrils. The muscle's contractile units, or sarcomeres, comprise the larger protein strands or myofibrils.

sugar. Any of several water-soluble carbohydrates. The two principal categories of sugars are monosaccharides and disaccharides. A monosaccharide is a single sugar such as glucose, fructose, or galactose. A disaccharide is a double sugar such as sucrose (table sugar) or lactose.

supine. Lying horizontally on the back.

thermogenesis. Production of heat, especially by the cells of the body.

thermoregulation. The control of heat production and heat loss, specifically the maintenance of body temperature through physiologic mechanisms activated by the hypothalamus.

thermoregulatory centers. Centers located in the hypothalamus concerned mainly with the regulation of heat production, heat inhibition, and heat conservation to maintain a normal body temperature. Kinds of thermoregulatory centers include: thermogenic center, thermoinhibitory center, and thermotaxic center.

viscera. The internal organs enclosed within a body cavity, primarily the abdominal organs.

Index

FREE Two-Week Membership

To receive your pass, or if you're already a member and you'd like to be part of the Gold's Gym information pipeline, complete and mail the coupon below.

Good luck from all of us at Gold's Gym Venice!

Offer good at participating Gold's Gym locations. For new members only. Must be 18 or older. Limit of one coupon per customer.

Please print clearly

Name: _____

Street: _____

Suite/PO Box: _____

City: _____

State: _____ Zip Code: _____

Country: _____

Mail to:
   Gold's Gym
   358 Hampton Drive
   Venice, CA 90291